NATIONAL ACADEMIES *Sciences Engineering Medicine*

NATIONAL ACADEMIES PRESS
Washington, DC

Charting a Path Toward New Treatments for Lyme Infection–Associated Chronic Illnesses

Kent Kester, Julie Liao, and Andrew March, *Editors*

Committee on The Evidence Base for Lyme Infection–Associated Chronic Illnesses Treatment

Board on Global Health

Board on Health Sciences Policy

Health and Medicine Division

Consensus Study Report

NATIONAL ACADEMIES PRESS 500 Fifth Street, NW Washington, DC 20001

This activity was supported by contracts between the National Academy of Sciences and the Steven & Alexandra Cohen Foundation. Any opinions, findings, conclusions, or recommendations expressed in this publication do not necessarily reflect the views of any organization or agency that provided support for the project.

International Standard Book Number-13: 978-0-309-73098-3
Digital Object Identifier: https://doi.org/10.17226/28578
Library of Congress Control Number: 2025938379

This publication is available from the National Academies Press, 500 Fifth Street, NW, Keck 360, Washington, DC 20001; (800) 624-6242; http://www.nap.edu.

The manufacturer's authorized representative in the European Union for product safety is Authorised Rep Compliance Ltd., Ground Floor, 71 Lower Baggot Street, Dublin D02 P593 Ireland; www.arccompliance.com.

Copyright 2025 by the National Academy of Sciences. National Academies of Sciences, Engineering, and Medicine and National Academies Press and the graphical logos for each are all trademarks of the National Academy of Sciences. All rights reserved.

Printed in the United States of America.

Suggested citation: National Academies of Sciences, Engineering, and Medicine. 2025. *Charting a path toward new treatments for Lyme infection-associated chronic illnesses*. Washington, DC: National Academies Press. https://doi.org/10.17226/28578.

The **National Academy of Sciences** was established in 1863 by an Act of Congress, signed by President Lincoln, as a private, nongovernmental institution to advise the nation on issues related to science and technology. Members are elected by their peers for outstanding contributions to research. Dr. Marcia McNutt is president.

The **National Academy of Engineering** was established in 1964 under the charter of the National Academy of Sciences to bring the practices of engineering to advising the nation. Members are elected by their peers for extraordinary contributions to engineering. Dr. John L. Anderson is president.

The **National Academy of Medicine** (formerly the Institute of Medicine) was established in 1970 under the charter of the National Academy of Sciences to advise the nation on medical and health issues. Members are elected by their peers for distinguished contributions to medicine and health. Dr. Victor J. Dzau is president.

The three Academies work together as the **National Academies of Sciences, Engineering, and Medicine** to provide independent, objective analysis and advice to the nation and conduct other activities to solve complex problems and inform public policy decisions. The National Academies also encourage education and research, recognize outstanding contributions to knowledge, and increase public understanding in matters of science, engineering, and medicine.

Learn more about the National Academies of Sciences, Engineering, and Medicine at **www.nationalacademies.org**.

Consensus Study Reports published by the National Academies of Sciences, Engineering, and Medicine document the evidence-based consensus on the study's statement of task by an authoring committee of experts. Reports typically include findings, conclusions, and recommendations based on information gathered by the committee and the committee's deliberations. Each report has been subjected to a rigorous and independent peer-review process and it represents the position of the National Academies on the statement of task.

Proceedings published by the National Academies of Sciences, Engineering, and Medicine chronicle the presentations and discussions at a workshop, symposium, or other event convened by the National Academies. The statements and opinions contained in proceedings are those of the participants and are not endorsed by other participants, the planning committee, or the National Academies.

Rapid Expert Consultations published by the National Academies of Sciences, Engineering, and Medicine are authored by subject-matter experts on narrowly focused topics that can be supported by a body of evidence. The discussions contained in rapid expert consultations are considered those of the authors and do not contain policy recommendations. Rapid expert consultations are reviewed by the institution before release.

For information about other products and activities of the National Academies, please visit www.nationalacademies.org/about/whatwedo.

COMMITTEE ON THE EVIDENCE BASE FOR LYME INFECTION-ASSOCIATED CHRONIC ILLNESSES TREATMENT

KENT E. KESTER (*Chair*), Coalition for Epidemic Preparedness Innovations
JOHN A. BRANDA, Harvard Medical School
BETTY A. DIAMOND, Feinstein Institute for Medical Research, Northwell Health
JESSE L. GOODMAN, Georgetown University
MIGUEL A. HERNÁN, Harvard T.H. Chan School of Public Health
ADRIAN F. HERNANDEZ, Duke School of Medicine; Duke Clinical Research Institute
BRANDON L. JUTRAS (*resigned from the committee September 2024*), Northwestern Feinberg School of Medicine
NICOLE MALACHOWSKI, Nicole Malachowski & Associates, LLC
CHERIE MARVEL, Johns Hopkins University School of Medicine
DEBJANI MUKHERJEE, Weill Cornell Medical College
LISE E. NIGROVIC, Boston Children's Hospital
SIMONE A. SEWARD, SUNY Upstate Medical University
ROBERT P. SMITH, MaineHealth Institute for Research; Tufts University School of Medicine
QING MEI WANG, Harvard Medical School
SUSAN J. WONG, Wadsworth Institute, New York State Department of Health (*retired June 2020*)

Study Staff

JULIE LIAO, Study Co-Director
ANDREW MARCH, Study Co-Director
EMILY MCDOWELL, Research Associate
RAYANE SILVA-CURRAN, Senior Program Assistant
REBECCA MORGAN, Senior Research Librarian
CAROLYN SHORE, Global Health Lead and Senior Program Officer (*as of January 2025*)
JULIE PAVLIN, Director, Board on Global Health
CLARE STROUD, Director, Board on Health Sciences Policy

Consultants

AMINA QUTUB, University of Texas, San Antonio
MAARTJE WOUTERS, Medical and Science Writer

Reviewers

This Consensus Study Report was reviewed in draft form by individuals chosen for their diverse perspectives and technical expertise. The purpose of this independent review is to provide candid and critical comments that will assist the National Academies of Sciences, Engineering, and Medicine in making each published report as sound as possible and to ensure that it meets the institutional standards for quality, objectivity, evidence, and responsiveness to the study charge. The review comments and draft manuscript remain confidential to protect the integrity of the deliberative process.

We thank the following individuals for their review of this report:

DAVID ALLISON, Indiana University
HUGH AUCHINCLOSS, National Institutes of Health (retired)
JOHN AUCOTT, Johns Hopkins University
JEANNE BERTOLLI, Centers for Disease Control and Prevention (retired)
CHARLES CHIU, University of California, San Francisco
CAROLYN COMPTON, Arizona State University
ROBERTA DEBIASI, Children's National Hospital
MAGDIA DE JESUS, Pfizer
MICHAEL IADEMARCO, U.S. Public Health Service (retired)
LORRAINE JOHNSON, LymeDisease.org
AKIKO IWASAKI, Yale University; Howard Hughes Medical Institute
SERENA SPUDICH, Yale University

Although the reviewers listed above provided many constructive comments and suggestions, they were not asked to endorse the conclusions or recommendations of this report, nor did they see the final draft before its release. The review of this report was overseen by **PAUL VOLDBERDING**, University of California, San Francisco, and **ENRIQUETA BOND**, Burroughs Wellcome Fund. They were responsible for making certain that an independent examination of this report was carried out in accordance with the standards of the National Academies and that all review comments were carefully considered. Responsibility for the final content rests entirely with the authoring committee and the National Academies.

Acknowledgments

The committee would like to express its gratitude to the many individuals and organizations that made this report possible. First, the committee would like to thank the Steven & Alexandra Cohen Foundation for sponsoring this study.

The committee is greatly indebted to the individuals who, through their generous contributions of time and expertise, informed this report over the course of the committee's open meetings. A full list of those individuals can be found in the meeting agendas, reproduced in Appendix A. The committee is particularly appreciative of the numerous individuals living with Lyme infection-associated chronic illnesses (IACI) and advocates who participated in the committee's meetings and had the impossible task of communicating the true toll of Lyme IACI.

The committee also thanks Amina Qutub for providing a critical analysis of the potential of artificial intelligence in advancing Lyme IACI research. The scoping review that the committee conducted would not have been possible without the methodological and operational guidance from the team at PICO Portal, including Eitan Agai, Renee Wilson, Alon Agai, Ahmed Elmoghazy, Rodrigo Conde, Stephanie Qureshi, Olabisi Oduwole, Ramesh Bhandari, and Riaz Qureshi.

Finally, this report is only possible thanks to the dedication of the staff at the National Academies of Sciences, Engineering, and Medicine. The study team of Julie Liao, Andrew March, Emily McDowell, and Rayane Silva-Curran provided the committee guidance and support throughout the process. Greysi Patton, finance business partner; Lori Brenig, editorial projects coordinator; Leslie Sim, senior report review officer; Taryn Young, report review associate; Marguerite Romatelli, communications specialist; and others in the Health and Medicine Division Executive Office, Office of the Chief Communications Officer, and Office of Congressional and Government Affairs assisted this study as well. And the committee extends its thanks to Maartje Wouters for her adept skills in contributing to the writing and editing of the report and to Robert Pool for his editorial assistance.

Contents

PREFACE	xvii
ACRONYMS AND ABBREVIATIONS	xxi
GLOSSARY	xxiii
SUMMARY	1

    Person-Centered, Symptom-Based Treatment Development, 4
    Shifting the Focus: Rigorous Clinical Trials That Target
        Symptoms, 5
    Broadening the Evidence Base: Collaboration Across Similar
        Conditions, 10
    Time for Action, 15

1 INTRODUCTION   17
    Study Context and Charge, 17
    Background, 19
    Committee Approach, 29
    References, 35

2 STATE OF THE EVIDENCE   41
    Operational Scope for Literature Review on Lyme IACI
        Research, 41
    Epidemiology of Lyme IACI, 44
    A Scoping Review of the Literature, 49

Evidence on the Treatment of Lyme IACI, 53
Evidence on the Mechanisms of Lyme IACI, 59
Evidence on the Diagnosis of Lyme IACI, 63
Key Questions for Future Research, 80
References, 84

3 **BUILDING ON RESEARCH FROM OTHER INFECTION-ASSOCIATED CHRONIC ILLNESSES**   93
Clinical Evidence on Symptom-Based Approaches to Treatments for IACI, 96
Opportunities for Translating Promising Approaches to Lyme IACI, 105
Lessons Learned, 116
References, 119

4 **INNOVATIVE APPROACHES TO ACCELERATING LYME IACI RESEARCH**   131
A Common Framework to Prioritize Lyme IACI Research, 131
Research Infrastructure, 136
Data Interpretation, 155
Considerations for Implementation, 163
References, 166

5 **RECOMMENDATIONS**   175
Research into New Treatments That Alleviate Symptoms, 176
Standardized Research Definitions and Metrics, 177
Improved Access to Biobanks and Registries, 182
Coordinated Research Funding and Collaboration Efforts, 183
Collaboration Across IACI Research, 184
Closing Thoughts, 187
References, 187

APPENDIXES
A Committee Meeting Agendas   189
B Committee Member and Staff Biographies   201
C Methodology of Literature Review   213

Boxes, Figures, and Tables

BOXES

S-1 Key Questions for Future Research, 5

1-1 Statement of Task, 18
1-2 Defining Lyme IACI, 24
1-3 Operational Scope of Lyme IACI, 25
1-4 A Critical Need and Opportunity, 27

2-1 Definition of Post-Treatment Lyme Disease Syndrome, 43

3-1 Developing Effective Treatments to Mitigate Symptoms: Case Study with Fibromyalgia, 106
3-2 Applying New Research Tools to Lyme IACI: A Case Study on Neuroscience, 110

4-1 Ongoing Longitudinal Observational Studies in Lyme IACI in the U.S., 141
4-2 Considerations for Multiplex Tick-borne Disease Diagnostics to Understand the Impact of Co-Infections on Lyme IACI, 153

5-1 Defining Research Funders, 176

FIGURES

S-1 Conceptual relationship among post-treatment Lyme disease syndrome (PTLDS), Lyme infection-associated chronic illnesses (IACI), and the broader IACI space, 3
S-2 Peer-reviewed Lyme IACI research, 1970–May 2024, 7
S-3 Framework for prioritization of potential Lyme IACI treatments for clinical trials, 9

1-1 Conceptual relationship among post-treatment Lyme disease syndrome (PTLDS), Lyme infection-associated chronic illnesses (IACI), and the broader IACI space, 30
1-2 Conceptual framework of the development and impact of Lyme IACI on the individual patient experience, 31
1-3 Relationship between the etiology, pathogenesis, and symptoms for Lyme IACI, 33

2-1 Flowchart of articles screened for and included in the scoping review, 51
2-2 Peer-reviewed research on mechanisms, diagnosis, or treatment of Lyme IACI between 1970 and May 2024, 52
2-3 Study designs of published Lyme IACI treatment trials, 55
2-4 Proposed mechanisms of Lyme IACI in published literature, 62

3-1 NIH funding for Lyme Disease research, 2008–2025, 118

4-1 Framework for research prioritization of Lyme IACI treatment interventions, 133
4-2 Types of patient-reported outcome tools used in Lyme IACI research articles identified in the committee's scoping review, 157

TABLES

2-1 Summary of Prospective Studies Reviewing the Prevalence of PTLDS, 46
2-2 Key Study Characteristics from Randomized Trials, 56
2-3 Study Designs of Publications in Scoping Review on Lyme IACI Mechanisms, 61
2-4 Potential Biomarkers and Other Diagnostic Approaches for Lyme IACI that Have Been Reported in the Literature, 67

3-1 Symptoms Commonly Reported for IACI, 95

4-1 Example of Applying Prioritization Assessment of Lyme IACI Treatment Interventions, 135

C-1 Keywords Used to Describe Lyme IACI for Title and Abstract Literature Search, 215
C-2 Inclusion and Exclusion Criteria for Abstracts Screening, 216
C-3 Inclusion and Exclusion Criteria for Full-Text Screening, 216
C-4 Data Extraction for Each Full Text Category, 217
C-5 Articles Included in Scoping Review, 217

Preface

While the causes of Lyme infection-associated chronic illnesses (IACI) remain uncertain, it is clear that patient symptoms are deserving of improved diagnosis and treatment, especially in this era of significant advances in medical science. This is the underlying reason for this consensus study—to evaluate and call attention to the existing evidence base associated with Lyme IACI and in doing so, help to frame the gaps in knowledge and the potential for innovative approaches to better understand, diagnose, and treat these diverse sequelae of Lyme disease.

In spite of myriad advances in the diagnosis and treatment of infectious diseases and their complications, Lyme disease, in many ways, remains an outlier. Whether related to an incomplete understanding of its epidemiology, imprecise and sometimes unvalidated diagnostic tests, or potentially suboptimal therapies for the infection, Lyme disease continues to bedevil clinicians and patients alike. A particularly important and poorly understood aspect of Lyme disease is its association with a variety of symptoms that persist post-infection and post-treatment, such as "brain fog" (characterized by difficulties in concentration and memory changes), sleep disturbances, systemic fatigue and weakness, or unexplained pain syndromes. Unfortunately, there is limited understanding of the pathophysiology of such persistent symptoms, and there are no validated diagnostic and therapeutic modalities. As a result, patients presenting with Lyme IACI and their health care providers lack access to well-defined, evidence-based, and commonly accepted standards to support either clear, consistent diagnosis or effective treatment.

This gap has led not only to continuing symptoms and disability for many people but also to a variety of unvalidated treatment regimens, some of which may carry great harm for patients. Owing to this, patients with Lyme IACI continue to be frustrated with uncertain or inconsistent diagnoses and treatments that in many cases do not improve their symptoms and quality of life. While there has been a fair amount of clinical research conducted into optimizing antibiotic treatment of well-defined Lyme disease entities associated with active infection, from erythema migrans to arthritis, much less effort and funding support has been dedicated to exploring the diverse Lyme IACI in terms of either diagnosis or treatment.

In the aftermath of the COVID-19 pandemic, we have seen the striking emergence of diverse symptoms and other findings considered under the umbrella of Long COVID in substantial numbers of patients after a SARS-CoV-2 infection. And while Long COVID may differ from Lyme IACI in many ways, there are a number of similar, overlapping symptoms, suggesting commonalities of the underlying pathophysiologic processes in the host. This parallel, along with other IACI syndromes, such as myalgic encephalomyelitis/chronic fatigue syndrome (ME/CFS), was the subject of a National Academies Forum on Microbial Threats workshop in 2023. The workshop highlighted data supporting hypotheses suitable for further investigation for understanding the pathophysiology of various IACI and exploring possible approaches to treatment. Notably, significant National Institutes of Health (NIH) funding has been allocated to study this newly recognized complication of SARS-CoV-2 infection. However, and in spite of the much longer timeline since the diverse chronic complications associated with Lyme disease were identified, limited NIH research support has so far been focused on Lyme IACI. Given the continued expansion of tick-borne disease across the United States, there is an urgent need for improved treatment of Lyme IACI. In this era of incredible technological advances in clinical medicine, the needed improvements are within our reach.

On behalf of the entire committee and the National Academies' project staff, I would like to thank the many patients, scientists, and advocates who provided input into this report. I especially want to highlight the role and contributions of patients with Lyme IACI, as they often continue to suffer persisting symptoms and, in many cases, work to call attention to the need for better treatments. We also thank the reviewers for their useful feedback as well as the monitor and coordinator who oversaw the report review.

This report would not have been possible without the incredible support of the talented National Academy staff, including the study co-directors Julie Liao and Andrew March, along with Emily McDowell, Rayane Silva-Curran, Rebecca Morgan, and Khiara Reed.

In the end, we hope that this report has real impact on the future of Lyme IACI research and the lives of people living with the syndrome. The goal of this report is to effectively highlight those areas of medical innovation that can be applied to address and ultimately treat the multitude of current and future patients who suffer with Lyme IACI. Our patients deserve better.

Kent E. Kester, M.D., *Chair*
Committee on the Evidence Base for Lyme
Infection-Associated Chronic Illnesses Treatment

Acronyms and Abbreviations

AHRQ	Agency for Healthcare Research and Quality
AI	artificial intelligence
CBT	cognitive behavioral therapy
CDC	Centers for Disease Control and Prevention
CDE	common data element
CDMRP	Congressionally Directed Medical Research Programs
CLIA	Clinical Laboratory Improvement Amendments
CNS	central nervous system
CSF	cerebral spinal fluid
CTN	Clinical Trials Network
ELISA	enzyme-linked immunosorbent assay
EM	erythema migrans
FDA	U.S. Food and Drug Administration
fMRI	functional magnetic resonance imaging
HHS	Department of Health and Human Services
IACI	infection-associated chronic illnesses
ICD	International Classification of Diseases
IDSA	Infectious Diseases Society of America
IND	investigational new drug
IRB	Institutional Review Board

LD	Lyme disease
LLM	large language model
MCID	minimal clinically important difference
ME/CFS	myalgic encephalomyelitis/chronic fatigue syndrome
ML	machine learning
NADH	Nicotinamide adenine dinucleotide (reduced)
NGS	next-generation sequencing
NIAID	National Institute of Allergy and Infectious Diseases
NIH	National Institutes of Health
NINDS	National Institute of Neurological Disorders and Stroke
PCORI	Patient-Centered Outcomes Research Institute
POTS	postural orthostatic tachycardia syndrome
PRO	patient-reported outcome
PTLDS	post-treatment Lyme disease syndrome
QoL	quality of life
RWD	real-world data
RWE	real-world evidence
STARI	southern tick-associated rash illness
TBDWG	Tick-Borne Disease Working Group
tDCS	transcranial direct current stimulation
VNS	vagus nerve stimulation

Glossary

Biobank: A collection of biological specimens and associated data suitable for research purposes.

Clinical trial: A study in which researchers assign individuals to specific interventions, which can be a therapeutic, diagnostic, medical device, or procedure to evaluate the safety and efficacy of the intervention.

Common data element (CDE): A standardized, precisely defined question that is paired with a set of specific allowable responses, that is then used systematically across different sites, studies, or clinical trials to ensure consistent data collection.

Control group: A group of individuals in a study who are assigned to receive a placebo or alternative treatment to the intervention of interest, or who do not exhibit a particular variable of interest. The control group serves as a comparison to the group receiving the intervention or the group exhibiting the particular variable of interest.

Etiology: The cause or origin of a disease.

Infection-associated chronic illnesses (IACI): Diseases or syndromes with a potential root cause in infections, encompassing some conditions where the etiology remains unknown but have been documented to include infectious triggers. Examples are Long COVID and myalgic encephalomyelitis/chronic fatigue syndrome (ME/CFS).

Lesion: An area of abnormal or damaged tissue caused by injury, infection, or disease. A lesion can occur anywhere in or on the body, such as the skin, blood vessels, brain, and other organs.

Negative predictive value: The probability that a negative test result correctly rules out the disease or condition for an individual in the given population.

Objective outcome measures: Quantifiable data that can be measured to minimize the potential influence of human bias from the study participant, researcher, or other observer. Objective measures are gathered using standardized tools and procedures. These may include laboratory tests, imaging studies and interpretations, physical examinations, and other clinical findings.

Observational studies: Studies in which researchers do not assign participants to receive interventions but rather observe the participants for outcomes of interest and compare them to participant factors, including use of a particular treatment. As a result, determining causation is difficult as outcomes could be due to the variable of interest, or to inherent participant factors that influence the distribution of the variable within the population.

Pathogenesis: The mechanisms by which a disease develops, progresses, and either persists or is resolved.

Pathophysiology: The functional and biochemical changes that are associated with or result from disease or injury.

Patient registry: An organized system that uses observational study methods to collect uniform data (clinical and other) to evaluate specified outcomes for a population defined by a particular disease, condition, or exposure, and that serves a predetermined scientific, clinical, or policy purpose.

Positive predictive value: The probability that a positive test result correctly identifies a case of the disease or condition in a given population.

Prospective studies: Studies in which data are collected in chronological order. All randomized trials are prospective studies.

Randomization: The process by which interventions are randomly assigned to study participants in a clinical trial to reduce the influence of inherent participant characteristics.

Rash: An area of the skin that has changes in texture or color and may look inflamed or irritated. The skin may be red, warm, scaly, bumpy, dry, itchy, swollen, or painful. It may also crack or blister. A rash can occur in one area of the body or all over the body and may look very different depending on the cause.

Retrospective studies: Data on treatments are collected after the outcomes have occurred. Some observational studies are retrospective.

Sensitivity: The sensitivity of a test refers to its ability to correctly identify individuals who have the target disease or condition. Few true positive cases are missed if a diagnostic test has high sensitivity.

Specificity: The specificity of a test refers to how likely it is to correctly return a negative result in people who do not have the target disease or condition. Tests with high specificity return few false-positive results.

Subjective outcome measures: Self-reported data obtained from study participants or researchers. These can be obtained using surveys or interviews and may include self-assessments of quality of life or pain severity.

Summary[1]

Tens of thousands of Americans develop Lyme infection-associated chronic illnesses (IACI) each year, a condition that can occur after acquiring Lyme disease and that often presents as debilitating physical symptoms including chronic fatigue, recurring pain, cognitive dysfunction such as "brain fog," and sleep disturbances despite antibiotic treatment for Lyme disease. Approximately 10–20 percent of the 476,000 individuals who develop Lyme disease each year following the bite of a tick infected with *Borrelia burgdorferi*, a spirochete bacteria, go on to develop Lyme IACI, which can lead to strains on interpersonal relationships, loss of careers, depression, anxiety, and other mental health conditions. People living with Lyme IACI also report being disbelieved by clinicians if objective clinical or laboratory findings are not able to substantiate the symptoms that they are experiencing. While some individuals eventually find relief through various interventions or return to functionality without treatment, many suffer from the condition for years. Much about Lyme IACI remains unknown. While there is a standardized diagnosis and treatment for Lyme disease, there are gaps in understanding the cause, diagnosis, and treatment for the persistent symptoms associated with Lyme IACI. Despite the need to better understand the disease, it is clear that Lyme IACI is debilitating to the health and well-being of tens of thousands of Americans. There is an urgent need for research to provide safe and effective treatments for Lyme IACI

---

[1] This summary does not include references. Citations for the information presented herein are provided in the main text.

that address the symptoms that affect the functionality and quality of life of those living with the condition.

There are no available treatments validated to safely and effectively cure or manage symptoms for those living with Lyme IACI. As a result, affected individuals may rely on word of mouth or trial and error in the hopes of relieving their symptoms with interventions of unknown safety and effectiveness. While clinicians have worked to better understand and treat Lyme IACI, research to develop and evaluate therapeutic interventions has received insufficient attention and investment, partially due to a lack of alignment on research priorities. To find better treatments for Lyme IACI, both increased research, and collaboration and coordination among researchers, clinicians, and patient communities are critical.

The broad recognition of Long COVID—a chronic condition associated with SARS-CoV-2 infection—has galvanized acceptance of Lyme IACI and promoted awareness that Lyme IACI and Long COVID are just two examples of chronic disease states with potential infectious triggers, referred to throughout this report as infection-associated chronic illnesses (IACI). The common threads among IACI are the similar chronic symptoms and the potential connection to an infectious trigger. These commonalities complicate the task of distinguishing individuals with Lyme IACI from individuals with any other IACI. Moreover, Lyme IACI has not been well defined as a condition as opposed to other IACIs such as Long COVID, though a subset of individuals who overlap with the Lyme IACI population has been defined as post-treatment Lyme disease syndrome (PTLDS) (Figure S-1). The population of people with Lyme IACI is heterogeneous: individuals with Lyme IACI differ in terms of symptom type and severity, and certainty of previous *B. burgdorferi* exposure. At the same time, the similarities among these various conditions present an opportunity, as researchers consider whether IACI may also share the same or similar underlying biological drivers or pathways. Until recently, however, there have not been concerted efforts to investigate these possible commonalities and translate knowledge across the silos of different disease areas to advance new treatments for Lyme IACI.

To address the lack of safe and effective treatments for Lyme IACI and to take advantage of the recent research advances stimulated by Long COVID, the Steven & Alexandra Cohen Foundation asked the National Academies of Sciences, Engineering, and Medicine (the National Academies) to assess the current evidence base for treatment of Lyme IACI and to identify priorities and new opportunities to advance treatment and diagnosis of this syndrome. Building on the recommendation in the 2022 report of the Tick-borne Disease Working Group, which called for a National Academies study to conduct a review on the basic science and clinical evidence for diagnosis and treatment that establishes "what is definitely known, what is partially understood, and what remains unknown"

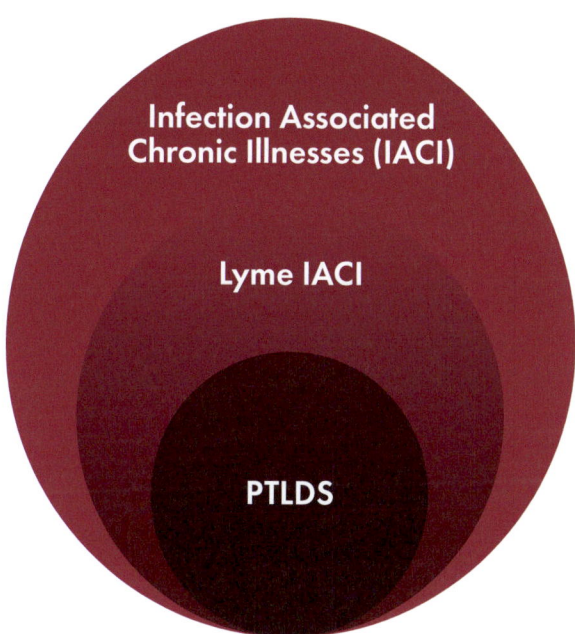

FIGURE S-1 Conceptual relationship among post-treatment Lyme disease syndrome (PTLDS), Lyme infection-associated chronic illnesses (IACI), and the broader IACI space.

for Lyme disease (covering early disease to the persistent symptoms), the current report reviewed the available evidence for treatment of Lyme IACI and for other similar conditions to illuminate a path toward advancing new treatments for Lyme IACI. An ad hoc committee consisting of experts in treating persistent symptoms associated with Lyme disease or similar conditions, clinical trials design and methodology, public health and epidemiology, neuroscience and infectious diseases research, health policy, medical ethics, community engagement, and individuals with lived experience with lingering symptoms associated with Lyme was assembled to respond to this request. To address this task, the committee reviewed the published literature on treatments for Lyme IACI and related conditions as well as the literature on the etiology and diagnosis of Lyme IACI. In addition to literature review, the committee carefully considered the perspectives shared by people affected by Lyme IACI and sought input from clinicians and researchers working to address Lyme and other IACI. The committee also gathered additional information through public presentations from researchers, technology developers, regulators, patients, and patient-led research organizations. A full discussion of the committee's approach to this study in provided in Chapter 1.

The recommendations in this report seek to address gaps in the evidence base for Lyme IACI treatments and diagnosis and can be classified into four themes: centering the lived experience, shifting to treatment research that focuses on addressing symptoms, broadening the evidence base to systematically draw lessons from similar syndromes, and developing a unifying vision for future research. Additional considerations for the implementation of the report's recommendations are discussed in Chapter 5.

PERSON-CENTERED, SYMPTOM-BASED TREATMENT DEVELOPMENT

In the absence of validated interventions for treating Lyme IACI, people living with this debilitating condition may try interventions that have not been adequately tested for safety or efficacy in the Lyme IACI population. The use of an untested treatment can put individuals living with Lyme IACI at risk of spending money on an ineffective product and of serious, unknown harm, particularly when multiple products are used in combination. Adults with capacity have the right to make their own health care decisions in consultation with a clinician. To support informed decision making, the efficacy, potential risks, benefits, and burdens of treatment need to be made clear through rigorous clinical evaluations. The discovery and development of safe and effective treatments has been slowed by the poor understanding of the biological mechanisms that lead to Lyme IACI. Ideally, curative treatments would be designed based on well-established disease mechanisms. However, full understanding of a disease's etiology is not a prerequisite for research and development on effective interventions that target what *is* known: symptoms that have uprooted people's lives. In the absence of clear mechanistic targets, it is imperative to pursue evidence-based interventions to relieve Lyme IACI symptoms and improve patients' quality of life, while continuing targeted mechanistic studies to uncover the underlying disease mechanisms and better target and design future treatments.

To move toward this goal, it is essential to adopt patient-centric approaches, by partnering with individuals with lived experience for their input in defining and executing research priorities for Lyme IACI. Their valuable insights on the disease experience can help in the formulation of research questions that address real-world impact, guide the overall research agenda, and inform the research strategy. Moreover, there are many patient-led groups and research initiatives interested in providing input, but their knowledge and networks are currently underused. Igniting this engagement has multiple benefits for people living with Lyme IACI, researchers, and funders, including improvement of research translation to clinical care, increased recruitment and retention of study participants, and more widespread dissemination of research findings. To promote ongoing patient-centeredness of Lyme IACI research, it will be necessary to seek and incorporate the input of individuals living with Lyme IACI in the implementation of the report's recommendations.

SHIFTING THE FOCUS: RIGOROUS CLINICAL TRIALS THAT TARGET SYMPTOMS

To review the current state of knowledge regarding clinical trials for the treatment of Lyme IACI, the committee conducted a scoping review of the published research to identify current evidence gaps and key questions to be addressed in future research. The scoping review also included existing literature on diagnosis and disease mechanisms since findings from these two research areas can inform treatment research. The scoping review excluded unpublished data, some of which are contained within patient registries and biobanks. However, these data are valuable, and the report addresses strategies to improve their use in research. Given the current state of the evidence, the committee identified several overarching questions relevant to planning future research and maximizing opportunities for success (Box S-1). Where supported by the available evidence, the committee has begun to address these questions throughout the report but acknowledges that researchers and funders will need to continue to grapple with these questions as the future of Lyme IACI research is charted.

The scoping review revealed 19 clinical trials that had been conducted for treatments of Lyme IACI, compared with 49 studies on disease mechanism (Figure S-2). In general, the number of publications related to potential disease mechanisms or diagnoses of Lyme IACI steadily grew in the past two decades, while the number of randomized controlled clinical trials for treatment stagnated despite the need for additional research. Many challenges have slowed progress in developing Lyme IACI treatments, including

---

BOX S-1
Key Questions for Future Research

1. How should Lyme IACI and potential subgroups of people with this condition be defined?
2. What are the pathogenesis mechanisms of Lyme IACI?
3. How should Lyme IACI be treated prior to a full understanding of its pathogenesis?
4. Which outcomes should be used to evaluate whether Lyme IACI treatments work?

the limited understanding of disease mechanisms that could guide the development of therapeutics.

Paucity of Rigorously Conducted Clinical Trials on Potential Treatments

Of the 19 publications on potential treatments for Lyme IACI, only five were randomized, controlled, and blinded clinical trials, and all five of those trials evaluated the effects of extended antibiotics regimens. A sixth randomized, controlled trial, which was not blinded, tested the benefit of yoga for Lyme IACI (Figure S-2). Taken together, the six randomized trials did not find consistent evidence of sustained benefits, and the antibiotic trials demonstrated some adverse effects. There have not been any randomized trials conducted in pediatric populations. The remaining 13 clinical trials evaluated a wider range of interventions, from antibiotics to electromagnetic radiation, exercise, immunosuppressants, dietary interventions, nutritional supplements, and cognitive behavioral therapies. However, these trials lacked important elements of rigorous study design, such as randomization or controls. Without rigorous methods in the study design, it is not possible to assess the scientific validity of the studies' outcomes.

Whether different approaches to the use of antibiotics could provide a benefit remains a point of scientific debate, but given the poor understanding of the many potential biological mechanisms in Lyme IACI, the near exclusive focus of the Lyme IACI research portfolio on antibiotic therapies lacks a clear scientific rationale. Antibiotics are only likely to be effective in treating Lyme IACI if the driver of symptoms were the persistence of *Borrelia spp.* despite the initial treatment of the infection. However, the pathogen persistence hypothesis is only one of many that have been proposed as the mechanism of chronic symptoms. Others include autoimmunity, central nervous system dysfunction, antigen persistence, metabolic changes, or microbiome changes. Given the current limited understanding of Lyme IACI mechanisms, it is premature to focus the conduct of randomized trials on interventions that target a single mechanism at the exclusion of others.

Moving Forward with Clinical Trials for Improving Symptoms

Ideally, knowledge of Lyme IACI disease mechanisms will make it possible to carry out more targeted research and development for treatments that act on specific disease pathways to alleviate symptoms or eventually find a cure. But as long as this knowledge is not available, it is critical to explore additional approaches to develop potential interventions that can address symptoms and improve people's quality of life even if the underlying disease process is not yet fully understood. Testing potential therapeutic

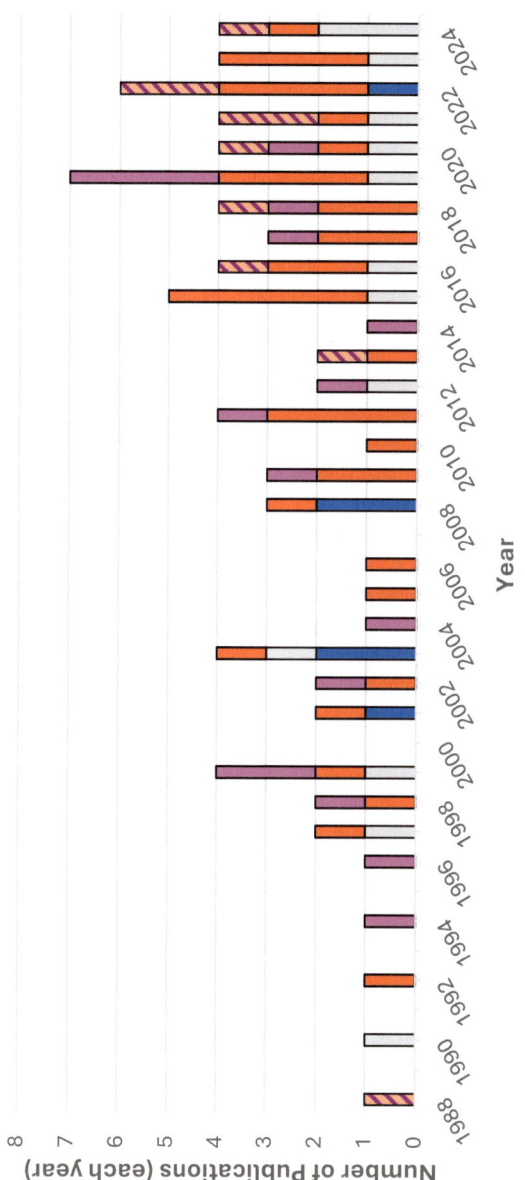

FIGURE S-2 Peer-reviewed Lyme IACI research, 1970–May 2024. The earliest publications that met the inclusion criteria for the scoping review was from 1988.
NOTE: IACI = infection-associated chronic illnesses; RCT = randomized controlled trial.

candidates to address Lyme IACI symptoms takes advantage of the existing evidence that can be drawn from other conditions with similar symptoms and the lived experience from individuals with this condition. There are many potential Lyme IACI treatments for which additional research may be warranted, including some currently in use by those living with the condition. Other potential treatments may be proposed by researchers and clinicians based on scientific evidence from Lyme IACI or other similar conditions.

A strategic assessment process is needed to evaluate and prioritize potential treatment candidates for clinical studies. The committee proposes a framework for this prioritization (Figure S-3) that strives to balance a systematic approach with the acknowledgment that different researchers or funders may have different interests that factor into the final decision-making. Potential treatments can be prioritized based on existing evidence, such as preclinical or clinical data demonstrating biological plausibility, safety, and efficacy for a similar symptom from a different condition. Lived experiences from people with Lyme IACI can guide researchers in determining those symptoms that, if addressed, will have the greatest impact on their lives.

Suggesting a shift in focus to clinical studies that address Lyme IACI symptoms does not mean that research on disease mechanisms should be abandoned. To the contrary, continued investigation into biological causes and disease pathways will be important to inform future research. Studies on the etiology and pathogenesis of Lyme IACI and a symptom-driven research agenda for treatments can be explored in a parallel and complementary fashion. To the extent possible, clinical studies evaluating potential treatments for Lyme IACI symptoms would also collect and share data or samples that help elucidate disease mechanisms. For example, clinical data on patient characteristics and disease manifestations or laboratory data, including potential diagnostic or prognostic biomarkers for Lyme IACI, can be collected from randomized, controlled trials for additional analyses.

> **RECOMMENDATION 1:** Research funders should prioritize improving the function and quality of life for people living with Lyme infection-associated chronic illnesses, including the relief of common symptoms, with scientifically supported interventions. To ensure these interventions are supported by robust evidence, clinical studies should be well-designed, randomized trials with appropriate control groups and, whenever possible, include collection of data to help further understanding of disease mechanisms.

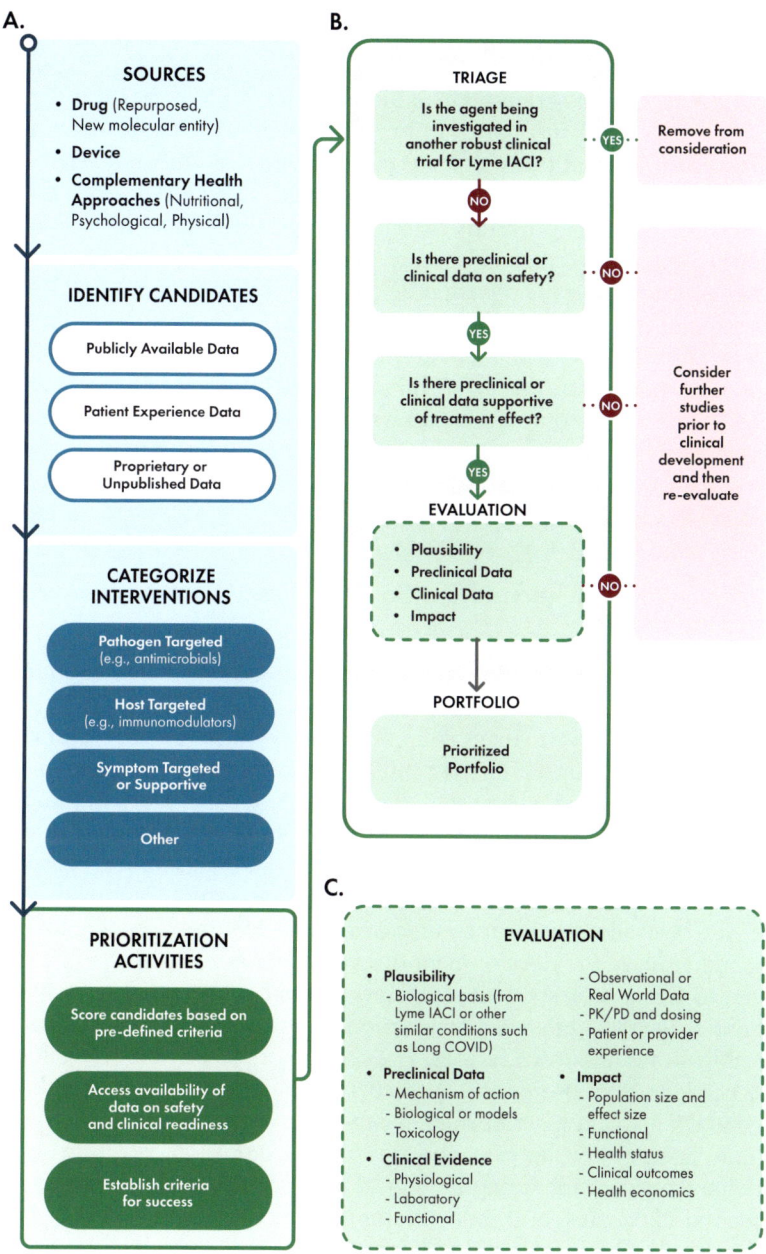

FIGURE S-3 Framework for prioritization of potential Lyme IACI treatments for clinical trials: (A) overall process for identification and prioritization of Lyme IACI treatment candidates, (B) decision framework for evaluating identified candidates. (C) Domains for evaluation of triaged candidates. Adapted from Buchman et al. (2021). NOTES: IACI = infection-associated chronic illness; IND = investigational new drug; PK/PD = pharmacokinetics and pharmacodynamics.

BROADENING THE EVIDENCE BASE: COLLABORATION ACROSS SIMILAR CONDITIONS

In this report, the committee explored potential lessons from the published scientific literature by examining systematic reviews on treatments for two chronic conditions that may be triggered by infection and share many symptoms and proposed mechanisms with Lyme IACI: Long COVID and myalgic encephalomyelitis/chronic fatigue syndrome (ME/CFS). The committee determined that for fatigue, pain, and cognitive dysfunction—the most common symptoms reported by people living with Lyme IACI—there were no interventions from Long COVID or ME/CFS treatment trials that warrant adoption as an immediate priority for Lyme IACI research given the unreplicated, inconsistent, or minor benefits reported in the literature. However, several lessons can be drawn to improve the current Lyme IACI research ecosystem, facilitate a coordinated approach to research between these similar conditions and Lyme IACI, and enable comparison or aggregate analyses of findings between IACI.

Standardize Definitions, Data Collection, and Outcome Measures

Research on ME/CFS and Long COVID has benefited from efforts to standardize clinical definitions and outcome measurements. Without a consensus definition or known diagnostics biomarkers for Lyme IACI, studies have often enrolled participant cohorts that may not be directly comparable to one another. A survey of over 3,000 affected individuals from a large, patient-led data registry reported fatigue, musculoskeletal pain, and cognitive impairment as the most frequent and severe symptoms, which are experienced by 30–62 percent of respondents. Other smaller, prospective observational trials have found similar patterns in symptom prevalence but have not been able to identify unique clinical features for diagnosis. For some individuals, the development of Lyme IACI symptoms may clearly be related to Lyme disease, while for other individuals, symptoms may occur without a clear diagnosis or connection to prior Lyme disease or may be caused by other unknown factors. The certainty of causation between someone's persistent symptoms and antecedent Lyme disease may depend on the individual's medical history, such as laboratory testing, previous erythema migrans rash, or recollection of a tick bite. In addition, research suggests that characteristics including biological sex, prior history of trauma, environmental exposures, and individual immunologic differences may be risk factors for developing Lyme IACI, but the degree to which they affect disease risk in all or a subset of individuals is not firmly established. Similarly, multiple mechanistic pathways may lead to persistent symptoms, and the pathways—or combinations of pathways—may differ within the Lyme IACI population.

The heterogeneity in disease symptoms and causal or risk factors for these symptoms suggests the existence of distinct subgroups within Lyme IACI that may inform disease course or treatment outcomes. PTLDS[2] is a definition that encompasses some people with persistent symptoms after Lyme disease, but its criteria for a well-documented diagnosis of Lyme disease and significant functional impairment excludes many whose symptom origins are unclear or who experience less severe symptoms but are still deserving of research and treatment. Furthermore, it is difficult to distinguish Lyme IACI from other conditions that share similar clinical presentation due to the emerging but unsettled evidence on diagnostic biomarkers to differentiate among these syndromes. Similar to the approach to defining Long COVID and ME/CFS, developing consensus definitions for Lyme IACI that (1) reflect the established evidence and remaining uncertainties regarding the heterogeneity of this condition, (2) include working definitions for subgroups that may be identified based on clinical or laboratory data, and (3) are reviewed and updated periodically to incorporate new findings are essential for overcoming these challenges and advancing research into this complex condition.

RECOMMENDATION 2: The U.S. Department of Health and Human Services (HHS) should develop consensus research definitions for Lyme infection-associated chronic illnesses (IACI) that address the different strata of the broad range of people living with Lyme IACI.
  a. HHS should develop a Lyme IACI definition and subgroup definitions that acknowledge the heterogeneity of these illnesses.
  b. HHS should establish a mechanism to regularly review the Lyme IACI literature and update the consensus research definition and subgroup definitions as new evidence emerges.
  c. The consensus research definition and subgroup definitions for Lyme IACI should be developed in such a way as to include a broad range of perspectives (e.g., lived experience, clinicians, researchers) and generally align with definitions for other similar conditions and facilitate coordination of research across the diseases.

In addition to helping develop a consensus definition for Lyme IACI, standardizing data collection and analyses could enable data interoperability and harmonize understanding of outcomes between different research

---

[2] Post-treatment Lyme disease syndrome has been used to describe people who experience persistent and debilitating symptoms for more than 6 months after completing appropriate treatment for a well-documented diagnosis of Lyme disease. This has been defined for research purposes and is not meant as a clinical case definition.

initiatives. Studies on Lyme IACI have not consistently captured the same outcomes or used the same measurement tools for those outcomes, complicating the comparison of results between trials. For example, at least four different tools have been used to measure fatigue in the Lyme IACI literature. One strategy to promote harmonization between studies would be to establish specific, actionable common data elements (CDEs), which would encourage alignment on minimum core datasets to collect in all trials, and also appropriate data-collection tools. As with the prioritization of clinical research candidates, it is important that the development of these research tools, metrics, and data standards include input from those living with Lyme IACI, including those currently underrepresented in research, such as children, so that research outcomes address the experience and goals of those affected by the condition.

> RECOMMENDATION 3: The National Institutes of Health (NIH), in coordination with the Centers for Disease Control and Prevention (CDC), should define a set of standard research tools and metrics to advance research and development of new treatments for Lyme infection-associated chronic illnesses (IACI). These include common data elements (CDEs), sensitive outcome measures, and terminologies that reflect the lived experience of people with Lyme IACI.
>
> a. NIH and CDC should assess, with participation of all interested parties, whether existing patient-reported outcome measurement tools reliably and accurately capture the priority outcomes for people with Lyme IACI, or if new tools and measures are needed. This should include determining if there are groups (e.g., children) for which existing reporting tools do not capture necessary Lyme IACI constructs.
> b. NIH and CDC should evaluate existing CDEs from myalgic encephalomyelitis/chronic fatigue syndrome (ME/CFS) and Long COVID for components that can be incorporated into Lyme IACI CDEs to enable knowledge sharing among IACI, including through comparative studies of multiple disease areas. This could include adopting a core set of clinical characteristics for study participants, study methodologies, and symptom reporting questionnaires that mirrors those already being used in ME/CFS or Long COVID research.

Expand Data Collection

The heterogeneity of Lyme IACI symptoms and potential pathophysiologies suggests that a large collection of useful data (e.g., epidemiologic, clinical, or laboratory findings from well-characterized treatment trials or prospective, longitudinal cohorts) is needed to untangle complex disease pathways or distinguish meaningful biological signals for disease prognosis and treatment response from background noise.

Sources for broadened data sampling that also improve the patient-centeredness of research endeavors would include patient registries that collect self-reported data directly from patients and biobanks that catalog biological material along with associated health information. Both patient registries and biobanks are underused in Lyme IACI research. Of 42 Lyme IACI research articles that mentioned the use of biological samples, just three reported obtaining those samples from a biobank. While data from patient registries and biobanks cannot substitute for randomized trials, the adoption of infrastructure and best practices to support the quality, standardization, and sustainability of these data streams would enable them to better complement clinical research. A coordinated research strategy between Lyme IACI and other similar conditions can also expand the pool of useful data across diseases with common symptoms, though careful data characterization and stratification will be critical to identify commonalities and differences among conditions. Artificial intelligence (AI) tools may be used to overcome challenges in analyzing the large volumes of data. For example, AI applications could be developed to analyze unstructured data from a patient registry and generate testable hypotheses on mechanistic pathways for Lyme IACI, or to predict subpopulations based on various sources of clinical and laboratory data.

RECOMMENDATION 4: To enhance impact in research, funders and managers of biobanks and patient registries for Lyme infection-associated chronic illnesses (IACI) should adopt the following practices that optimize the sustainability of these resources and the accessibility, quality, and utility of their samples.
    a. Biobanks should promote awareness, coordination, governance, accessibility, sustainability, and standardization of data and samples from participants with Lyme IACI and those serving as appropriate control groups, including healthy controls and participants with other similar conditions or symptoms.
    b. Biobanks and patient registries should refine and make public the data domains they capture to increase accessibility and spur collaboration. In sample and data collection, the samples should be characterized in a manner that promotes data quality

and confidence in their use. Biological collections associated with individual research studies should follow a standardized set of basic data and metadata domains to facilitate use across studies.
c. Biobanks and patient registries should develop and communicate protocols that describe the intended use of collected samples and data for participants who contribute their data and samples.

Collaborate and Coordinate

Lyme IACI research currently does not have a coordination mechanism. This inhibits both collaboration and the effective sharing of information and resources across research sites. The expansion of trial networks will be important to developing a concerted strategy within Lyme IACI research and to connecting with research advances in other similar conditions, but supporting such an expansion will require significant infrastructure. An effective model that has been applied to ME/CFS and Long COVID research is a data-coordinating center that promotes collaboration, improves interoperability, and reduces administrative burden on investigators in complex and interdisciplinary research.

RECOMMENDATION 5: Research funders should support the development and sustainment of a Lyme infection-associated chronic illnesses (IACI) research data-coordinating center that facilitates resource and knowledge sharing across programs conducting Lyme IACI clinical research and incorporates input from people living with Lyme IACI.
a. To further the visibility of biobank resources, the research data coordinating center should collaborate with biobanks on the development of a central repository that catalogues the location and characteristics of available samples and data.

There is an unrealized opportunity for researchers, clinicians, and people living with Lyme IACI and other conditions with similar clinical features to share knowledge, best practices, and other learnings to understand and address what may be common mechanistic pathways or effective treatments across the different syndromes. Pooling research efforts to examine biological processes that may be at the root of these similar conditions can streamline the discovery, validation, and translation of findings to maximize impact from the available funding and resources. For example, this coordinated approach could identify new treatments that are effective in treating symptoms shared by more than one condition (e.g., an anti-inflammatory drug that works for fatigue in ME/CFS and Lyme IACI) while reducing the inefficiencies of conducting individual, sequential studies for each disease. These studies need to be designed carefully to ensure scientific rigor and patient-centeredness, with an appropriate stratification of the study participants for meaningful and robust analyses of the specific pathogen trigger, additional risk factors, or host characteristics.

> RECOMMENDATION 6: The Department of Health and Human Services (HHS) should develop an integrated strategic plan for infection-associated chronic illnesses (IACI) research that facilitates collaboration across the different disease research efforts. The strategic plan should improve the understanding of commonalities among IACI and identify and advance interventions to address specific conditions, including Lyme IACI. The strategic plan should balance the need for clinical research on treatments, basic and clinical research on disease mechanisms, and incorporation of real-world evidence (RWE).
> a. The strategic plan should prioritize the development and support of substantive efforts to improve the treatment and management of IACI symptoms.
> b. The strategic plan should include continued investment in large-scale, prospective, multicenter observational studies designed to generate evidence on the mechanistic similarities and differences between Lyme IACI and other IACI, including clinical and laboratory characteristics.
> c. To complement prospective studies, the strategic plan should address the opportunity to use RWE, including information based on patient registry data and findings from observational studies.

TIME FOR ACTION

As this report lays out, the current understanding of the causes and mechanisms of Lyme IACI and how to best treat the disease state remain unclear. Yet there is urgency to proceed with research to identify and develop safe and effective treatments that can restore functionality and quality of life despite these uncertainties, as many people continue seeking relief from debilitating symptoms of Lyme IACI in the vacuum of evidence-based treatments for this condition. Research capable of delivering effective Lyme IACI treatments can be conducted now. However, there needs to be a paradigm shift in how researchers, clinicians, and funders navigate the uncertainties and complexities within this field: specifically, researchers should prioritize the investigation of treatments to address the symptoms of

Lyme IACI, while investigations of the disease mechanism occur in parallel with or as a complement to the treatment-oriented efforts. The Lyme IACI field should take advantage of this paradigm shift to enhance standardization and coordination among its dedicated researchers, clinicians, people living with Lyme IACI, and funders for these efforts. Furthermore, there is a critical opportunity to advance Lyme IACI research through enhanced collaboration with related disease areas such as Long COVID and ME/CFS. The committee's six recommendations chart the path to concerted action on research that will benefit the individuals living with Lyme IACI.

1

Introduction

Lyme disease, or Lyme borreliosis, is the most common vector-borne disease in the United States (Rosenberg et al., 2018). While limitations in diagnosis and reporting continue to make accurate surveillance for Lyme disease difficult, estimates suggest that an average of 476,000 cases of Lyme disease were diagnosed each year between 2010 and 2018 (Kugeler et al., 2021). This represented a significant increase in the number of cases over the previous decade, which had an estimated 329,000 cases per year from 2005 to 2010 (Nelson et al., 2015). With effective antibiotic treatment, most people with Lyme disease recover. However, some individuals who have Lyme disease and receive the recommended antibiotic treatment still experience prolonged symptoms, sometimes for years, limiting the individual's function and quality of life (Aucott et al., 2022). The presence of these symptoms following Lyme disease and corresponding antibiotic treatment is referred to in this report as Lyme infection-associated chronic illnesses (IACI). There are no accepted, standardized, or proven treatments for Lyme IACI, despite the significant burden of the condition for those living with it.

STUDY CONTEXT AND CHARGE

To explore opportunities for new treatments that could address this unmet need, the Steven & Alexandra Cohen Foundation asked the National Academies of Sciences, Engineering, and Medicine to assess the evidence base for the etiology and treatment of Lyme IACI and to clarify a pathway toward identifying and developing interventions for this disease state. In accordance with standard procedures, the National Academies formed an independent ad hoc committee of 14 volunteer experts with the requisite knowledge and experience to address the five aspects of this challenging issue outlined in the statement of task (Box 1-1). The Committee on the Evidence Base for Lyme Infection-Associated Chronic Illnesses Treatment consisted of individuals with expertise in treating persistent symptoms associated with Lyme disease or similar conditions, clinical trials design and methodology, public health and epidemiology, neuroscience and infectious diseases research, health policy, medical ethics, community engagement, and individuals with lived experience with lingering symptoms associated with Lyme disease. This committee conducted a careful review of the current evidence, considered the perspectives shared by people affected by Lyme IACI, and sought input from clinicians and researchers working to address

---

BOX 1-1
Statement of Task

An ad hoc committee under the auspices of the National Academies of Sciences, Engineering, and Medicine will conduct a study of the evidence base for Lyme infection-associated chronic illnesses (Lyme IACI) treatment. Specifically, the committee will:

- Review current knowledge and gaps regarding research into the etiology of Lyme IACI and clinical trials for its treatment;
- Examine what is known regarding co-infection with multiple tick-borne pathogens, and consider implications for research and development of Lyme IACI diagnostics and treatment;
- Consider how emerging lessons learned from Long COVID and other infection-associated chronic conditions may be applied to advancing Lyme IACI treatment;
- Explore advances in medicine and biotechnology that may hold promise for accelerating Lyme IACI treatment; and
- Identify priorities for additional research to advance Lyme IACI diagnostics and treatment.

The study is intended to focus on diagnostics and treatment of Lyme IACI symptoms and not to improve diagnostics and treatment for acute Lyme disease. As such, the prevention of Lyme disease transmission or onset, including development and use of vaccines or other prophylactic drugs, is also outside the scope of this study. Based on its review of the literature and input from a public workshop, the committee will develop a report with its findings, conclusions, and recommendations for advancing Lyme IACI treatment.

Lyme and other IACI. The recommendations in this report are focused on providing a research framework for timely advancement of new treatment options for Lyme IACI by learning from similar conditions, incorporating lived experience, and shifting the current paradigm to prioritize clinical trials for treatments.

BACKGROUND

Diagnosis and Epidemiology of Lyme Disease

Lyme disease is caused by members of the *Borrelia burgdorferi* sensu lato species complex, a group of spirochetal bacteria found in arthropod and vertebrate reservoirs and transmitted to humans via arthropod bites.[1] Lyme disease is endemic throughout many regions in Europe, Asia, and North America, with environmental factors expected to drive further expansion (Stone et al., 2017). In the United States, *Borrelia burgdorferi* sensu stricto (i.e., *B. burgdorferi*) is the most common causative pathogen, though a handful of cases have been attributed to *Borrelia mayonii* since 2013.[2,3] Clinical manifestations may differ between Lyme disease acquired in Europe and in the United States (Marques et al., 2021). The primary vectors transmitting *B. burgdorferi* to humans in North America are the black-legged ticks, *Ixodes scapularis* and *Ixodes pacificus* (Brown and Lane, 1992; Kilpatrick et al., 2017). Notably, not all *Ixodes* spp. ticks are infected with the *Borrelia* spp. bacteria (Tokarz et al., 2019). *Ixodes* species that are infected can carry various genotypes of *B. burgdorferi*, which may contribute to heterogeneity in the clinical presentation of Lyme disease (Crowder et al., 2010; Lemieux et al., 2023; Tyler et al., 2018), and may carry multiple

---

[1] There is controversy as to whether the existing *Borrelia* genus should be split into two genera: *Borrelia* and *Borreliella* (Winslow and Coburn, 2019). In the new classification, Lyme borreliosis-causing bacteria would fall into the latter. Given the unresolved controversy and historical association with Lyme disease and established literature, this report will use the *Borrelia* genus name throughout.

[2] *Borrelia burgdorferi* sensu stricto will be referred to as simply *Borrelia burgdorferi* or *B. burgdorferi* throughout this report.

[3] Based on currently available epidemiology data, *B. mayonii* remains a rare cause of Lyme disease that appears to be limited to the upper Midwest. To date, eight cases of *B. mayonii* have been reported in the literature, and none have been associated with chronic sequelae (McGowan, 2023). Public health surveillance from Wisconsin and Minnesota have identified one to three cases each year since the pathogen was first identified in 2013 (Minnesota Department of Health, 2022; Wisconsin Department of Health Services, 2024). Reference to *Borrelia spp.* that cause Lyme disease throughout the report is based on data reported for *B. burgdorferi* unless otherwise specified. Furthermore, the report refers to findings, conclusions, and recommendations related to chronic sequelae associated with Lyme disease attributed to *B. burgdorferi* with the intention that they may also apply to Lyme IACI resulting from *B. mayonii* infections.

other pathogens that can cause human disease (e.g., *Anaplasma phagocytophilum*, *Babesia spp.*, *Borrelia miyamotoi*, deer tick virus) (Caulfield and Pritt, 2015). Acknowledging the differences between Lyme disease outside of and originating in the United States, the committee focused its efforts primarily on reviewing the available evidence for *B. burgdorferi* sensu stricto while also considering important information from relevant non-U.S. studies when appropriate.

Lyme disease was first described in the United States in the late 1970s (Steere et al., 1977), the U.S. Centers for Disease Control and Prevention began surveillance of the disease by 1982, and it was designated as a nationally reportable disease in 1990 (Orloski et al., 2000). Despite the recognition of its public health importance and efforts to address its impact, the accuracy of the surveillance for Lyme disease continues to be challenged by several limitations in diagnosis and reporting.

Early Lyme disease often presents with a characteristic erythema migrans (EM) rash or lesion, which may be accompanied by general symptoms including fever, sweats and chills, headache, fatigue, muscle and joint pain, and swollen lymph nodes (Steere, 2001; Steere et al., 2003; Wormser, 2006). The presence of an EM can serve as a highly suggestive clinical diagnostic sign during early disease. In an endemic region, a clinical diagnosis may be made for individuals presenting with a characteristic EM and a possible tick exposure (Eldin et al., 2019; Lantos et al., 2021). However, 20–30 percent of people with Lyme disease who are seeking care may not present with a rash, and the EM lesion does not always appear in its typical form, leading to missed diagnoses and resulting in later manifestations such as Lyme arthritis, (Schwartz et al., 2017; Steere et al., 2003). When no EM is observed, diagnosis may be delayed or missed before the development of additional clinical symptoms or biomarkers (Lantos et al., 2021). Further complicating the clinical diagnosis, a similar rash is present in the southern tick-associated rash illness (STARI), which may follow bites by lone star ticks (*Amblyomma americanum*) but which is not caused by *B. burgdorferi* and not associated with Lyme IACI (Philipp et al., 2006; Wormser et al., 2005). While the geographic distribution of STARI and Lyme disease are generally separate, anthropogenic environmental changes have led to expansions in the range of these vectors that threaten to create increasing overlap between the two along the Atlantic coast and into the Midwestern states (Springer et al., 2015).

Laboratory evidence to support the diagnosis of infectious diseases can be categorized as direct or indirect detection. Direct detection assays determine the presence of a specific disease pathogen using methods such as detection of whole organisms (e.g., via culture or microscopy) or antigens or nucleic acids from the organism. Indirect detection assays measure different components of the host response to the pathogen or disease state (e.g., antibodies). While *B. burgdorferi* may be cultivated or detected by methods such as poLymerase chain reaction, these methods are not sufficiently sensitive and reliable for clinical use. Other direct detection approaches, such as culturing bacteria from tissue biopsies, have also not yielded validated clinically assays, though readouts from a recent clinical trial for xenodiagnoses, a unique approach with proof-of-concept data, have not been released (Marques et al., 2014; NIAID, 2024). Support for the diagnosis of Lyme disease relies on testing for *B. burgdorferi* antibodies, an indirect diagnostic approach. Despite continued improvements to serologic assay methods, there are inherent limitations to serodiagnosis that affect clinical accuracy (see Glossary) (Branda and Steere, 2021). Because it takes a few weeks for the body to generate antibodies after infection, these tests have limited sensitivity during this early period of infection when people with EM typically seek medical evaluation. In addition, early antibiotic treatment may alter the kinetics and character of antibody response. People receiving antibiotics due to recognition of EM may produce overall lower levels of *B. burgdorferi* antibodies, may only produce antibodies against a limited repertoire of *Borrelia* antigens, and may have impeded IgM-to-IgG isotype switching. This may lead to false-negative serologic results during the acute clinical phase when the EM is apparent and occasionally even during the convalescent (post-treatment) phase of illness. Compared with individuals who received antibiotic treatment early in the disease course, those treated for late or disseminated Lyme disease typically mount a more robust antibody response and remain seropositive for longer despite a resolution of their symptoms. In such individuals the antibody response—even the IgM isotype—may persist, for up to 10–20 years after treatment. Thus, positive serologic tests, including for IgM, cannot reliably distinguish between a prior exposure to *B. burgdorferi* and an ongoing infection or determine the recency of an infection (Kalish et al., 2001). A number of active research efforts are underway to identify and develop new diagnostic approaches for Lyme disease, including detection of the host response through transcriptomics, proteomics, and metabolomics (Bockenstedt and Belperron, 2024; LymeX Innovation, 2025).

Treatment of Lyme Disease

Recommended antibiotic treatment for early Lyme disease typically includes the use of oral doxycycline or amoxicillin. For some patients with neurological involvement, intravenous ceftriaxone or oral doxycycline is recommended (Lantos et al., 2021). If untreated, early Lyme disease symptoms may resolve or may progress and later present with neurologic, cardiac, or joint involvement or some combination of the three (Steere et al., 2016). While neurologic or cardiac disease usually occurs relatively early in the course of Lyme disease, sometimes overlapping with the presence of EM, Lyme arthritis typically occurs months to years after the untreated initial infection. Most people with either early or late Lyme disease recover after recommended antibiotic treatment, but a subset of individuals experience long-lasting and debilitating symptoms that may last months, years, or even decades.

Lyme Infection-Associated Chronic Illnesses

The estimated prevalence of Lyme IACI varies widely. It is challenging to estimate how many people are living with Lyme IACI without a consensus case definition for the syndrome, especially given the subjective symptoms that overlap with those of similar conditions. The commonly referenced estimate of the proportion of individuals experiencing protracted symptoms after standard antibiotic treatment of Lyme disease is 10–20 percent, a range that was drawn from prospective studies where the reported prevalence ranges from 0 to 36 percent (Aucott, 2013b; Aucott et al., 2022; Weitzner 2015; Wormser et al., 2020). On the other hand, 61 percent of participants in the MyLymeData patient registry self-reported as having chronic Lyme disease (Johnson, 2019).[4] The wide range in prevalence estimated from the aforementioned studies and the patient may be attributed to a few reasons, including the inherent difference between the participants captured by prospective cohort studies and those from a retrospectively surveyed, patient-driven disease registry. For the pediatric population, one publication suggests that some children and adolescents experience persistent symptoms, but this was a retrospective survey study, and prospective studies are needed to further examine the prevalence in this population (Monaghan et al., 2024). Data from these studies are discussed in more detail in Chapter 2.

The most common long-term, unrelenting post-treatment symptoms that patients have reported include persistent fatigue, cognitive issues (so-called "brain fog," which includes difficulties with concentration, memory, and word finding), sleep quality disturbances, and recurring pain, which may include headache, joint pain, and other musculoskeletal pain.[5] Mood disturbances and orthostatic intolerance, which may be related to postural orthostatic tachycardia syndrome (POTS) or other forms of autonomic dysfunction, have also been observed (Rebman and Aucott, 2020). All of these symptoms may occur alone or in combination and may fluctuate in intensity over time. For example, one randomized trial of individuals with

---

[4] LymeDisease.org, the home organization of the MyLymeData registry, defines "chronic Lyme disease" as remaining ill for ≥ 6 months after treatment with antibiotics for 10–21 days.

[5] Other symptoms have been reported in the MyLymeData patient registry and in peer-reviewed studies.

Lyme IACI found that commonly reported symptoms at baseline ranged in prevalence from less than half of individuals experiencing headache or dysesthesia (painful or burning sensation) to as high as 92 percent for arthralgia or myalgia (Klempner et al., 2001).

Controversy and disagreement remain over the terminology used to describe the collection of these debilitating symptoms. The terms "chronic Lyme disease" and "persistent Lyme disease," which are adapted and preferred by various organizations, have evolved to take on implications of disease etiology, for which there is no scientific consensus (i.e., unsupported implications that chronic or persistent *B. burgdorferi* infection is the cause of these symptoms). Individuals experiencing persistent and debilitating symptoms may be characterized as having post-treatment Lyme disease syndrome (PTLDS) (Aucott et al., 2013a; Wormser et al., 2006). Developed for research purposes, PTLDS requires a well-documented diagnosis of Lyme disease, a set of subjective symptoms based on patient reports, and significant impact of the symptoms on daily activities for 6 or more months after completing recommended treatment for Lyme disease (see Chapter 2). There are clear advantages to having a precise definition of the study population in conducting research. The trade-off for this stringency is the exclusion of people with these symptoms who may not have clinical or serologic evidence to meet the PTLDS criteria but whose conditions still need understanding and treatment (Aucott et al., 2012, 2013a; Rebman and Aucott, 2020).

The recognition of Long COVID as "an infection-associated chronic condition that occurs after SARS-CoV-2 infection" (NASEM, 2024a) has focused attention on the legitimacy and importance of post-acute infection syndromes that have been documented following a number of viral, bacterial, and parasitic diseases (Choutka et al., 2022). In 2023, the National Academies held a public workshop on advancing a common research agenda for these post-infection syndromes, referred to as "infection-associated chronic illnesses" (NASEM, 2024b). Following the increasing acceptance and use of the terms "infection-associated chronic illnesses (or conditions)"[6] to describe persistent symptoms with a potential infectious trigger, the committee adapted "Lyme IACI" as an umbrella term to, for the purposes of this study, encompass the broad group of illnesses that have been previously described under a variety of terminologies, including PTLDS, chronic Lyme disease, persistent Lyme disease, and others. As with Long COVID, the use of this term affirms the authenticity and impacts of the symptoms experienced by people but does not carry any proven implications with respect to disease etiology or pathogenesis.

---

[6] See Key Terms below.

Unlike the case for Long COVID, a working definition of Lyme IACI has not yet been established, and this committee was not charged with defining the condition (Box 1-2). However, the committee has been asked to examine the current knowledge on the etiology and clinical trials for treatment of Lyme IACI. In the absence of a consensus definition of Lyme IACI, the committee developed an operational scope for the limited purpose of conducting the necessary literature review (Box 1-3). As with Long COVID and other infection-associated chronic illnesses, a full understanding of the pathogenesis of Lyme IACI remains elusive, and hypothesized disease mechanisms have ranged from the persistence of pathogens or antigens to host responses such as microbiome alterations, autoimmunity, or other immune dysregulation (Bobe et al., 2021; Marques et al., 2021). Similarly, while there are diagnostic procedures to detect the initial infection (i.e., *B. burgdorferi* infection in the case of Lyme IACI), there are currently no known or validated objective biomarkers, clinical examinations, or laboratory findings to define or diagnose Lyme IACI, monitor treatment

---

BOX 1-2
Defining Lyme IACI

There are many ways to characterize diseases for specific applications, from criteria that guide research enrollment or stratification to case definitions that can be used in clinical care, epidemiological surveillance, or benefit claims. These different descriptions are developed for different use cases: more detailed or narrower definitions ensure accuracy of conclusions that can be drawn from research results, whereas a broader clinical definition can be necessary for diagnosis and access to care. Feasibility of use is also considered in development of these specific definitions (e.g., case definition for epidemiological surveillance would be hard to operationalize if it requires use of highly specialized methods or equipment that are not readily available to sources that track or report the disease).

A consensus definition for Lyme IACI can serve as the basis for these derivative definitions and applications. In that case, it is clear that the consensus definition needs to be developed through thorough and careful considerations of the potential downstream use cases, perspectives of the users (e.g., people living with Lyme IACI, clinicians who treat this disease, researchers, among others), and how to balance between these different elements. While the necessary time for extensive engagement and requisite expertise to conduct this deliberation could not be a part of this study process, this report does issue recommendations to guide future efforts in defining Lyme IACI.

response, or indicate cure. No prognostic factors have been consistently shown to predict the risk of developing Lyme IACI after the initial disease, and no validated treatments are available, though research remains ongoing for future diagnosis and therapeutic options. Objective indicators and diagnostic procedures for Lyme IACI may yet be identified in the future, as exploratory research has reported potentially promising findings. Chapter 2 summarizes the committee's review of the existing evidence from published literature on Lyme IACI etiology, diagnosis, and treatment.

Impact of Disease

It is clear that Lyme IACI, even when limited to the minority of individuals who meet the criteria for PTLDS, have significant health and economic impacts on society. Based on the current estimates of prevalence from prospective observational studies, tens of thousands of people may develop Lyme IACI in the United States each year,[7] while a simulation model that assumes linear growth of Lyme disease diagnosis from year to year suggests that a cumulative count of nearly 2 million people in the United States may have experienced PTLDS at some point in their lifetime between 1980 and 2020 (DeLong et al., 2019). In Europe, cumulative or societal cost-of-illness has been reported to be over 170 million euros for PTLDS in Belgium and between 5.2 million and 6.3 million euros for persistent symptoms related to Lyme disease in the Netherlands (approximately 27 percent of the 19.3–23.5 million euro total societal cost associated with Lyme disease) (van den Wijngaard et al., 2017; Willems et al., 2023). While there have not been

---

BOX 1-3
Operational Scope of Lyme IACI

For the purpose of this study, the committee carried out a review of the literature under the following operational scope: that "Lyme infection-associated chronic illnesses" includes an illness with otherwise unexplained symptoms that persist for at least 6 months following antibiotic treatment for either proven or presumed infection with *Borrelia spp.* that cause Lyme disease. See Chapter 2 for details.

---

[7] Calculated based on the average estimated prevalence of PTLDS following Lyme disease diagnosis from the studies discussed earlier in the chapter (range between 14–20 percent depending on interpretation of Wormser et al., 2020) and the currently reported annual prevalence of Lyme disease of 476,000.

specific attempts to estimate the financial costs of Lyme IACI in the United States, the aggregated cost-of-illness for Lyme disease in the United States was estimated to range from $345 million to over $900 million dollars each year (in 2016) and projected to continue increasing (Hook et al., 2022).

Without specific diagnostic tools for Lyme IACI, patients and care providers rely on symptom reports coupled with diagnostics for the initial *Borrelia spp.* infection, some of which may be derived from methods or facilities whose performance has not been validated (Fallon et al., 2014; Waddell et al., 2016). The lack of diagnostic tools and the subjective nature of the persistent symptoms have often led to stigmatization and dismissal of people living with Lyme IACI by the health care system, as these individuals and their illnesses do not match well-established disease narratives besides "medically unexplained symptoms" (Ali et al., 2014). As with other complex chronic conditions of unclear cause (e.g., Long COVID), and absent well-documented effective interventions, the U.S. medical system is not geared to provide effective longitudinal—and perhaps multidisciplinary—care and support for these people.

Studies have shown that patient suffering is high, with health-related quality of life being lower compared with control populations and with individuals with some other chronic diseases (Johnson et al., 2014; Rebman et al., 2017). Further, depression rates in this group of patients are estimated as being between 8 and 45 percent, and these individuals are at increased risk for suicide (Doshi et al., 2018; Fallon et al., 2021). A study of individuals diagnosed with PTLDS found that they exhibited an increased prevalence of depression and sleep disturbance compared to healthy controls (Rebman et al., 2017). In another study of individuals reporting persistent symptoms after diagnosis and treatment of Lyme disease, this group was more likely to report concentration problems and receive a diagnosis of major depressive disorder and generalized anxiety disorder when compared to healthy controls and controls with other chronic conditions (Hassett et al., 2008).

Due to the physical and mental toll of living with Lyme IACI and the lack of available treatments, people living with Lyme IACI are in urgent need for therapies to alleviate their symptoms, improve quality of life, or cure the underlying disease state. As there are no therapies demonstrated to be safe and effective through clinical research, patients and their treating clinicians seek out approaches or treatments that are deemed to have the potential to address their symptoms based on clinical experience or experience in illnesses with similar symptoms. Since these treatments are not approved for this condition, patients often have to pay out of pocket for expensive care and treatments of unknown safety and effectiveness (Box 1-4). Among patients diagnosed with Lyme disease, those subsequently diagnosed with PTLDS-related conditions were found to have medical

> **BOX 1-4**
> **A Critical Need and Opportunity**
>
> Adults with capacity have the right to make their own health care decisions in consultation with a clinician, yet for these decisions to be well informed, the efficacy, potential risks, benefits, and burdens of treatment need to be made clear. In the absence of evidence-based treatments that effectively alleviate persistent symptoms, those living with Lyme IACI have reported trying various interventions, many of which have not been rigorously evaluated in clinical research for this population. Clinicians are also unable to discuss the scientific evidence regarding potential risks and benefits in relation to the individual's experiences, values, and preferences. Rigorous clinical evaluations of possible interventions are therefore key to informing the public about the potential risks and benefits of using an intervention.
>
> Six randomized trials have been conducted on potential treatments for Lyme IACI, but no intervention has been found to lead to sustained benefit for people living with Lyme IACI. Many possible interventions, including those that patients currently use, have never been tested through rigorous clinical evaluations. While some interventions used by people living with Lyme IACI may not have sufficient scientific rationale to merit their evaluation in randomized trials, others may represent scientifically plausible interventions that lack empirical data. Researchers must embrace opportunities to partner with the Lyme IACI community—including people with Lyme IACI, clinicians who treat this disease, and other caregivers—throughout the entire research process, with attention to the patient voice in identifying symptoms of greatest concern and developing clinically meaningful outcome measures. Moreover, given the lack of options for people seeking symptom relief from Lyme IACI, interventions shown to be effective in similar conditions, such as Long COVID, may also be effective at treating symptoms of Lyme IACI. These critical opportunities will be explored throughout the report.

costs that were nearly twice that of patients with Lyme disease but without persistent symptoms (Adrion et al., 2015).[8] Up to half of the illness-related costs are borne out-of-pocket, as people living with Lyme IACI often sought complementary therapies to alleviate their symptoms that have not been

---

[8] Since there is no standard clinical definition or medical record coding for PTLDS, this study used *International Classifications of Diseases* codes corresponding to symptoms covered under PTLDS and referred to these as "PTLDS-related conditions." These include debility and undue fatigue, musculoskeletal signs and symptoms, peripheral neuropathy or neuritis, arthropathy, and nonspecific signs and symptoms.

validated in clinical research for Lyme IACI. The financial burden might be even higher for those without insurance, as the majority of participants in available studies had health insurance coverage (70 percent in Hook et al., 2022, and 100 percent in Adrion et al., 2015).

A robust patient community has developed to share resources and information, often based on their individual experiences navigating the medical system and trying various therapies. However, given the nature of protracted symptoms experienced by people living with Lyme IACI and the paucity of efficacious treatments supported by evidence generated through clinical studies, profiteering entities have also emerged to exploit this prolonged unmet needs by promoting products and procedures that are costly, may not work, and may cause harm (Sakizadeh et al., 2025).

Context of Other Infection-Associated Chronic Illnesses

Shortly after the start of the COVID-19 pandemic, some individuals started reporting persisting, often long-term, symptoms after acute SARS-CoV-2 infection. This condition is now named Long COVID. The large scale of the COVID-19 pandemic has raised awareness in the medical and scientific world, as well as for the public, that acute infections can trigger chronic illness.

However, chronic illness after infections has been described for decades. Various viral pathogens have been associated with IACI, including not just SARS-CoV-2 but Ebola virus, dengue viruses, poliovirus, chikungunya virus, Epstein-Barr virus, enteroviruses, and West Nile virus as well as several nonviral pathogens, including *Coxiella burnetti* (the bacterial causative agent of Q fever) and *Giardia lamblia* (the protozoan causative agent of giardiasis) (Choutka et al., 2022). Also described as "post-acute infection syndromes," these conditions are generally characterized by chronic, nonspecific symptoms that remain or develop following an acute infection and typically lack objective markers to aid in diagnosis. The committee uses the term "IACI" throughout this report to refer to chronic illnesses with a potential infectious trigger and encompass some conditions, like myalgic encephalomyelitis/chronic fatigue syndrome (ME/CFS) or fibromyalgia, where the etiology remains unknown but have been documented to include infectious triggers (Hickie et al., 2006; Magnus et al., 2015; Hanson, 2023). ME/CFS is referenced throughout this report, although the committee does not intend to imply that infections are the only root cause of ME/CFS.

A clear overlap in symptoms can be identified among many IACI, including ME/CFS, Long COVID, and Lyme IACI (Bai and Richardson, 2023; Komaroff and Lipkin, 2023). The symptoms described in the literature that overlap for Lyme IACI, ME/CFS, and Long COVID include fatigue, musculoskeletal pain, sleep disorders, and cognitive issues.[9] There are some symptoms associated frequently with ME/CFS but rarely in the other two conditions (painful lymph nodes, chemical sensitivities, and tinnitus) and others that are associated primarily with Long COVID but not ME/CFS or Lyme IACI (e.g., decreased smell and taste, rash, and hair loss) (Komaroff and Lipkin, 2023). However, the overlapping symptoms (fatigue, pain, cognitive dysfunction) are also the ones most commonly reported by those with Lyme IACI. The degree to which these symptoms overlap with other similar conditions, along with the lack of specific biomarkers for each condition, makes it difficult to diagnose the root cause of an individual's symptoms, particularly with the near ubiquitous exposure to SARS-CoV-2 (Figure 1-1; see Chapter 3).

In addition to the similarities in symptoms and hypothesized underlying disease mechanisms, people living with these illnesses also often share the common experience of not being believed to be ill if diagnostic testing for general disease biomarkers are not able to substantiate the real, even if subjective, symptoms that they have. Taken together, Lyme IACI and at least two other similar conditions, Long COVID and ME/CFS, are connected in the lack of understanding by health care practitioners, the lack of effective interventions, and the marginalization and suffering of people living with these illnesses.

COMMITTEE APPROACH

To reinforce a person-centered conceptualization of the nuanced and multifactorial components of Lyme disease and the development of Lyme IACI, the committee developed a conceptual framework to visualize the various elements and their potential interactions in the development and treatment of Lyme IACI. This conceptual framework (Figure 1-2) specifically highlights the individual factors that may affect one's ability to navigate their illness trajectory. The framework does not purport to encompass a universal experience and instead serves as a general outline of the factors surrounding the development and experience of Lyme IACI.

Committee's Interpretation of the Task and Approach

While the prevention of Lyme disease is the most straightforward way to reduce the burden of Lyme IACI, effective prevention likely requires sustained education initiatives directed at the public and clinicians, which are outside the purview of this committee but has been addressed in other

---

[9] Post-exertional malaise is reported by some as a symptom of Lyme IACI but has not been evaluated separately from measures of fatigue in studies on Lyme IACI.

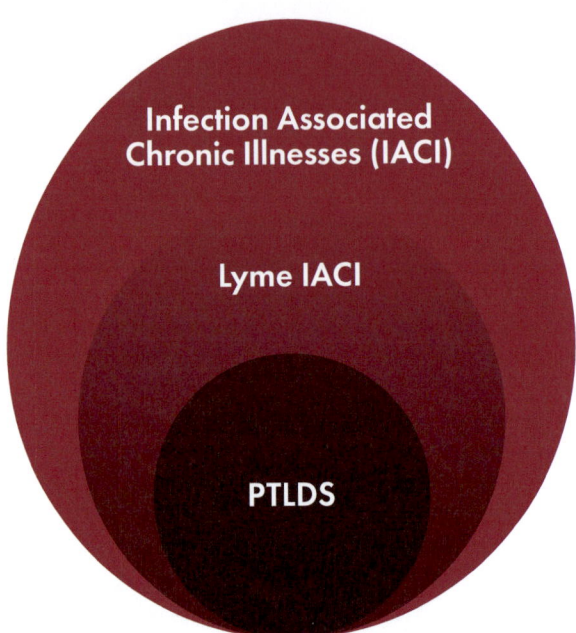

FIGURE 1-1 Conceptual relationship among post-treatment Lyme disease syndrome (PTLDS), Lyme infection-associated chronic illnesses (IACI), and the broader IACI space.
NOTES: The largest oval includes individuals with syndromes likely triggered by non-Lyme infections, including Long COVID, and other chronic conditions such as ME/CFS with potential infectious triggers, known and unknown. The two embedded ovals indicate a subset that includes people with a possible diagnosis of Lyme IACI (i.e., not meeting the criteria for PTLDS and may have a Lyme-related IACI or may have illness triggered by non-Lyme factors) and, within that group, those with well-documented prior *B. burgdorferi* infection (i.e., meeting criteria for PTLDS) and others. The blurring between Lyme IACI and larger IACI ovals represents the challenges in distinguishing etiology between the groups, given both uncertainties in diagnosis of Lyme IACI and the widespread presence of other IACI, including Long COVID. This figure is a general depiction of the relationship between the three populations and the difficulty in distinguishing between them.

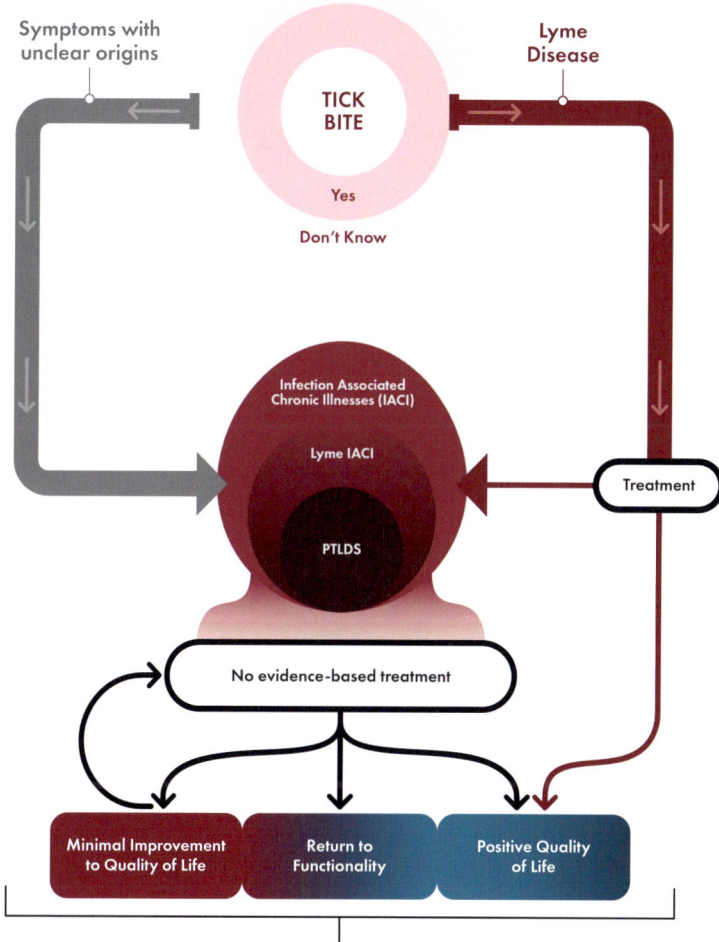

FIGURE 1-2 Conceptual framework of the development and impact of Lyme IACI on the individual patient experience.
NOTES: Not all individuals who are bitten by ticks will develop Lyme disease, and not all individuals with Lyme disease will develop Lyme IACI. This figure is focused on the trajectories and experiences of individuals with Lyme IACI. Scenarios in which Lyme IACI is absent are not depicted. IACI = infection-associated chronic illnesses; PTLDS = post-treatment Lyme disease syndrome.

reports (TBDWG, 2018, 2020). Preventive measures, including post-tick bite prophylaxis to prevent development of Lyme disease or progression to Lyme IACI, were also not considered to be within scope for this study. Clinical care and management guidelines or recommendations, explored in the aforementioned reports, do not fall within the committee's charge to examine current scientific evidence and research priorities to advance new treatments. Identifying new treatments that are ready for clinical use and evaluating their integration into the practice of evidence-based medicine are also beyond the scope of this report. The focus of this report is on generation of research evidence on Lyme IACI treatments, which is part of an evidence-based medicine framework, but the other components of this framework (patient values and clinician judgment in the context of clinical decisions) are not within the charge to this committee.

In examining the evidence base, the committee determined that the study would focus on persistent symptoms associated with prior Lyme disease in the United States, while acknowledging that there may be findings from research in Europe that could inform the committee's task. The committee decided that general findings from studies based in Europe that are relevant to the committee's review could be incorporated into the report. The committee also interpreted the scope of literature review on treatments to include both curative interventions, if any are reported, and those that manage or improve symptoms, while excluding publications that solely comment on the provision of care. Similarly, the committee decided that while the report might include consideration of medical ethics in conducting future research, the role of medical ethics in clinical practice was out of scope for this study. The committee focused its efforts on the examining the uncertainties and knowledge gaps in the current evidence base, interpreted as limited to biomedical and clinical research. Aspects of implementation research (e.g., economics, health systems, or disability research) were considered out of scope for this study. Given that the overarching focus of the study is on treatments for Lyme IACI, the committee interpreted the statement of task (Box 1-1) such that the examination of diagnostics and etiology literature would be framed through its role in advancing new treatments that benefit people who are living with these chronic symptoms. Accordingly, the committee focused its literature search on the pathogenic mechanisms of Lyme IACI (Figure 1-3).

The committee also focused on Long COVID and ME/CFS as two conditions with similar symptoms and potential infectious triggers and, given the significant research efforts and available literature, as a basis for expanding the literature review for lessons learned that could inform future Lyme IACI research. However, the committee focused its efforts on identifying recommendations for future Lyme IACI research rather than on conducting an exhaustive review of the existing literature for Long COVID, ME/CFS, and other similar conditions.

INTRODUCTION

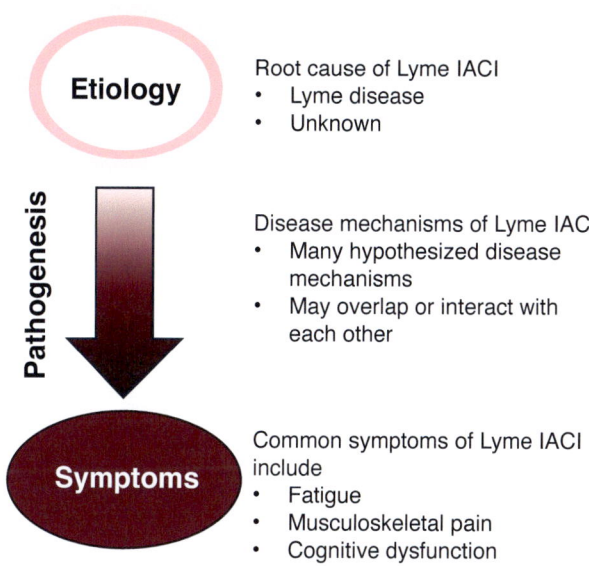

FIGURE 1-3 Relationship between the etiology, pathogenesis, and symptoms for Lyme IACI.
NOTES: IACI = infection-associated chronic illnesses.

To address its task, the committee held three public, in-person or virtual information-gathering sessions with invited presentations from researchers, technology developers, regulators, people living with Lyme IACI, and patient-led research organizations. One hybrid (in-person and virtual) information-gathering session, held on July 11, 2024, was a public workshop, Research for Lyme Infection-Associated Chronic Illnesses Treatment: Broadening the Lens. Over the course of the study, the committee met eight times in closed session. Agendas for these meetings can be found in Appendix A.

In addition, the committee conducted a scoping review of the literature on the mechanisms, treatment, and diagnosis of Lyme IACI to gain insight into the research that has been conducted in understanding these aspects of the disease state and to identify potential knowledge gaps. While it was not within the scope of the study to put forth a consensus definition for Lyme IACI, the committee broadly considered Lyme IACI to be a condition in which an individual has persistent symptoms following Lyme disease with or without a prior Lyme disease diagnosis (see Chapter 2 for details). A detailed protocol and methodology for the scoping review is provided in Appendix C. The committee also commissioned a paper on potential artificial intelligence applications in Lyme IACI. The findings from that paper are summarized in Chapter 4.

Based on the evidence reviewed, the committee did not attempt to identify or rank specific treatments as future research priorities. However, key actions that need to be taken to advance Lyme IACI research were identified, and a framework to help enable stakeholders to assess and prioritize potential candidate interventions is presented.

Key Terms

A glossary of common scientific terminology that is used throughout the report is provided at the beginning of this report. The committee also considered and used additional key terms that the committee describes for the purposes of this report, which are detailed below.

Different terms have been used to describe the population or subpopulations living with nonspecific chronic symptoms associated with Lyme disease that share some similarities with other conditions. Some of these terms include long Lyme, chronic Lyme disease, persistent Lyme disease, and PTLDS. This study has adopted "Lyme infection-associated chronic illnesses" (Lyme IACI) to encompass these different terms. Coined at the June 2023 National Academies workshop (NASEM, 2024b), "infection-associated chronic illnesses" are characterized by similar sets of persistent, multisystem symptoms that may share common pathophysiology. This report refers to ME/CFS and Long COVID as part of this group of infection-associated chronic illnesses.

Alternatively, a related term, "infection-associated chronic conditions," has been used, sometimes interchangeably with IACI, in the emerging research literature. In health care and medicine, the term "condition" often refers to a diagnosable, billable, or defined state of health (e.g., the *International Classification of Diseases* [ICD] is a catalog of codes for health conditions that is widely used for health records and medical billing). Thus, use of the term may inadvertently exclude infection-associated chronic syndromes that currently do not have a diagnostic test or definition and may not yet be included in coding systems for payers. To avoid this unintended exclusion, this report uses the term "illnesses" to recognize these collections of infection-associated chronic syndromes. In some instances, the report also applies the colloquial use of the term "diseases" to describe IACI.

The committee recognizes that a consensus definition for Lyme IACI does not exist. For the literature review, the committee described an intentionally inclusive operational scope of this condition to address the broader need for treatment and research, regardless of the certainty with which symptoms can be attributed to Lyme disease. Differences in patient subgroups—and the potential for resulting differences in response to therapies—can be subsequently addressed through appropriate stratification in research.

Organization of the Report

This report is divided into five chapters. Chapter 2 discusses the current evidence base on Lyme IACI, including its prevalence, treatment, mechanisms, and diagnosis. The chapter culminates with key research questions that require investigation to address the gaps in the evidence base. Chapter 3 draws on insights gleaned from research on conditions similar to Lyme IACI, such as Long COVID and ME/CFS, and assesses how lessons learned from these conditions could be used in Lyme IACI research. In Chapter 4, the committee proposes a framework to prioritize Lyme IACI treatment candidates for clinical research and highlights approaches to research infrastructure, data interpretation, and research implementation that can improve the efficiency of future Lyme IACI research. The report concludes with the committee's six recommendations, which are described in Chapter 5.

REFERENCES

Adrion, E. R., J. Aucott, K. W. Lemke, and J. P. Weiner. 2015. Health care costs, utilization and patterns of care following Lyme disease. *PLOS One* 2(10):e0116767.

Ali, A., L. Vitulano, R. Lee, T. R. Weiss, and E. R. Colson. 2014. Experiences of patients identifying with chronic Lyme disease in the healthcare system: A qualitative study. *BMC Family Practice* 15(1):79.

Aucott, J. N., A. Seifter, and A. W. Rebman. 2012. Probable late Lyme disease: A variant manifestation of untreated *Borrelia burgdorferi* infection. *BMC Infectious Diseases* 12(1):173.

Aucott, J. N., L. A. Crowder, and K. B. Kortte. 2013a. Development of a foundation for a case definition of post-treatment Lyme disease syndrome. *International Journal of Infectious Diseases* 17(6):e443–e449.

Aucott, J. N., A. W. Rebman, L. A. Crowder, and K. B. Kortte. 2013b. Post-treatment Lyme disease syndrome symptomatology and the impact on life functioning: Is there something here? *Quality of Life Research* 22(1):75–84.

Aucott, J. N., T. Yang, I. Yoon, D. Powell, S. A. Geller, and A. W. Rebman. 2022. Risk of post-treatment Lyme disease in patients with ideally-treated early Lyme disease: A prospective cohort study. *International Journal of Infectious Diseases* 116:230–237.

Bai, N. A., and C. S. Richardson. 2023. Posttreatment Lyme disease syndrome and myalgic encephalomyelitis/chronic fatigue syndrome: A systematic review and comparison of pathogenesis. *Chronic Diseases and Translational Medicine* 9(3):183–190.

Bockenstedt, L. K., and A. A. Belperron. 2024. Insights from omics in Lyme disease. *Journal of Infectious Disease* 230(Supplement_1):S18-s26.

Bobe, J. R., B. L. Jutras, E. J. Horn, M. E. Embers, A. Bailey, R. L. Moritz, Y. Zhang, M. J. Soloski, R. S. Ostfeld, R. T. Marconi, J. Aucott, A. Ma'ayan, F. Keesing, K. Lewis, C. Ben Mamoun, A. W. Rebman, M. E. McClune, E. B. Breitschwerdt, P. J. Reddy, R. Maggi, F. Yang, B. Nemser, A. Ozcan, O. Garner, D. Di Carlo, Z. Ballard, H. A. Joung, A. Garcia-Romeu, R. R. Griffiths, N. Baumgarth, and B. A. Fallon. 2021. Recent progress in Lyme disease and remaining challenges. *Frontiers in Medicine (Lausanne)* 8:666554.

Branda, J. A., and A. C. Steere. 2021. Laboratory diagnosis of Lyme borreliosis. *Clinical Microbiology Reviews* 34(2):e00018-19.

Brown, R. N., and R. S. Lane. 1992. Lyme disease in California: A novel enzootic transmission cycle of *Borrelia burgdorferi*. *Science* 256(5062):1439–1442.

Caulfield, A. J., and B. S. Pritt. 2015. Lyme disease coinfections in the United States. *Clinics in Laboratory Medicine* 35(4):827–846.

Choutka, J., V. Jansari, M. Hornig, and A. Iwasaki. 2022. Unexplained post-acute infection syndromes. *Nature Medicine* 28(5):911–923.

Crowder, C. D., H. E. Matthews, S. Schutzer, M. A. Rounds, B. J. Luft, O. Nolte, S. R. Campbell, C. A. Phillipson, F. Li, R. Sampath, D. J. Ecker, and M. W. Eshoo. 2010. Genotypic variation and mixtures of Lyme *Borrelia* in *Ixodes* ticks from North America and Europe. *PLOS One* 5(5):e10650.

DeLong, A., M. Hsu, and H. Kotsoris. 2019. Estimation of cumulative number of post-treatment Lyme disease cases in the U.S., 2016 and 2020. *BMC Public Health* 19(1):352.

Doshi, S., J. G. Keilp, B. Strobino, M. McElhiney, J. Rabkin, and B. A. Fallon. 2018. Depressive symptoms and suicidal ideation among symptomatic patients with a history of Lyme disease vs. two comparison groups. *Psychosomatics* 59(5):481–489.

Eldin, C., A. Raffetin, K. Bouiller, Y. Hansmann, F. Roblot, D. Raoult, and P. Parola. 2019. Review of European and American guidelines for the diagnosis of Lyme borreliosis. *Médecine et Malaladies Infectieuses* 49(2):121–132.

Fallon, B. A., M. Pavlicova, S. W. Coffino, and C. Brenner. 2014. A comparison of Lyme disease serologic test results from 4 laboratories in patients with persistent symptoms after antibiotic treatment. *Clinical Infectious Diseases* 59(12):1705–1710.

Fallon, B. A., T. Madsen, A. Erlangsen, and M. E. Benros. 2021. Lyme borreliosis and associations with mental disorders and suicidal behavior: A nationwide Danish cohort study. *American Journal of Psychiatry* 178(10):921–931.

Hanson, M. R. 2023. The viral origin of myalgic encephalomyelitis/chronic fatigue syndrome. *PLoS Pathogen* 19(8):e1011523.

Hassett, A. L., D. C. Radvanski, S. Buyske, S. V. Savage, M. Gara, J. I. Escobar, and L. H. Sigal. 2008. Role of psychiatric comorbidity in chronic Lyme disease. Arthritis Rheumatism 59(12):1742-1749.

Hickie I., T. Davenport, D. Wakefield, U. Vollmer-Conna, B. Cameron, S. D. Vernon, W. C. Reeves, A. Lloyd, and Dubbo Infection Outcomes Study Group. 2006. Post-infective and chronic fatigue syndromes precipitated by viral and non-viral pathogens: prospective cohort study. *BMJ* 16;333(7568):575.

Hook, S. A., S. Jeon, S. A. Niesobecki, A. P. Hansen, J. K. H. Bjork, F. M. Dorr, H. J. Rutz, K. A. Feldman, J. L. White, P. B. Backenson, M. B. Shankar, M. I. Meltzer, and A. F. Hinckley. 2022. Economic burden of reported Lyme disease in high-incidence areas, United States, 2014–2016. *Emerging Infectious Diseases* 28(6):1170–1179.

Johnson, L. 2019. *MyLymeData 2019 chart book*: figshare. https://figshare.com/articles/book/MyLymeData_2019_Chart_Book/8063039/1?file=17413562 (accessed February 1, 2025).

Johnson, L., S. Wilcox, J. Mankoff, and R. B. Stricker. 2014. Severity of chronic Lyme disease compared to other chronic conditions: A quality of life survey. *PeerJ* 2:e322.

Kalish, R. A., G. McHugh, J. Granquist, B. Shea, R. Ruthazer, and A. C. Steere. 2001. Persistence of immunoglobulin M or immunoglobulin G antibody responses to *Borrelia burgdorferi* 10–20 years after active Lyme disease. *Clinical Infectious Diseases* 33(6):780–785.

Kilpatrick, A. M., A. D. M. Dobson, T. Levi, D. J. Salkeld, A. Swei, H. S. Ginsberg, A. Kjemtrup, K. A. Padgett, P. M. Jensen, D. Fish, N. H. Ogden, and M. A. Diuk-Wasser. 2017. Lyme disease ecology in a changing world: Consensus, uncertainty and critical gaps for improving control. *Philosophical Transactions of the Royal Society B: Biological Sciences* 372(1722):20160117.

Klempner, M. S., L. T. Hu, J. Evans, C. H. Schmid, G. M. Johnson, R. P. Trevino, D. Norton, L. Levy, D. Wall, J. McCall, M. Kosinski, and A. Weinstein. 2001. Two controlled trials of antibiotic treatment in patients with persistent symptoms and a history of Lyme disease. *New England Journal of Medicine* 345(2):85–92.

Komaroff, A. L., and W. I. Lipkin. 2023. ME/CFS and Long COVID share similar symptoms and biological abnormalities: Road map to the literature. *Frontiers in Medicine (Lausanne)* 10:1187163.

Kugeler, K. J., A. M. Schwartz, M. J. Delorey, P. S. Mead, and A. F. Hinckley. 2021. Estimating the frequency of Lyme disease diagnoses, United States, 2010–2018. *Emerging Infectious Diseases* 27(2):616–619.

Lantos, P. M., J. Rumbaugh, L. K. Bockenstedt, Y. T. Falck-Ytter, M. E. Aguero-Rosenfeld, P. G. Auwaerter, K. Baldwin, R. R. Bannuru, K. K. Belani, W. R. Bowie, J. A. Branda, D. B. Clifford, F. J. DiMario, J. J. Halperin, P. J. Krause, V. Lavergne, M. H. Liang, H. C. Meissner, L. E. Nigrovic, J. J. J. Nocton, M. C. Osani, A. A. Pruitt, J. Rips, L. E. Rosenfeld, M. L. Savoy, S. K. Sood, A. C. Steere, F. Strle, R. Sundel, J. Tsao, E. E. Vaysbrot, G. P. Wormser, and L. S. Zemel. 2021. Clinical practice guidelines by the Infectious Diseases Society of America, American Academy of Neurology, and American College of Rheumatology: 2020 guidelines for the prevention, diagnosis, and treatment of Lyme disease. *Neurology* 96(6):262–273.

Lemieux, J. E., W. Huang, N. Hill, T. Cerar, L. Freimark, S. Hernandez, M. Luban, V. Maraspin, P. Bogovic, K. Ogrinc, E. Ruzic-Sabljic, P. Lapierre, E. Lasek-Nesselquist, N. Singh, R. Iyer, D. Liveris, K. D. Reed, J. M. Leong, J. A. Branda, A. C. Steere, G. P. Wormser, F. Strle, P. C. Sabeti, I. Schwartz, and K. Strle. 2023. Whole genome sequencing of *Borrelia burgdorferi* isolates reveals linked clusters of plasmid-borne accessory genome elements associated with virulence. *bioRxiv* [Preprint]. Feb 27:2023.02.26.530159. Update in: *PLOS Pathogens,* 2023, 19(8):e1011243.

LymeX Innovation. 2025. *Announcing the phase 3 winners.* https://www.Lymexdiagnosticsprize.com/announcing-the-phase-3-winners/ (accessed March 14, 2025).

Magnus, P., N. Gunnes, K. Tveito, I. J. Bakken, S. Ghaderi, C. Stoltenberg, M. Hornig, W. I. Lipkin, L. Trogstad, and S. E. Håberg. 2015. Chronic fatigue syndrome/myalgic encephalomyelitis (CFS/ME) is associated with pandemic influenza infection, but not with an adjuvanted pandemic influenza vaccine. *Vaccine* 17;33(46):6173-6177.

Marques, A., S. R. Telford, 3rd, S. P. Turk, E. Chung, C. Williams, K. Dardick, P. J. Krause, C. Brandeburg, C. D. Crowder, H. E. Carolan, M. W. Eshoo, P. A. Shaw, and L. T. Hu. 2014. Xenodiagnosis to detect *Borrelia burgdorferi* infection: A first-in-human study. *Clinical Infectious Diseases* 58(7):937–945.

Marques, A. R., F. Strle, and G. P. Wormser. 2021. Comparison of Lyme disease in the United States and Europe. *Emerging Infectious Diseases* 27(8):2017–2024.

McGowan, M. S., T. M. Kalinoski, and S. E. Hesse. 2023. Acute Lyme disease with atypical features due to *Borrelia mayonii*. *Open Forum Infectious Diseases* 10(11):ofad524.

Minnesota Department of Health. 2022. *Borrelia mayonii disease statistics* https://www.health.state.mn.us/diseases/bmayonii/statistics.html (accessed January 27, 2025).

Monaghan, M., S. Norman, M. Gierdalski, A. Marques, J. E. Bost, and R. L. DeBiasi. 2024. Pediatric Lyme disease: Systematic assessment of post-treatment symptoms and quality of life. *Pediatric Research* 95(1):174–181.

NASEM (National Academies of Sciences, Engineering, and Medicine). 2024a. *A Long COVID definition: A chronic, systemic disease state with profound consequences.* Washington, DC: The National Academies Press.

NASEM. 2024b. *Toward a common research agenda in infection-associated chronic illnesses: Proceedings of a workshop.* Washington, DC: The National Academies Press.

Nelson, C. A., S. Saha, K. J. Kugeler, M. J. Delorey, M. B. Shankar, A. F. Hinckley, and P. S. Mead. 2015. Incidence of clinician-diagnosed Lyme disease, United States, 2005–2010. *Emerging Infectious Diseases* 21(9):1625–1631.

NIAID (National Institute of Allergy and Infectious Diseases. 2024. *Xenodiagnosis after antibiotic treatment for Lyme disease*. https://www.clinicaltrials.gov/study/NCT02446626 (accessed January 27, 2025).

Orloski, K. A., E. B. Hayes, G. L. Campbell, and D. T. Dennis. 2000. Surveillance for Lyme disease—United States, 1992-1998. *Morbidity and Mortality Weekly Report* 49(SS03):1-11.

Philipp, M. T., E. Masters, G. P. Wormser, W. Hogrefe, and D. Martin. 2006. Serologic evaluation of patients from Missouri with erythema migrans-like skin lesions with the C6 Lyme test. *Clinical and Vaccine Immunolology* 13(10):1170–1171.

Rebman, A. W., K. T. Bechtold, T. Yang, E. A. Mihm, M. J. Soloski, C. B. Novak, and J. N. Aucott. 2017. The clinical, symptom, and quality-of-life characterization of a well-defined group of patients with posttreatment Lyme disease syndrome. *Frontiers in Medicine (Lausanne)* 4:224.

Rebman, A. W., and J. N. Aucott. 2020. Post-treatment Lyme disease as a model for persistent symptoms in Lyme disease. *Frontiers in Medicine (Lausanne)* 7:57.

Rosenberg, R., N. P. Lindsey, M. Fischer, C. J. Gregory, A. F. Hinckley, P. S. Mead, G. Paz-Bailey, S. H. Waterman, N. A. Drexler, G. J. Kersh, H. Hooks, S. K. Partridge, S. N. Visser, and C. B. Beard. 2018. Vital signs: Trends in reported vectorborne disease cases — United States and territories, 2004–2016. *Morbidity and Mortality Weekly Report* 67(17):496-501.

Sakizadeh, J. R., M. K. Rothenberger, and J. D. Alpern. 2025. Characteristics of clinics offering nontraditional Lyme disease therapies in Lyme endemic states of the United States. *Open Forum Infectious Diseases* 12(3).

Schwartz, A. M., A. F. Hinckley, P. S. Mead, S. A. Hook, and K. J. Kugeler. 2017. Surveillance for Lyme disease—United States, 2008-2015. *MMWR Surveillance Summaries* 66(22):1–12.

Springer, Y. P., C. S. Jarnevich, D. T. Barnett, A. J. Monaghan, and R. J. Eisen. 2015. Modeling the present and future geographic distribution of the Lone Star tick, *Amblyomma americanum* (Ixodida: Ixodidae), in the Continental United States. *American Journal of Tropical Medicine and Hygiene* 93(4):875–890.

Steere, A. C. 2001. Lyme disease. *New England Journal of Medicine* 345(2):115–125.

Steere, A. C., S. E. Malawista, D. R. Snydman, R. E. Shope, W. A. Andiman, M. R. Ross, and F. M. Steele. 1977. Lyme arthritis: An epidemic of oligoarticular arthritis in children and adults in three Connecticut communities. *Arthritis & Rheumatology* 20(1):7–17.

Steere, A. C., A. Dhar, J. Hernandez, P. A. Fischer, V. K. Sikand, R. T. Schoen, J. Nowakowski, G. McHugh, and D. H. Persing. 2003. Systemic symptoms without erythema migrans as the presenting picture of early Lyme disease. *American Journal of Medicine* 114(1):58–62.

Steere, A. C., F. Strle, G. P. Wormser, L. T. Hu, J. A. Branda, J. W. R. Hovius, X. Li, and P. S. Mead. 2016. Lyme borreliosis. *Nature Reviews Disease Primers* 2(1):16090.

Stone, B. L., Y. Tourand, and C. A. Brissette. 2017. Brave new worlds: The expanding universe of Lyme disease. *Vector Borne Zoonotic Diseases* 17(9):619–629.

TBDWG (Tick-Borne Disease Working Group). 2018. *Tick-Borne Disease Working Group 2018 report to Congress*. https://www.hhs.gov/sites/default/files/tbdwg-report-to-congress-2018.pdf (accessed November 27, 2024).

TBDWG. 2020. *Tick-Borne Disease Working Group 2020 report to Congress*. https://www.hhs.gov/sites/default/files/tbdwg-2020-report_to-ongress-final.pdf (accessed November 27, 2024).

Tokarz, R., T. Tagliafierro, S. Sameroff, D. M. Cucura, A. Oleynik, X. Che, K. Jain, and W. I. Lipkin. 2019. Microbiome analysis of *Ixodes scapularis* ticks from New York and Connecticut. *Ticks and Tick-Borne Diseases* 10(4):894–900.

Tyler, S., S. Tyson, A. Dibernardo, M. Drebot, E. J. Feil, M. Graham, N. C. Knox, L. R. Lindsay, G. Margos, S. Mechai, G. Van Domselaar, H. A. Thorpe, and N. H. Ogden. 2018. Whole genome sequencing and phylogenetic analysis of strains of the agent of Lyme disease *Borrelia burgdorferi* from Canadian emergence zones. *Science Reports* 8(1):10552.

van den Wijngaard, C. C., A. Hofhuis, A. Wong, M. G. Harms, G. A. de Wit, A. K. Lugnér, A. W. M. Suijkerbuijk, M. J. Mangen, and W. van Pelt. 2017. The cost of Lyme borreliosis. *European Journal of Public Health* 27(3):538–547.

Waddell, L. A., J. Greig, M. Mascarenhas, S. Harding, R. Lindsay, and N. Ogden. 2016. The accuracy of diagnostic tests for Lyme disease in humans: A systematic review and meta-analysis of North American research. *PLOS One* 12(11):e0168613.

Weitzner, E., D. McKenna, J. Nowakowski, C. Scavarda, R. Dornbush, S. Bittker, D. Cooper, R. B. Nadelman, P. Visintainer, I. Schwartz, and G. P. Wormser. 2015. Long-term assessment of post-treatment symptoms in patients with culture-confirmed early Lyme disease. *Clinical Infectious Diseases* 61(12):1800–1806.

Willems, R., N. Verhaeghe, C. Perronne, L. Borgermans, and L. Annemans. 2023. Cost of illness in patients with post-treatment Lyme disease syndrome in Belgium. *European Journal of Public Health* 33(4):668–674.

Winslow, C., and J. Coburn. 2019. Recent discoveries and advancements in research on the Lyme disease spirochete *Borrelia burgdorferi*. *F1000Res* 8:F1000 Faculty Rev-763.

Wisconsin Department of Health Services. 2024. *Lyme disease: Wisconsin data*. https://www.dhs.wisconsin.gov/tick/Lyme-data.htm (accessed January 27, 2025).

Wormser, G. P. 2006. Early Lyme disease. *New England Journal of Medicine* 354(26):2794–2801.

Wormser, G. P., E. Masters, J. Nowakowski, D. McKenna, D. Holmgren, K. Ma, L. Ihde, L. F. Cavaliere, and R. B. Nadelman. 2005. Prospective clinical evaluation of patients from Missouri and New York with erythema migrans-like skin lesions. *Clinical Infectious Diseases* 41(7):958–965.

Wormser, G. P., R. J. Dattwyler, E. D. Shapiro, J. J. Halperin, A. C. Steere, M. S. Klempner, P. J. Krause, J. S. Bakken, F. Strle, G. Stanek, L. Bockenstedt, D. Fish, J. S. Dumler, and R. B. Nadelman. 2006. The clinical assessment, treatment, and prevention of Lyme disease, human granulocytic anaplasmosis, and babesiosis: Clinical practice guidelines by the Infectious Diseases Society of America. *Clinical Infectious Diseases* 43(9):1089–1134.

Wormser, G. P., D. McKenna, C. L. Karmen, K. D. Shaffer, J. H. Silverman, J. Nowakowski, C. Scavarda, E. D. Shapiro, and P. Visintainer. 2020. Prospective evaluation of the frequency and severity of symptoms in Lyme disease patients with erythema migrans compared with matched controls at baseline, 6 months, and 12 months. *Clinical Infectious Diseases* 71(12):3118–3124.

2

State of the Evidence

The committee was charged with reviewing the current gaps in knowledge regarding the etiology and treatment of Lyme infection-associated chronic illnesses (IACI). The committee addressed this charge in two components. First, to understand the link between *Borrelia* infection and Lyme IACI, the committee reviewed evidence on the prevalence of persistent, generalized symptoms (e.g., fatigue, pain, brain fog) among U.S. individuals who had Lyme disease compared with those without previous Lyme disease. This knowledge is foundational to the interpretation of findings on the disease's etiology and to inform future study design. Second, the committee examined the evidence concerning treatment effectiveness and potential disease mechanisms, as well as diagnostic tools for Lyme IACI, given their critical role as part of disease treatment and etiology research. This was accomplished through a scoping review of the peer-reviewed literature. Both components were complicated by the absence of a consensus definition or diagnostic biomarkers for Lyme IACI. This chapter starts with describing an operational scope of the committee's literature review, which is followed by an assessment of the published evidence.

OPERATIONAL SCOPE FOR LITERATURE REVIEW ON LYME IACI RESEARCH

For this literature review, the committee considered the scope of "Lyme IACI" to include an illness with otherwise unexplained symptoms that persist at least 6 months following antibiotic treatment for either proven or presumed infection with *Borrelia spp.* that cause Lyme disease. Due to the lack of a gold standard diagnostic for Lyme IACI and the heterogeneity with which the population of interest has been reported in the existing literature, the committee's consideration of Lyme IACI included both individuals with a known association with an initial infection by *Borrelia spp.* and those with an unproven but possible association to these infections. Inclusion under this operational scope was dependent on the study population as described in the research publications (i.e., studies of unexplained fatigue conducted in Lyme disease endemic areas but without a description of Lyme disease history or connection were not sought out or included).

The first group under the operational scope consists of individuals with confirmed Lyme disease based on a history of an erythema migrans (EM) or other clinical findings consistent with Lyme disease and positive two-tier Lyme disease serology, and persistent illness for 6 months following antibiotic treatment. This is similar to the case definition of post-treatment Lyme disease syndrome (PTLDS; Box 2-1) and the criteria for Group 1 from a recently proposed research classification for studying Lyme IACI (Fallon et al., 2025).

The second group comprises individuals who were treated for suspected Lyme disease but experience persistent symptoms without a confirmed previous *Borrelia spp.* infection (i.e., without a history of observed EM or documented confirmatory two-tier seropositivity), have possible epidemiologic exposure to infected ticks (i.e., reside, work, or visit in a Lyme disease endemic area), and for whom alternative diagnoses have been excluded. This group may include individuals with delayed Lyme disease diagnosis, such as those who may have limited knowledge of the disease and those who may not have had access to adequate tests or medical care (Gould et al., 2024; NCFH, 2023). This group may also capture individuals with similar symptoms whose illness is not directly related to prior *Borrelia spp.* infection, including other infectious or noninfectious etiologies. It is important that a comprehensive evaluation be undertaken to exclude alternative diagnoses and to minimize the improper inclusion of individuals with a known cause of their symptoms that is not Lyme IACI in this second group. Given the uncertain etiology in this group, the degree of comprehensiveness in clinical evaluation may vary significantly, contributing to the challenges in studying this heterogeneous group.

As many chronic illnesses with a potential infectious trigger share similar symptoms with Lyme IACI, attribution of an individual's symptoms to a specific infectious agent may not always be possible. The nearly universal exposure to SARS-CoV-2 and the potential consequences of Long COVID further complicates this issue of attribution.[1] Chapter 3 will explore con-

---

[1] This challenge also highlights the critical role of biobanks, particularly the collection and maintenance of pre-COVID-19 samples that can serve as important experimental controls. See Chapter 4 for more discussion on biobanks.

BOX 2-1
Definition of Post-Treatment Lyme Disease Syndrome

The Infectious Diseases Society of America offers the following inclusion and exclusion criteria for PTLDS (edited for brevity).

Inclusion criteria:

An adult or child with documented Lyme disease fulfilling the case definition of the Centers for Disease Control and Prevention. If based on an erythema migrans lesion, the diagnosis must be made and documented by an experienced health care practitioner.

After treatment with a generally accepted treatment regimen, there is resolution or stabilization of the objective manifestation(s) of Lyme disease.

Onset of any of the following symptoms within 6 months after the diagnosis of Lyme disease and persistence of continuous or relapsing symptoms for at least a 6-month period after completion of antibiotic therapy:

1. Fatigue
2. Widespread musculoskeletal pain
3. Complaints of cognitive difficulties
4. Symptoms result in substantial reduction in previous levels of occupational, educational, social, or personal activities.

Exclusion criteria:

An active, untreated, well-documented co-infection, such as babesiosis.

The presence of objective abnormalities on physical examination or on neuropsychologic testing that may explain the patient's complaints. For example, a patient with antibiotic-refractory Lyme arthritis would be excluded. A patient with late neuroborreliosis associated with encephalopathy who has recurrent or refractory objective cognitive dysfunction would be excluded.

Alternative diagnoses prior to Lyme disease: fibromyalgia or chronic fatigue syndrome [or a history of] undiagnosed or unexplained somatic complaints.

Alternative diagnosis, laboratory or imaging abnormalities that can explain the patient's symptoms.

SOURCE: Wormser et al. (2006).

nections between research on Lyme IACI and research on similar chronic conditions, including how the investigation of such similar conditions may identify common treatment approaches for Lyme IACI and these conditions.

EPIDEMIOLOGY OF LYME IACI

The association between Lyme disease and persistent, multisystem symptoms has been described in research publications and reaffirmed by the Tick-Borne Disease Working Group, a federal advisory committee of the Department of Health and Human Services (Aucott et al., 2013; TBDWG, 2018, 2020, 2022; Wormser et al., 2006).[2,3] However, the prevalence of symptoms in individuals who have been infected by *Borrelia spp.* compared with those without infection is also important to establish. The risk for contracting Lyme disease fluctuates based on environmental and behavioral factors (e.g., where one lives or visits, what one does for work or recreation), and people are not routinely tested for Borrelia infections unless they exhibit symptoms. In addition, many conditions with similar symptoms are relatively common in the U.S. population—the prevalence of myalgic encephalomyelitis (ME/CFS) and fibromyalgia, two such conditions that may present the same symptoms as Lyme IACI, have been reported as 0.9 percent and 2 percent, respectively—potentially contributing to the misattribution of Lyme IACI in epidemiologic studies (American College of Rheumatology, 2023; Choutka et al., 2022; IOM, 2011).[4]

---

[2] The Tick-borne Disease Workgroup is a federal advisory committee established from the 21st Century Cures Act and was active from 2016 to 2022. Its formation follows a federal advisory committee on ME/CSF, whose work spanned from 2002 to 2018. A federal advisory committee on Long COVID was established in August 2023 and disbanded by Executive Order in February 2025. See: *Renewal of Charters for Certain Federal Advisory Committees,* 81 Fed Reg. 74456. (October 26, 2016), *Establishment of the Office of Long COVID Research and Practice,* 88 Fed Reg. 50159. (August 1, 2023); *Commencing the Reduction of the Federal Bureaucracy,* 90 Fed Reg. 10577. (February 25, 2025), and "Chronic Fatigue Syndrome Advisory Committee," U.S. Department of Health and Human Services, archived January 28, 2019, at https://wayback.archive-it.org/org-745/20190128204246/https:/www.hhs.gov/ash/advisory-committees/cfsac/index.html.

[3] While this study was not conducted in response to the recommendation in the 2022 report of the Tick-borne Disease Working Group, which called on the National Academies to review the evidence for diagnosis and treatment to establish "what is definitely known, what is partially understood, and what remains unknown" for Lyme disease, with emphasis on early disease and the persistent symptoms, the current report includes a review of the scientific and clinical evidence on causes, disease mechanisms, diagnosis, and treatment of Lyme IACI. In addition, this report includes a review of the clinical evidence in treating other IACI to illuminate a path toward advancing new treatments for Lyme IACI.

[4] Some cases of ME/CFS and fibromyalgia may stem from Lyme disease and would be considered as part of Lyme IACI (see Hu et al., 2025, and Gluckman et al., 2025).

Prospective Studies

The ideal method to accurately determine the incidence of Lyme IACI would be a prospective cohort study that tracks individuals from the time of Borrelia infection compared with control groups to compare the incidence of persistent symptoms that arise between infected and uninfected individuals. In a prospective cohort of 1,135 patients in The Netherlands with Lyme disease treated with recommended antibiotics as well as two control groups (Ursinus et al., 2021), the cumulative incidence of symptoms (fatigue, pain, or cognitive impairment) that persisted for at least 6 months was 27.2 percent in the Lyme disease group and 34.3 percent in the subgroup that had disseminated Lyme disease. However, these symptoms were quite common in the controls as well—21.2 percent in healthy controls and 23.3 percent in the tick bite only group. The relatively small difference in the frequency of symptoms between the Lyme disease group and the control groups demonstrates the importance of including appropriate comparator groups. The National Institutes of Health has committed funding for a similar prospective study to take place in the United States over the next 4.5 years (NIH Reporter, 2025).

PTLDS is a stringent but consistent research definition that allows for comparisons between studies. This definition has been used in small-scale prospective studies in the United States to estimate the rate of developing persistent symptoms associated with Lyme disease. These studies found that the portion of adults with confirmed Lyme disease who develop PTLDS ranges from 5 to 36 percent, leading to an often-cited figure of an average 10–20 percent (Aucott et al., 2013; Aucott et al., 2022; Weitzner et al., 2015; Wormser et al., 2015, 2020). This wide range can be explained by differences in inclusion criteria, study designs (e.g., clinical studies versus database studies), and data sources (e.g., health records, insurance claims, patient-led data registries). Table 2-1 summarizes the findings from studies that have measured the prevalence of PTLDS in various patient populations in the United States.

Retrospective Studies

Electronic health records and insurance claims can be used to assemble large cohorts. Their utility, however, is limited by a lack of patient-level information, including details of Lyme disease diagnosis, comorbidities, and symptoms. A study that analyzed records from 48,596 adults who sought medical attention and received the Lyme disease diagnostic code found that 3.1 percent had symptoms matching PTLDS criteria in the 2 years after the Lyme disease diagnosis (Chung et al., 2023).

There is limited evidence of the prevalence of persistent symptoms in children after Lyme disease. In the only published study of persistence of

TABLE 2-1 Summary of Prospective Studies Reviewing the Prevalence of PTLDS

Study	PTLDS symptom(s) defined and assessed by study	Study groups		PTLDS prevalence (n)	
		Lyme disease	Control (type)	Lyme disease group	Control group
Wormser et al. (2020)	At least one of the following symptoms through self-report: fatigue, headache, stiff neck, joint pain, muscle pain, decreased appetite, difficulty with concentration/memory, feeling feverish/chilly, dizziness, tingling/abnormal sensation, nausea or vomiting, cough	52	104 (healthy, LD-negative, recruited from same primary care site as LD group)	• Enrollment: 25.0% (13/52) • 6-month follow-up: 39.1% (18/46) • 12-month follow-up: 55.1% (27/49)	• Enrollment: 1.0% (1/104) • 6-month follow-up: 51.6% (49/95) • 12-month follow-up: 51.0% (50/98)
Wormser et al. (2015)	Persistent fatigue (score ≥ 4.0 on the 11-Item Fatigue Severity Scale, FSS-11) coincident with onset of Lyme disease, lasted at least 6 months in the first year after treatment, had no other known explanation other than history of Lyme disease, and persisted at least intermittently until the time of the visit	100	N/A	• None, based on FSS-11 scoring and defined criteria (based on clinical assessment, 3 may have post-Lyme disease fatigue despite FSS-11 score < 4	N/A
Aucott et al. (2013)	Operationalized definition of PTLDS: self-reported presence of new-onset fatigue, widespread musculoskeletal pain, or neurocognitive difficulties	71	14 (healthy, LD-negative, recruited from same primary care site as LD group, matched to LD cases based on age, sex, and time of enrollment)	• 6-month follow-up: 37% (26/71)	• 6-month follow-up: 0% (0/14)

Study	Definition	N	Controls	PTLDS cases	
Aucott et al. (2022)	Operationalized definition of PTLD fulfills either symptoms or both criteria at least one of the two follow-ups (6-month, 12-month): • Symptoms: fatigue, pain, and/or cognitive symptoms at moderate or severe level of the Post-Lyme Questionnaire of Symptoms • Functional impact: average composite score of four specific norm-based subscales on the SF-36 is 0.5 standard deviation below population mean	234	49 (no clinical or serologic history of Lyme disease, no overlapping symptoms with PTLDS, recruited from same primary care site as LD group)	• 12-month follow-up: 13.7% (32/234)	• 12-month follow-up: 4.1% (2/49)
Weitzner et al. (2015)	Symptoms that were otherwise unexplained within 6 months after diagnosis of Lyme disease and lasted for at least 6 months following the completion of antibiotic therapy	128	N/A	• Over 11- to 20-year follow-up range: 10.9% met PTLDS criteria (14/128) • By last study visit: 4.7% met PTLDS criteria (6/128)	N/A

NOTE: LD = Lyme disease; N/A = not applicable; PTLDS = post-treatment Lyme disease syndrome.

symptoms after Lyme disease in the pediatric population is a retrospective survey. In it, 402 children and adolescents were identified for enrollment based on a review of the available electronic health records. Of these, 102 participants were confirmed as eligible for inclusion and consented to enroll in the study. Questionnaires were completed, on average (mean), 2 years after initial diagnosis. Among the respondents, 13 percent experienced persistent symptoms although most did not recall an impact on function (Monaghan et al., 2024). Prospective studies to further examine the frequency and severity of persistent symptoms after Lyme disease in the pediatric population are needed.

Modeling Studies

Simulation or other modeling studies can be a helpful adjunct to estimating disease prevalence, which does not require extensive coordination and data reporting from public health jurisdictions around the country. However, the accuracy of projections from simulations are highly dependent on the quality of data that define the parameters of the underlying model. A simulation of six scenarios based on different estimates of Lyme disease incidence and the likelihood of developing PTLDS (an assumption of either 10 percent or 20 percent) have reported estimated prevalent cases of PTLDS by 2020 to range widely from 69,011 to 1,944,189 (DeLong et al., 2019). However, this simulation had to make key assumptions to address the lack of available data. For example, the model does not include a rate of recovery from PTLDS. It also assumes, in the scenario with the highest prevalence estimate, a linear growth of Lyme disease incident cases from 329,000 cases in 2005 continuing until 2020. The need to use various assumptions in key parameters of this model underscores the need for data in this field. As more knowledge on the development and disease course of Lyme IACI emerges, simulations can be refined to provide more precise estimates on the disease prevalence.

Risk Factors for Developing Lyme IACI

Characteristics that have been associated with an increased likelihood of developing persistent symptoms following Lyme disease include previous traumatic life events (Aucott et al., 2022; Mustafiz et al., 2022; Solomon et al., 1998), female sex (Johnson et al., 2023), and delayed initial antibiotic treatment (Asch et al., 1994; Shadick et al., 1994). Notably, the association between persistent symptoms and female sex is based on data from a majority female patient registry (85 percent female, 15 percent male), and individuals who have persistent symptoms are likely to be overrepresented in a self-reported registry. Furthermore, associations with certain characteristics may not suggest causation or indicate that the characteristics identified through association are indeed risk factors for developing Lyme IACI. However, sex-based differences in responses to infectious diseases as well as in diagnosis and care have been well documented (Klein and Flanagan, 2016; Mauvais-Jarvis et al., 2020; Sun et al., 2023), and females are also disproportionately affected in other similar chronic conditions with unknown etiology, such as ME/CFS (Bretherick et al., 2023; Faro et al., 2016).

Individual immunologic differences in the human host may predict the development of PTLDS (Aucott et al., 2016; Bouquet et al., 2016); on the other hand, no relationship has been found between *B. burgdorferi* genotype and the risk of developing PTLDS (Lemieux et al., 2023). While there may be certain occupations at higher risk for Lyme disease or tick-borne diseases in general (Adjemian et al., 2012; Piacentino and Schwartz, 2002), no association between occupation and risk of Lyme IACI has been documented. Environmental risk factors or triggers including exposure to chemical contaminants have been associated with Gulf War illness, another chronic condition with multisystem symptoms overlapping with Lyme IACI, but they have not been reported in association with Lyme IACI (Elhaj and Reynolds, 2023; Haley et al., 2022).

Additional prospective studies are needed to determine the prevalence and likelihood of developing Lyme IACI in the United States, including in the pediatric population. Regardless, findings to date support the hypothesis that individuals with Lyme disease, even after antibiotics treatment, are more likely to develop persistent, multi-system symptoms. It is not possible to determine whether these symptoms stem from Lyme disease or another cause (e.g., Long COVID, ME/CFS, fibromyalgia).

Conclusion 2-1: A subset of individuals who are infected with and treated for Borrelia spp. *subsequently develop persistent symptoms that can often be debilitating.*

Conclusion 2-2: The lack of a consensus definition for Lyme IACI makes it difficult to accurately determine the population prevalence.

A SCOPING REVIEW OF THE LITERATURE

The committee arranged for a scoping review of the literature to be conducted in order to assess the breadth of the available published research on the treatment, mechanisms, and diagnosis of Lyme IACI. The scoping review included peer-reviewed research published between January 1970 and May 2024. The review exclusively covered studies that were conducted within or used samples from North America, based on previously described differences in Lyme disease by geographic region. A summary of this scoping review findings are provided below.

Scoping Review Methods

The methodology used for the scoping review is described in detail in Appendix C and summarized here. Search terms were chosen to be broadly descriptive and reflect the Lyme IACI operational scope. The preliminary literature search was conducted in PubMed, Medline (Ovid), Embase (Ovid), and Scopus databases by a research librarian at the National Academies. Two supplemental searches were conducted to identify articles that may not have been captured by the initial database searches. The first was a manual review of the references from the 10 most recent review articles addressing Lyme IACI. The second expanded the search terms used in the preliminary search to include older publications, which used index terms not initially considered (e.g., neuroborreliosis) in PubMed and Embase.

The initial screening of article titles and abstracts was performed by two reviewers (National Academies staff), and conflicts were adjudicated by a third National Academies staff member. Included abstracts were categorized as addressing research questions related to the treatment, diagnosis, or mechanisms (or some combination thereof) of Lyme IACI and subsequently screened for full-text review based on predefined inclusion and exclusion criteria. A final screening of full-text articles was conducted by two methodology consultants from PICO Portal and a National Academies staff member. Review of and data extraction from included full-text articles were performed by one consultant methodologist and verified by a second methodologist.

The diagnostic status (i.e., clinical or laboratory documentation of Lyme disease using approved test methods, or whether someone met the PTLDS definition) of participants in clinical studies or samples derived from volunteers that are used in basic science studies is a critical piece of information for interpretation of the research results. However, the degree of detail reported among the literature varies greatly. Most studies affirm that patients or study participants have clinical or laboratory documentation of Lyme disease as described in the PTLDS definition.

The Evidence Landscape

After de-duplication, the combined primary and supplemental literature search yielded 824 unique abstracts (Figure 2-1). Initial screening with the dual review resulted in 232 records for full-text retrieval. One publication could not be retrieved, and 146 articles were excluded after full-text review, resulting in 85 articles that were ultimately included in the scoping review. Notably, the publications used inconsistent definitions of Lyme IACI. Some of the terms used included post-treatment Lyme disease, persistent Lyme encephalopathy, chronic Lyme disease, and post-Lyme disease syndrome.

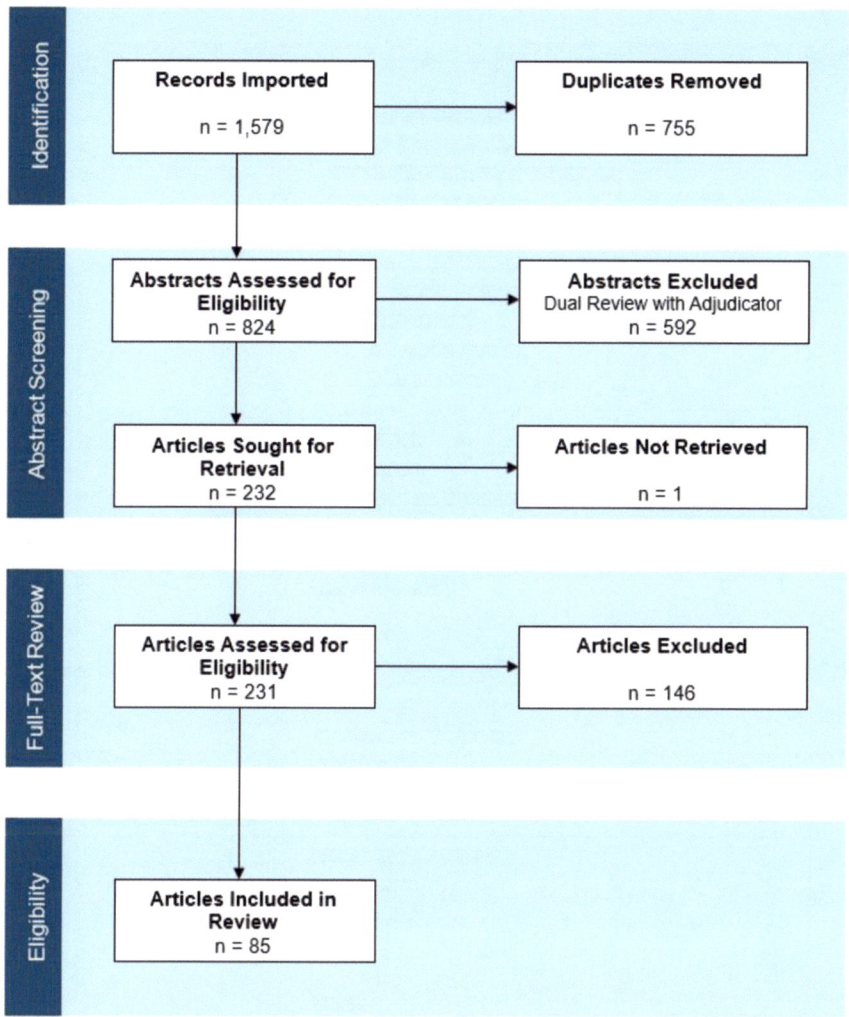

FIGURE 2-1 Flowchart of articles screened for and included in the scoping review.
NOTE: n = number.

Of the 85 manuscripts included in the scoping review, 49 reported on concepts related to the potential disease mechanisms for Lyme IACI, 19 studies evaluated Lyme IACI treatments, and 27 addressed findings related to Lyme IACI diagnosis (Figure 2-2). Ten articles reported on more than one of the three categories. The majority of manuscripts reported findings from observational studies except when the goal was to evaluate treatments.

Next, the committee summarizes findings for the treatment, mechanisms, and diagnosis of Lyme IACI.

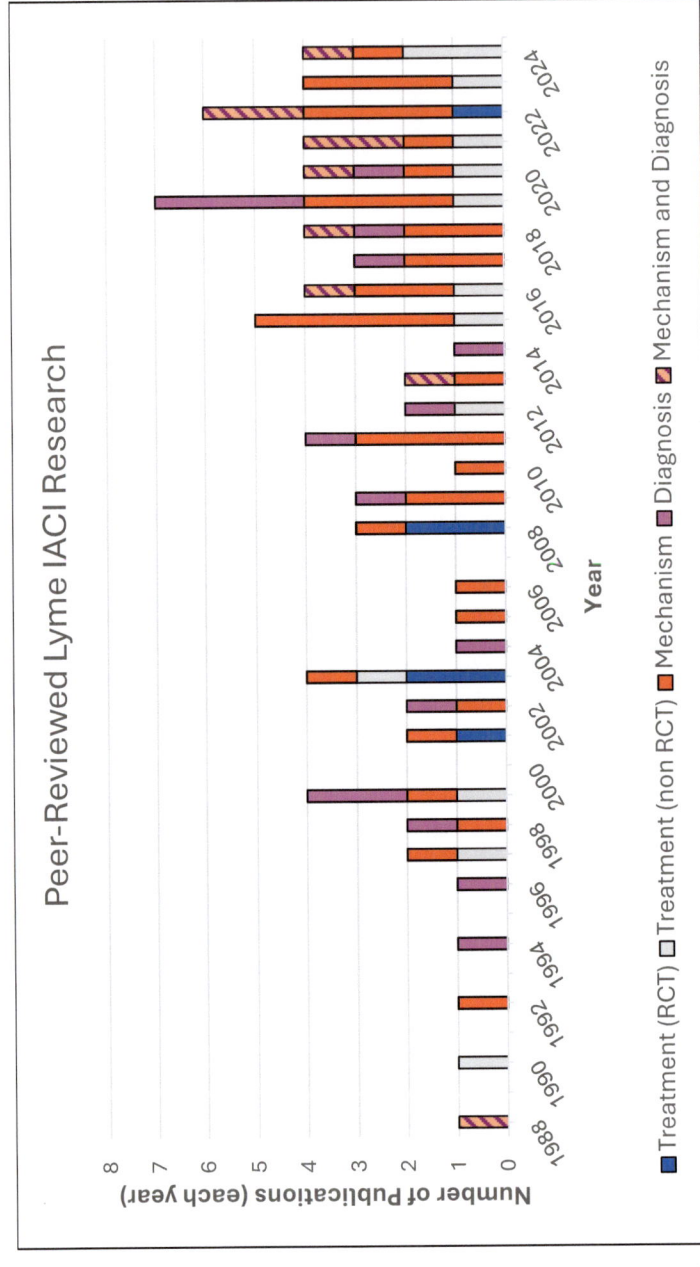

FIGURE 2-2 Peer-reviewed research on the mechanisms, diagnosis, or treatment of Lyme IACI between 1970 and May 2024.
NOTES: IACI = infection-associated chronic illness; RCT = randomized controlled trial.

EVIDENCE ON THE TREATMENT OF LYME IACI

Randomized trials are the preferred design for determining the effectiveness of medical treatments. Well-designed randomized trials include clearly specified eligibility criteria, treatment strategies, and outcomes of interest. The population(s) eligible for a trial will depend on the study's goals. In the case of Lyme IACI, eligibility for a trial could be narrow (e.g., PTLDS) or broad (e.g., persistent symptoms after a tick bite).

In randomized trials, participants are randomly assigned to one of several treatment strategies and followed for a prespecified time with periodic measures of the outcomes of interest. Outcome measures can include clinical findings evaluated by medical professionals, patient-reported outcomes (PROs) measured by validated tools, or changes in particular biomarkers determined through laboratory tests. Currently, clinical findings and some PROs are used in Lyme IACI studies, but there are no laboratory biomarkers that are validated for the measurement of Lyme IACI disease course or treatment response.

Selecting appropriate outcome measures is critical for randomized trials. Failing to measure outcomes that may be affected by the intervention being tested could lead to inaccurate results and incorrect conclusions. Studies may examine the effects of a treatment on many outcome measures or may be directed at specific symptoms with limited outcome measures. The choice for outcomes measures may be informed by what is known of the disease etiology and pathogenesis, the intervention's mechanism of action, and patients' lived experience. Due to the subjective aspects of several symptoms in Lyme IACI (e.g., pain, fatigue, and cognitive function), PROs are necessary to capture findings that are important to people living with Lyme IACI. Research funders and regulatory agencies have also increasingly supported the inclusion of PROs in clinical research and product development. For example: the National Institutes of Health (NIH) developed the Patient-Reported Outcomes Measurement Information System, a large, public reporting system of PROs (NIH, 2025), and the Food and Drug Administration has published guidance documents for industry (HHS et al., 2009).

Since many different existing tools are used to measure clinical outcomes in studies, it can complicate comparisons between studies (Mayo-Wilson et al., 2017). To measure outcomes that matter to people living with Lyme IACI, researchers need assessment instruments that are valid (i.e., accurately measure the intended construct), reliable (i.e., free of measurement error), responsive (i.e., can detect change in the outcome), and interpretable (i.e., can connect with clinically meaningful changes).

Another critical aspect of randomized trials is that they are informative when they provide effect estimates that are sufficiently precise. Take, for example, a randomized trial testing the effect of a certain treatment on a specific outcome estimates a relative risk of 0.8 with a 95 percent confidence interval from 0.4 to 2.2 (a relative risk of 1 indicates no effect). The boundary of the confidence interval is interpreted to mean that any values between a 60 percent lower risk and more than twofold higher risk are compatible with the study data. Under this interpretation with conventional statistical criteria, the result is too imprecise to confidently determine that the treatment should not be further investigated. That is, this hypothetical trial does not provide adequate information to guide decisions. Given that randomized trials require a substantial investment of societal resources, trials must be properly designed to provide informative results, which requires that a sufficient number of participants be enrolled. In fact, in a functioning research system, small trials are infeasible for ethical reasons: institutional review boards would not approve human experimentations that are not expected to result in helpful findings, and potential participants might refuse to enroll when the expected imprecise results are disclosed during the informed consent process.

Studies based on observational data may be used in attempts to emulate randomized trials. Explicit target trial emulations, in which the concepts of clinical trials are applied to observational studies eliminate common biases in observational research (e.g., biases that arise from selection of participants or from attempting to recall past events). However, unlike in a randomized trial, the factors that determine the receipt of a particular treatment in the real world may themselves be prognostic factors. If these confounders are not appropriately measured and adjusted for, observational emulations of target trials may be subject to residual confounding bias.

The committee also considered the heterogeneity of the population of people living with Lyme IACI and the implications for assessing the efficacy and safety of potential treatments. Ideally, studies to evaluate efficacy and safety for new treatments would be designed and conducted with clearly defined patient populations to monitor beneficial or adverse effects of the intervention in patients. Therefore, studies assessing variably defined populations may be hard to compare, and results may not apply to the entire Lyme IACI population.

Summary of Current Evidence

Of the 19 primary research studies with human participants assessing treatments for Lyme IACI, six were randomized controlled trials of variable methodological quality (Cameron, 2008; Fallon et al., 2008; Kaplan et al., 2003; Klempner et al., 2001; Krupp et al., 2003; Murray

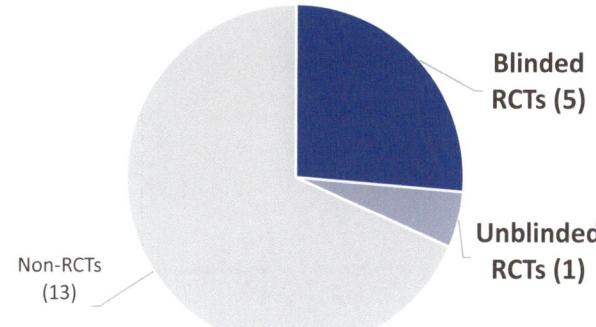

FIGURE 2-3 Study designs of published Lyme IACI treatment trials.
NOTES: IACI = infection-associated chronic illnesses; RCT = randomized controlled trial.

et al., 2022).[5] The remainder were observational studies or single-arm interventional studies enrolling people living with Lyme IACI at a single medical center (Figure 2-3).

The interventions in five of the six randomized trials were antibiotic treatments, and the remaining randomized trial evaluated yoga. Alternative medicine treatments that people with Lyme IACI have reported using (e.g., herbal therapies and acupuncture) have not been rigorously investigated in randomized trials. No randomized trials have been conducted in the pediatric population. Table 2-2 summarizes the design and outcomes of the six randomized trials.

Extended courses (up to 3 months) of antibiotics known to be effective for acute *B. burgdorferi* infection have been studied in five well-designed randomized trials. Two of these trials studied 30 days of intravenous ceftriaxone followed by 60 days of oral doxycycline, one study assessed 28 days of intravenous ceftriaxone, one study evaluated 3 months of oral amoxicillin, and the fifth study assessed 10 weeks of intravenous ceftriaxone. Taken together, these randomized controlled trials did not demonstrate a sustained benefit from treatment with extended courses of antibiotics. Furthermore, while one study did not report safety monitoring, the other four studies all reported adverse effects associated with the treatment. There remains ongoing debate over the trial designs and outcomes, as discussed through extensive reanalyses of the available data (Delong et al., 2012; Fallon et al., 2012; Klempner et al., 2013) and in summaries in the TBDWG reports (TBDWG, 2020, 2022).

---

[5] Klempner et al. (2001) and Kaplan et al. (2003) review the same two randomized trials.

TABLE 2-2 Key Study Characteristics from Randomized Trials

Study	Klempner et al. (2001)[1] Seropositive study	Klempner et al. (2001)[1] Seronegative study	Krupp et al. (2003)	Cameron (2008)	Fallon et al. (2008)	Murray et al. (2022)
Sample size	78	51	55	86	37	29
Eligibility	Positive Western blot for IgG antibodies against *B. burgdorferi*; and at least 1 of the following symptoms that interfered with function: musculoskeletal pain, cognitive impairment, radicular pain, or abnormal burning or itching sensation	Documentation of EM rash and negative Western blot; and at least 1 of the following symptoms that interfered with function: musculoskeletal pain, cognitive impairment, radicular pain, or abnormal burning or itching sensation	Documented EM rash or CDC-defined late manifestation of Lyme validated by positive ELISA or Western blot, completion of standard antibiotic treatment at least 6 months prior to enrollment; and current severe fatigue	Recurrence of Lyme disease symptoms after initial successful treatment; no specific symptoms were reported as inclusion criteria, but fatigue, stiff or painful joints, headaches, poor concentration, muscle soreness, sleep disturbances were present in more than 80% of participants at baseline	Documented EM rash or CDC-defined manifestation of Lyme disease and positive or equivocal ELISA confirmed by Western blot, current positive IgG Western blot, at least 3 weeks IV ceftriaxone treatment for Lyme at least 4 months before enrollment; and subjective and objective memory impairment starting after Lyme onset	Clinician diagnosis of Lyme disease at least 6 months prior to enrollment, received IDSA-recommended antibiotic treatment for Lyme; have symptoms starting within 6 months after Lyme onset and persisting at least 6 months; pain or fatigue as primary symptom complaint
Intervention	Antibiotic (30 days of IV ceftriaxone [2g/day] followed by 60 days of oral doxycycline [100mg twice/day])	Antibiotic (30 days of IV ceftriaxone [2g/day] followed by 60 days of oral doxycycline [100mg twice/day])	Antibiotic (28 days of IV ceftriaxone [2g/day])	Antibiotic (3 months of oral amoxicillin [3g/day])	Antibiotic (10 weeks of IV ceftriaxone [2g/day])	Kundalini yoga (8 weeks of a 90-min session once/week in groups of 4–6 participants)
Control	Placebo	Placebo	Placebo	Placebo	Placebo	Waitlist control
Blinding	Double blinded	Double blinded	Double blinded	Double blinded	Double blinded	Unblinded

Outcomes	Health-related quality of life at 180 days; cognitive function, pain, role functioning, neuropsych-ological test scores, and mood at 60 and 180 days	Health-related quality of life at 180 days; cognitive function, pain, role functioning, neuropsych-ological test scores, and mood at 60 and 180 days	Fatigue, mental speed, OspA antigen clearance at 6 months	Quality of life at 6 months	Neuro-psychological symptoms at 24 weeks	Pain, pain interference, fatigue, and global health at 8 weeks
Results	13 participants (37%) assigned to the intervention showed improved quality of life compared with 14 participants (40%) in the placebo group. 12 participants (34%) in both the intervention and placebo groups had worsened quality of life.	10 participants (45%) assigned to the intervention showed improved quality of life compared with 7 participants (30%) in the placebo group. 6 participants (27%) in the intervention group and 8 participants (35%) in the placebo group had worsened quality of life.	18 participants (64%) in intervention group had reduced fatigue compared with 5 participants (19%) in the placebo arms. Two participants in both the intervention and placebo arms had increased mental speed, reflecting 8% and 9%, respectively. OspA antigen was only present in 9 participants at baseline. At follow-up, 4 participants that received the intervention were negative for OspA, and 3 of 4 participant in the placebo arm were negative.	46% of participants randomized to intervention had improved quality of life compared with 18% of those assigned to placebo. In a subset of 48 participants who completed the trial, average improvement in the mental component of quality of life (measured by SF-36 score) was 14.4 in intervention arm vs. 6.2 in placebo arm. Average improvement in the physical component of quality of life was 8.5 in intervention arm vs. 7 in placebo arm.	According to predefined effect size cutoffs for small, moderate, and large improvement of 0.2, 0.5, and 0.8, respectively, the intervention group demonstrated a large improvement (effect size = 1.1) in cognitive index compared with a moderate improvement in the group receiving placebo (effect size = 0.72).	Pain decreased by an average of 1.37 points (on 10-point scale) in both the intervention and control arms. Pain interference decreased by 4.44 points in intervention group vs. 2.96 in control. Fatigue improved by 4.54 points in intervention arm and 0.41 points in control arm. And global health increased in the intervention arm by 0.72 points compared with 0.37 points in the control arm.

[1] The results from the Kaplan et al., 2003 are not included in this table because the data in that article are a combination of results from the seropositivity and seronegativity study together.

NOTE: EM = erythema migrans; CDC = Centers for Disease Control and Prevention; ELISA = enzyme-linked immunosorbent assay; IDSA = Infectious Diseases Society of America; IgG = immunoglobulin G; IV = intravenous; OspA = outer surface protein A.

Randomized controlled trials remain the preferred method to determine efficacy of an intervention, but even well-designed trials may be limited by the available methods or tools (Bauchner et al., 2019). Although the results of the antibiotic trials to date are disappointing, it is important to note that they address only one of a number of hypothesized mechanisms for persistent illness in persons with Lyme IACI. To date, there is only one randomized trial that addresses symptom relief through other potential disease mechanisms. There is currently insufficient evidence of benefit from a small study evaluating the effect of Kundalini yoga, but it is a generally safe intervention (Murray et al., 2022). The discovery of biomarkers or other more precise measures of efficacy could lead to additional trials of extended antibiotic treatment or to combinations of interventions targeting plausible mechanisms for persistent illness, as suggested in the 2022 TBDWG. It is important to build on the existing evidence and the incorporation of new findings as they become available through ongoing research into the pathogenesis of Lyme IACI and similar conditions to direct future research (see Chapters 3 and 4). The current evidence affirms that new approaches for treatment of persons suffering with Lyme IACI are needed.

In contrast to the results from the randomized controlled trials, 52 percent of the respondents in the MyLymeData patient registry reported taking antibiotics to manage their symptoms, and, of those, 38 percent self-reported the treatment as being moderately or very effective (MyLymeData, 2019). The reason for this discrepancy in reported effectiveness of antibiotic treatment between randomized trials and patient registry survey have not been explored, but there are generally limitations to using and interpreting retrospective registry data, including the need to control or account for bias in the data and, similar to randomized controlled trials, the challenges in controlling for placebo effects in the use and interpretation of the data. The choice of antibiotics as treatment is predicated on the assumption that persistent infection is the cause of Lyme IACI, although some antibiotics such as doxycycline and ceftriaxone also have anti-inflammatory activity that may have had a role in alleviating symptoms. However, as will be discussed later in this chapter, the pathogenesis of Lyme IACI remains poorly understood.

The methodological rigor of the 13 observational or single-arm studies was generally low. These studies, by design, do not include randomization or blinding but could include controls. However, none of the studies included a control or comparator group. In clinical studies, the use of controls, randomization, and blinding are important to increase the confidence in the results by accounting for the previously demonstrated placebo effect, in which individuals who received no active treatment reported improvement in their symptoms (Marques, 2008). These studies have evaluated a variety of interventions, including antibiotics, anti-infective agents, electromagnetic radiation, exercise, immunosuppressants, dietary interventions, nutritional supplements, and mind–body interventions (D'Adamo et al., 2015; Derderian and Otenbaker, 2024; Donta, 1997, 2003; Fallon et al., 1999; Horowitz and Freeman, 2016, 2019; Horowitz et al., 2023; Jernigan et al., 2021; Logigian et al., 1990; Johnson et al., 2020; Nicolson et al., 2012; Shere-Wolfe et al., 2024). However, the methodological limitations of these studies prevented the committee from interpreting their outcomes.

Outcome measures varied between studies. The majority assessed fatigue, cognitive function, or musculoskeletal pain or some combination of those, while a few studies also assessed neuropathy, psychiatric, gastrointestinal, and cardiac symptoms. The 36-Item Short Form Survey (SF-36) was the most frequently used outcome measurement tool. However, there was a high degree of variability in the tools used in the studies, including general tools such as the SF-36 and disease-specific tools such as the General Symptom Questionnaire-30 (GSQ-30). Standardization of the outcome measurement tools used in Lyme IACI research is a prerequisite for reproducible research and comparability between studies.

Conclusion 2-3: Results from studies that are conducted without randomization, controls, or blinding provide insufficient evidence to guide patients and clinicians in treatment decisions.

Conclusion 2-4: Many studies in the Lyme IACI literature have small sample sizes that limit the accuracy of their results.

Conclusion 2-5: Patient-reported symptoms have not been consistently or always adequately addressed in published treatment trials for Lyme IACI.

Conclusion 2-6: No safe and effective therapies for the treatment of Lyme IACI have been identified through clinical research.

EVIDENCE ON THE MECHANISMS OF LYME IACI

An understanding of disease pathogenesis can help in identifying new targets for treatment or diagnosis, inform trials to evaluate treatments and diagnostics, and ultimately lead to effective interventions. Multiple mechanisms of Lyme IACI have been proposed, including immune dysregulation and autoimmunity, pathogen or antigen persistence, central nervous system dysfunction, metabolomic changes, and microbiome changes (Marques, 2022). Studies that contribute to the understanding of disease mechanisms range from in vitro research that generates evidence to explain observed phenotypes to prospective cohort studies that observe select characteristics in participants over time. However, preclinical and observational studies may be insufficient for moving from hypothesis generation to establishing a clear understanding of the mechanistic processes that lead to disease. This is particularly true for Lyme IACI, which may present with different symptoms in different individuals and appears to affect various pathways or systems in the body, perhaps in overlapping ways that remain difficult to untangle (Rebman and Aucott, 2020). Existing knowledge gaps in how host, pathogen, and environmental factors may influence disease development and progression further hinder the understanding of mechanistic pathways and the development of treatments for Lyme IACI.

Understanding potential disease mechanisms is complicated by the challenge of diagnosing and classifying people living with Lyme IACI. Many of the symptoms reported by individuals with Lyme IACI are common to other IACI (Choutka et al., 2022; Rebman and Aucott, 2020). While the presence of antibodies to *B. burgdorferi* may indicate prior or current infection, they may persist for years and do not indicate active infection (Glatz et al., 2006).

There is no widely accepted animal model for Lyme IACI. Due to the subjective nature of Lyme IACI symptoms, no well-validated approaches currently exist to assess if animals experience these symptoms. Animal models can provide insights into immunologic interactions between host and pathogen and address the potential of pathogen or antigen persistence as well as the presence or absence of associated pathologic sequelae (Crossland et al., 2018; Hodzic et al., 2014; Pavia and Wormser, 2014). The heterogeneity of the population of people living with Lyme IACI, the lack of pathologic biomarkers, and the potential for several mechanistic pathways greatly complicate the interpretation of animal model studies for Lyme IACI (Verschoor et al., 2022). The extrapolation of findings from animal studies is further complicated by immunologic adaptations in animals that serve as natural reservoirs for *B. burgdorferi* (i.e., many small rodent species) (Brisson et al., 2008). However, animal models may provide additional insights if objective biomarkers are identified. Well-designed human studies have the highest likelihood of yielding new insights and are important for evaluating hypotheses generated in vitro or in animal models.

Large cohorts of people living with Lyme IACI are needed to identify patterns and correlations that can be examined for causal relationships. First, large prospective cohorts of adults and children with acute *B. burgdorferi* infection will allow researchers to identify patient and pathogen factors associated with the development of Lyme IACI. Second, data from individuals with Lyme IACI compared to individuals without Lyme IACI can allow "deep phenotyping." This strategy has been employed to explore mechanisms behind ME/CFS (Walitt et al., 2024), which will be discussed in more detail in Chapter 3. These prospective approaches are better suited than retrospective designs for identifying potential causative factors that can illuminate disease mechanisms. Ultimately, interventional studies can provide confirmatory evidence for mechanistic hypotheses.

Summary of Current Evidence

The committee reviewed the published, peer-reviewed evidence on the mechanisms of Lyme IACI to identify opportunities for future research that could advance treatments for people with Lyme IACI. In developing the scoping review methodology on mechanisms, the committee aimed to identify articles that could provide information on the possible causes, processes, and pathways of Lyme IACI.

The scoping review identified 49 publications relating to the potential mechanisms of Lyme IACI. Of these references, two publications exclusively examined Lyme IACI in children, while an additional three included both children and adults. Table 2-3 outlines the study designs of the included publications. The majority of the publications reported on the results of observational studies. Ten publications reported on prospective studies, consisting of the sole interventional study, seven cohort studies, and two case-control studies.

The 49 included articles cover various themes related to mechanisms of disease, including etiology, symptomology, biomarkers, risk factors, and patient subgroups. Many publications addressed multiple of these themes within a single paper.

Twenty-three manuscripts addressed potential pathogenesis of Lyme IACI (Figure 2-4). These publications vary greatly in the degree to which they investigated potential etiologies, from studies with the express objective of observing particular characteristics related to a specific proposed mechanism to studies that discussed their findings in the context of several potential mechanisms. Most of the 23 studies narrowly focused their

TABLE 2-3 Study Designs of Publications in Scoping Review on Lyme IACI Mechanisms

Interventional	
Nonrandomized	1
Observational	
Cohort	10
Case–control	37
Cross-sectional	1
TOTAL	49

NOTE: IACI = infection-associated chronic illnesses.

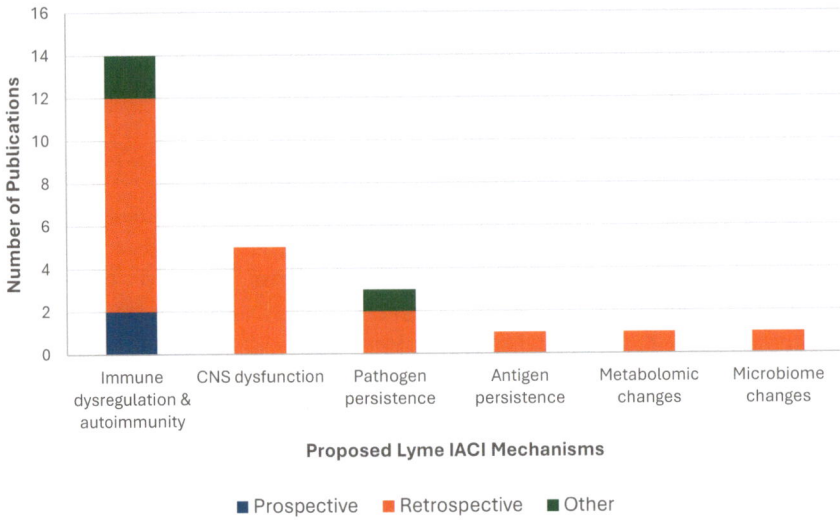

FIGURE 2-4 Proposed mechanisms of Lyme IACI in published literature.
NOTES: Some publications address multiple potential mechanisms and appear twice in the chart. "Other" includes studies that use a combination of prospective and retrospective data and studies that do not sufficiently describe their methodology. CNS = central nervous system; IACI = infection-associated chronic illnesses.

investigations on a specific characteristic or biomarker. This targeted approach to studying disease etiology may hinder the identification of potentially overlapping and interacting mechanisms. Likewise, the heterogeneity of people with Lyme IACI may complicate the interpretation of results from such studies, given that any particular characteristic or biomarker may only be present in a subset of individuals.

Two prospective studies exploring potential disease mechanisms included 149 people with Lyme disease of which at least 40 developed prolonged symptoms.[6] One was a prospective cohort study of immune markers (Clarke et al., 2021), and one was a prospective case–control study of differential gene expression (Aucott et al., 2016). As demonstrated in Figure 2-4, many potential mechanisms of Lyme IACI have not been examined in prospective studies. Interventional studies—which are also inherently prospective studies—illuminate components of the disease mechanistic pathway by testing the effect of a small molecule, natural product, biologic, or medical device on observable symptoms or surrogate markers of disease pathogenesis. Additionally, well-designed and controlled prospective studies

---

[6] One of the prospective studies did not identify the precise number of participants with Lyme IACI within the Lyme disease cohort (Clarke et al., 2021).

can provide strong evidence to support causation, unlike retrospective studies, which can only identify associations.[7]

Finally, while many interventional studies were summarized in the earlier section on treatments, these trials can also provide insight into disease mechanisms. As noted earlier, most of the treatment trials examine antibiotics, which presumes that the cause of Lyme IACI is the persistence of *Borrelia* in the body. Other potential mechanisms have rarely been evaluated through interventional studies. The lack of demonstrated effectiveness of various extended antibiotic regimens in these randomized trials suggests that pathogen persistence is not a primary driver of Lyme IACI. However, the current evidence is insufficient to entirely rule out the possibility that bacterial persistence might occur in a subset of people living with Lyme IACI. For example, case reports have suggested detection of the bacteria in postmortem human samples and in primate models that simulate the delayed treatment of Lyme disease. These and other work with uncontrolled, non-randomized studies in small cohorts or animal models cannot provide conclusive findings for Lyme IACI disease mechanisms due to their inherent methodologic limitations, but they could indicate potential future research directions.

Conclusion 2-7: Full understanding of Lyme IACI disease mechanisms remains elusive and is unlikely to be resolved in the next few years, while people living with Lyme IACI continue to suffer from chronic symptoms. Treatments trials that aim to mitigate Lyme IACI symptoms are needed while research on the disease mechanisms continues.

EVIDENCE ON THE DIAGNOSIS OF LYME IACI

Diagnostic or prognostic applications play a critical role in designing robust treatment studies to measure the effectiveness of interventions. Accurate diagnosis is essential to identify appropriate participants for enrollment (e.g., those with or without the disease). Diagnostic or prognostic tests could be used to differentiate or characterize in more detail potential subpopulations among study participants and to monitor their response to treatment. Stratifying the study population (e.g., by biomarkers, symptoms, or other phenotypes) could help reveal interventions that benefit different clusters or subgroups and build evidence for clinical tools that can be tailored for individualized care plans. This approach of using symptom clusters to manage the heterogeneity of clinical presentation and individual experience for research is being explored in Long COVID and ME/CFS (Asprusten et al.,

---

[7] Causation is used in the statistical meaning here, and not in reference to the etiology or root cause of Lyme IACI.

2021; Vaes et al., 2023; Zhang et al., 2023a). However, while there are existing diagnostic methods and ongoing efforts to improve them for Lyme disease, there are no validated and approved diagnostic or prognostic tools for Lyme IACI. The lack of consensus definitions for Lyme IACI is a critical barrier in diagnosis. There are also no broadly accepted biomarkers for Lyme IACI. Though some candidates and associated preliminary data have been described in the research literature, there are many potential pitfalls in translation from discovery to the successful development of diagnostic assays that can be used for clinical care and research.

It is possible that there are no unique objective biomarkers or clinical features to distinguish Lyme from other IACI. It is also possible that future research will identify effective interventions for shared symptoms and mechanisms for Lyme and other IACI, bypassing the importance of differentiating each disease to guide treatment decisions. However, given the current knowledge gaps regarding these diseases, it is through efforts to achieve diagnostic certainty that discoveries will be made in identifying the shared and unique elements between Lyme and other IACI.

Diagnostic tests can be broadly categorized into non–laboratory-based and laboratory-based. The former can be administered without trained laboratorians, such as point-of-care tests given by a physician, at-home tests taken by an individual, or other over-the-counter tests sold at neighborhood pharmacies. While these tests are easy and rapid to perform outside the laboratory setting, they may lack the accuracy of traditional in vitro diagnostics. Laboratory-based tests are performed in certified clinical laboratories, with samples either collected by patients (e.g., natural secretions such as sputum or urine) or by health professionals (e.g., blood). Additionally, diagnostic tests can be categorized as in vitro diagnostics, which are required to go through rigorous review by the Food and Drug Administration (FDA) for approval, or laboratory-developed tests, which in most instances have only had the validation reviewed by the developer laboratories. Quality standards for testing human specimens in clinical laboratories are regulated through the Clinical Laboratory Improvement Amendments (CLIA). Ultimately, diagnostic tests used for Lyme IACI must be fit for purpose, whether it is for clinical diagnostics or research.

For some diseases or conditions, a diagnosis can be made through distinct clinical signs, observations, and other objective findings. Clinical diagnosis must rely on physician review of signs, symptoms, and available laboratory data. Symptom or health questionnaires can be used to collect self-reported information for screening (which may be part of the clinical diagnosis) or for research purposes, but they are rarely used on their own to make a diagnosis. In the research scenario, clinical trial participants may be enrolled using a set of symptom questionnaires and clinical evaluation scales that define the study inclusion criteria, and measure and track outcomes as part of the study. Without a consensus definition for Lyme IACI, it is not possible to develop clinical diagnosis criteria or guidelines for the condition.

Diagnostic tests for Lyme IACI aim to discriminate this disease from other IACI with similar clinical presentations and possibly similar pathophysiology, a challenge compounded by the now near-universal exposure of humans to SARS-CoV-2. New approaches for Lyme IACI diagnosis that can achieve this differentiation will likely rely on identification of biomarkers that account for the potential impact of concurrent or sequential co-infections, such as markers of autoimmunity or immune dysfunction that may be unique to Lyme IACI and are altered by co-infections. Biomarkers are observable and measurable characteristics that can indicate pathology or response to an intervention (Califf, 2018). Biomarkers could have potential for diagnostic (identify cases) or prognostic (identify those individuals at highest risk) use and can sometimes be obtained from minimally invasive biological samples (e.g., serum, urine, oral, or nasal swabs) but may require more challenging and riskier samples (e.g., tissue biopsies, cerebrospinal fluid). Readily available and easily obtained specimens that do not require highly specialized personnel or equipment will be the most valuable in research to identify Lyme IACI biomarkers and also in the translation of these discoveries to practical diagnostic assays, as accessibility considerations can enable broader participation in research, especially in multi-center trials. Individuals with Lyme IACI also often seek care at primary care clinics and may not always have access to larger medical centers where complex tests are carried out. Development of an FDA-cleared in vitro diagnostic test can facilitate adoption of a standardized diagnostic. Laboratory-developed tests are not transferable from one study site to another without a complete re-validation at each new site. In addition, trial results will likely be more useful if the study participants were characterized using a single test for which clinical validity was endorsed by a neutral third party such as the FDA.

Researchers need to approach the development of diagnostic tests for Lyme IACI cautiously given the lack of knowledge on both the pathogenesis of these IACI and Lyme IACI-specific biomarkers, particularly with laboratory-developed tests that are not subject to the extensive regulatory oversight that the FDA exercises over in vitro diagnostic tests.[8] Less oversight on

---

[8] In 2024, the FDA finalized a new rule that would phase in laboratory-developed tests under a similar level of regulatory oversight as in vitro diagnostics, including requirements for quality compliance and pre-market review. However, this is a 4-year phase-in process where enforcement actions on quality and review begin in stage 3, and at the time of this report's publication, there have been legal challenges to the regulatory authority of the FDA to enact and enforce the rule (Aaron et al., 2024). See *Ass'n for Molecular Pathology v. U.S. Food & Drug Admin.*, Nos. 4:24-CV-479-SDJ & 4:24-CV-824-SDJ (E.D. Tex. Mar. 31, 2025).

laboratory-developed tests thus far opens the possibility that inadequately validated tests that produce unreliable results might be used, which would then become a confounding factor in the participant enrollment, stratification, and data analysis of clinical trials (e.g., uncertainty about whether a given participant actually had an initial *Borrelia* infection).

Summary of Current Evidence

From the scoping review, the committee highlighted opportunities for further investigation based on promising findings and gaps in the existing literature. The committee's summary of current approaches reported from in vivo studies is summarized below. Some studies briefly mention examples of laboratory tests that have been used as part of the diagnosis without providing a comprehensive list of these tests. In the findings below, details on laboratory tests used in diagnosis are only noted if available.

Since there are no validated diagnostic tests or methods for identifying Lyme IACI, the committee broadened the inclusion criteria for full-text review of diagnosis-related research compared with that for the treatment- and mechanism-related publications in order to capture potentially promising observations that could be considered for future research directions. As a result, case studies and case reports related to potential diagnosis applications were included for review. The review included publications on the development of symptom surveys and clinical scoring models for categorizing the condition. Objective biomarkers can be an important component in the diagnosis of Lyme IACI, together with careful clinical assessment and patient history. Thus, the review also included studies that assessed and correlated objective findings with symptoms reported by study participants, with the acknowledgement that research on potential disease mechanisms may uncover promising diagnostic biomarkers, and vice versa.

In all, 27 full-text articles related to the diagnosis of Lyme IACI were included in the scoping review (Table 2-4). Of these, only one study was focused on the pediatric population, and three studies included both adults and children. The diagnosis approaches or methods are categorized into three groups: questionnaires or clinical evaluation scales, direct detection, and indirect detection.

There are five publications of symptom questionnaires: two of these evaluated the same Multiple Systemic Infectious Disease Syndrome questionnaire as a clinical diagnostic instrument (Citera et al., 2017; Horowitz and Freeman, 2018), one documented the use of the Post-Lyme Questionnaire of Symptoms as a research tool to differentiate between individuals who developed PTLDS and those who have not (Aucott et al., 2022), one assessed the General Symptom Questionnaire (GSQ-30) as a tool to reflect symptom burden and track changes over time (Fallon et al., 2019), and

TABLE 2-4 Potential Biomarkers and Other Diagnostic Approaches for Lyme IACI that Have Been Reported in the Literature

Study	Description			Study size	
	Sample type	Biomarker type	Test		Control

Symptom Questionnaires or Clinical Evaluation Scales

Questionnaire

Study	Sample type			Test	Control
Aucott et al., 2022		Not applicable (longitudinal prospective study for risk of developing PTLDS)		243 adults with history of Lyme disease	49 adults without history of Lyme disease
Citera et al., 2017[1]		Not applicable Study 1: evaluate use of symptom questionnaire to identify symptoms reported by patients currently being treated for Lyme disease Study 2: validate use of symptom questionnaire in capturing health status of self-identified Lyme disease patients Study 3: validate use of symptoms questionnaire in distinguishing patients currently being treated for Lyme disease		Study 1: 537 individuals (mean age, 45) currently being treated for Lyme disease Study 2:[2] 782 individuals (mean age 50) self-identified with active symptoms of Lyme disease Study 3: 236 individuals (mean age 47) currently being treated for Lyme disease (subset from same cohort as Study 1)[3]	Study 1: none Study 2:[4] 217 individuals (mean age 53) self-identified as healthy Study 3: 568 individuals (mean age 49) self-identified as healthy (did not reuse cohort from Study 2 control group)
Fallon et al., 1999		Not applicable (use of existing objective treatment response measurement tools [Short Form 36 Functional Status Questionnaire, Zung Anxiety Scale, Beck Depression Inventory, Wechsler Adult Intelligence Scale, Wechsler Memory Scale, Controlled Oral Word Association Test])		23 adults with previously diagnosed Lyme disease, treated between 4 to 16 weeks with intravenous antibiotics, and persistent cognitive symptoms	None
Fallon et al., 2019		Not applicable (development of a patient-reported measure of symptom burden)		PTLDS: 124 adults Early Lyme disease: 94 adults	Depression: 36 adults Traumatic brain injury: 51 adults Healthy control: 37 adults

continued

TABLE 2-4 Continued

	Description		Study size	
Study	Sample type	Biomarker type	Test	Control
Horowitz and Freeman, 2018	Not applicable (patient symptom survey and retrospective chart review)		Medical records from 200 adults with history of Lyme disease based on clinical findings and/or laboratory testing, and experience persistent symptoms after prior antibiotic treatment[5]	None

Clinical evaluation scale

Bransfield et al., 2020	Not applicable (retrospective chart review)		Medical records from 100 patients (mean age 38, range 6–89) with history of Lyme disease based on CDC's 2011 case definition and documented psychiatric findings	None
Turk et al., 2019	Not applicable (developing statistical model of objective outcome measures to characterize and monitor symptom severity, using existing tools [Short Form 36 version 2, Fatigue Severity Scale, Patient Self-report Survey for the Assessment of Fibromyalgia, Neuro-QoL Cognition Function SF v2.0, Neuro-QoL Fatigue SF v1.0, Neuro-QoL Sleep Disturbance SF v1.0, Neuro-QoL Anxiety SF v1.0, Neuro-QoL Ability to Participate in Social Roles and Activities SF v1.0, Neuro-QoL Emotional and Behavioral Dyscontrol SF v1.0, Neuro-QoL Positive Affect and Well-Being SF v1.0, Neuro-QoL Satisfaction with Social Roles and Activities SF v1.1])		Development cohort: 15 adults with PTLD symptoms Validation cohort: 10 adults with PTLD symptoms	Development cohort: 14 adults recovered from Lyme disease Validation cohort: 13 adults recovered from Lyme disease

TABLE 2-4 Continued

	Description			Study size	
Study	Sample type	Biomarker type	Test		Control
Wormser et al., 2021	Not applicable: analysis of a subset from previous published prospective study of adults with erythema migrans		37 adults with EM		None

Direct Detection

Molecular detection

Sapi et al. (2019)	Autopsy tissues from brain, heart, kidney, liver	Whole cell pathogen, alginate exopolysaccharide	1 adult (case report) with no history of EM or tick bite and negative on thorough evaluation for Lyme disease, received empirical treatment for Lyme disease[6]	None
Bayer et al. (1996)	Urine	DNA	97 adults with documented EM, completed recommended antibiotics treatment, and have persistent symptoms	62 healthy adults from same regions with no history of Lyme disease

Culture

Phillips et al. (1998)	Blood	Live pathogen	47 individuals with prior diagnosis of Lyme disease, between 6 weeks to 6 months of intravenous antibiotics, and persistent symptoms[7]	23 individuals with unspecified chronic illnesses from regions not endemic for Lyme disease

continued

TABLE 2-4 Continued

	Description		Study size	
Study	Sample type	Biomarker type	Test	Control
Xenodiagnosis				
Marques et al. (2014)	Skin	Live pathogen	26 adults • 10 with high C6 antibody levels[8] • 10 with PTLDS • 5 with EM after completion of antibiotic treatment • 1 with EM and currently being treated with antibiotics	10 adults with no history of Lyme disease and seronegative by commercially available C6 ELISA
Indirect Detection				
Autoimmune markers				
Miller et al. (2024)	Serum	Anti-annexin A2 antibody	303 • 44 adults with EM >5 cm in diameter that have not started or received less than 72 hours of antibiotics at enrollment, no prior Lyme disease history and symptoms were not present for more than 3 months[9] • 281 individuals with PTLD[10]	94 healthy individuals without history of autoimmune disease (not screened for prior history of Lyme disease)
Greco et al. (2011)	Serum	Antiphospholipid antibody	106 individuals (mean age 43) with suspected, diagnosed, or treated persistent symptoms with history of positive Lyme disease immunoassay[11]	None

TABLE 2-4 Continued

	Description		Study size	
Study	Sample type	Biomarker type	Test	Control
Jacek et al. (2013)	Serum	Anti-neural antibody	19 individuals (mean age 42 ± 13.9) as a subset from a previously published study, with history of Lyme disease and objective memory impairment[12] • 14 received 10 weeks of intravenous ceftriaxone • 5 received 10 weeks of placebo treatment	11 individuals previously treated for early Lyme disease (localized or disseminated) with no persistent symptoms after treatment 20 healthy individuals with no history or serologic evidence of Lyme disease
Pathogen-specific markers				
Coyle et al. (1994)	Serum, cerebrospinal fluid	Anti-borrelial antibodies	13 individuals with history of Lyme disease and persistent fatigue after antibiotic treatment	12 individuals with unexplained persistent fatigue without history of *B. burgdorferi* infection or treatment for Lyme disease
Jacek et al. (2013)	Serum	Anti-borrelial antibodies	See above.	See above.
Fleming et al. (2004)	Serum	Anti-borrelial antibody	129 adults with Lyme disease and persistent symptoms after antibiotics treatment, same cohort as previously published trials on extended antibiotics treatment[13] • 78 were seropositive at enrollment of treatment trial • 51 were seronegative at enrollment of treatment trial	None

continued

TABLE 2-4 Continued

	Description		Study size	
Study	Sample type	Biomarker type	Test	Control
Other immune markers				
Uhde et al. (2016)	Serum	C-reactive protein, serum amyloid A level	90 individuals with early to late Lyme disease, same cohort as previously published trials on extended antibiotics treatment[14] • Early localized: 18 (mean age 46.5±14.3) • Early disseminated: 17 (mean age 47.1±16.4) • Early neurologic: 16 (mean age 46.3±9.6) • Late neurologic: 16 (mean age 52.5±16.9) • Antibiotic-responsive arthritis: 12 (mean age 45.5±15.5) • Antibiotic-refractory arthritis: 11 (mean age 52.5±20.9) 74 individuals (mean age 56.0±12.6) with PTLDS	67 healthy individuals (mean age 47.6±12.1) without history or serologic evidence of Lyme disease from the same geographic regions. 68 individuals (mean age 53.0±14.9) with history of Lyme disease but no persistent symptoms after completion of treatment.

TABLE 2-4 Continued

Study	Sample type	Biomarker type	Test	Control
		Description		Study size
Dattwyler et al. (1988)	Blood	T cell proliferation from *B. burgdorferi* whole cell stimulation	17 individuals (age range 10–65) with clinical history consistent with Lyme disease (EM or history of tick bite preceding symptoms of Lyme disease), seronegative at time of initial diagnosis, persistent symptoms after antibiotics treatment.	18 individuals (age range 16–72) with similar clinical history as the test group except seropositive by ELISA. 17 healthy individuals with no history of Lyme disease or other rheumatic or immune disorders.
Jacek et al. (2013)	Serum	Interferon alpha	See above.	See above.
Stricker et al. (2009)	Plasma	C3a and C4a complement protein	445 individuals (mean age 45.1±15, range 7–86) with positive western blot and persistent symptoms lasting more than 3 months[15]	29 healthy controls (mean age 45.3±17, range 8–75)[16] 11 adults (mean age 43.3±19, range 18–68) with systemic lupus erythematosus 6 adults (mean age 57.2±8, range 51–72) with AIDS
Stricker et al. (2002)	Blood	CD57	1 adult with history of tick bite, no recollection of EM, symptoms consistent with Lyme disease, and positive western blot.	None (case report)

continued

TABLE 2-4 Continued

	Description		Study size	
Study	Sample type	Biomarker type	Test	Control
Molecular biomarker				
Fitzgerald et al. (2021)	Serum	Metabolite signature	Cohort 1, archived serum samples from patients presenting with EM and skin culture positive for *B. burgdorferi*:[17] • 11 adults (mean age 48±13, range 32–70) who went on to develop PTLDS Cohort 2, archived serum samples from patients presenting with EM and diagnosis of Lyme disease:[18] • 13 adults (mean age 44±16, range 20–75) who went on to develop PTLDS	Cohort 1, archived serum samples from patients presenting with EM and skin culture positive for *B. burgdorferi*: • 10 adults (mean age 50±11, range 26–64) who did not experience persistent symptoms after treatment Cohort 2, archived serum samples from patients presenting with EM and diagnosis of Lyme disease: • 13 adults (mean age 50±14, range 25–73) who did not experience persistent symptoms after treatment

TABLE 2-4 Continued

		Description		Study size	
Study	Sample type	Biomarker type	Test		Control
Morrissette et al. (2020)	Stool	Microbiome signature	87 individuals with PTLDS (mean age 48.3±14.7) from an existing cohort[19]		292 • 17 healthy donor not currently and did not take antibiotics within two weeks of sample collection • 152 samples randomly selected from the American Gut Project healthy subset • 123 critically ill ICU patients from four sites across the U.S.
Neuroimaging					
Coughlin et al. (2018)	In vivo	Translocator protein (TSPO) level using [11C]DPA-713 radiotracer and PET scan	12 adults with history of probable or confirmed Lyme disease based on CDC's 2011 case definition, completed recommended antibiotic treatment, and experience PTLD symptoms of any duration. Exclusion criteria for control group also apply to the test group.		19 healthy adults (historic control from two prior studies) in stable health, without recent infections other than Lyme disease; history of neurological condition not associated with Lyme disease; clinical abnormality on blood, urine, or electrocardiogram screening; substance abuse; contraindication to imaging; or use of benzodiazepine, anti-inflammatory medication, or minocycline

continued

TABLE 2-4 Continued

		Description		Study size	
Study	Sample type	Biomarker type	Test		Control
Donta et al. (2012)	In vivo	Brain structure and function using technetium-99m SPECT	183 individuals with exposure or risk of exposure to deer ticks in a Lyme disease endemic region, and have at least two of the following symptoms: unexplained fatigue, musculoskeletal pain, neurocognitive dysfunction for at least 6 months[20]		None
Plutchok et al. (1999)	In vivo	Brain structure and function using technetium-99m SPECT	19 individuals with a diagnosis of chronic Lyme disease (mean age 35.6, standard error 2.8)[21]		14 individuals (mean age 46, range 29–47) with recent SPECT imaging in the same department and chief diagnosis was not Lyme disease[22]
Marvel et al. (2022)	In vivo	Brain structure and function with fMRI and diffusion tensor imaging	12 adults with PTLD and no comorbidities having symptom overlap with PTLD (fibromyalgia, chronic fatigue syndrome, major psychiatric disease excepting non-suicidal depression manifesting after Lyme disease), malignancy, autoimmune disease) and no history of Lyme disease vaccine, sleep apnea, cirrhosis, hepatisis B/C, HIV, dementia, cancer (in the past 2 years), substance abuse (illicit or prescription drugs, alcohol)		18 healthy adults without comorbidities having symptom overlap with PTLD and no past diagnosis of Lyme disease

TOTAL = 27

TABLE 2-4 Continued

[1] The three studies reported in this publication did not use the same symptom scales. Differences between the symptom scales used are detailed by the authors in the article.

[2] 84.1% of the self-identified Lyme disease patient group met or partially met the case definition for Lyme disease surveillance based on the 2011 CDC criteria.

[3] This study reported some of participants have documented positive laboratory results as part of their Lyme disease diagnosis using tests that include immunofluorescent antibodies, polymerase chain reaction, and an IgG/IgM immunoblot. Not all these tests are FDA cleared, and accuracy likely varies among them.

[4] 30% of self-identified healthy cohort met or partially met the case definition for Lyme disease surveillance based on the 2011 CDC criteria.

[5] This study reported some of participants have documented positive laboratory results as part of their Lyme disease diagnosis using tests that include immunofluorescent antibodies, polymerase chain reaction, IgG/IgM immunoblot, and enzyme linked immunospot assay. Not all these tests are FDA cleared, and accuracy likely varies among them.

[6] See publication for thorough clinical history for this case report.

[7] Lyme disease was diagnosed clinically, though ELISA and immunoblots with IgG and IgM were reported for some individuals.

[8] High C6 antibody level defined as having C6 antibody index >3 for at least 6 months after completion of antibiotics treatment.

[9] See Aucott et al., 2022.

[10] See Rebman et al., 2017.

[11] Referred to as 'purported chronic Lyme disease' in the publication. Immunoassays for Lyme disease included ELISA and immunoblots with IgG and IgM.

[12] See Fallon et al., 2008.

[13] See Klempner et al., 2001.

[14] See Klempner et al., 2001.

[15] See publication for detailed characterization of study participants and treatment.

[16] Additional clinical history or characteristics for this control group were not described in the publication.

[17] See Weitzner et al., 2015.

[18] See Aucott et al., 2016.

[19] Samples are from the SLICE cohort, see Rebman et al., 2017

[20] Age of the study participants were not included in the publication.

[21] Specific criteria for the chronic Lyme disease diagnosis were not described in the publication.

[22] Past history or prior test results for Lyme disease, if performed, is unknown.

NOTE: AIDS = acquired immunodeficiency syndrome; CD = cluster of differentiation; ELISA = enzyme-linked immunosorbent assay; EM = erythema migrans; fMRI = functional magnetic resonance imaging; ICU = intensive care unit; PET = positron emission tomography; PTLD = post-treatment Lyme disease; PTLDS = post-treatment Lyme disease syndrome; QoL = quality of life; SPECT = single-photon emission computed tomography.

one examined the use of a modified Fibromyalgia Impact Questionnaire to evaluate the functional impairment in PTLDS (Fallon et al., 1999). The range of applications reported for the symptom questionnaires is notable. Validation assessment has been described for GSQ-30, a PTLDS-specific instrument that was able to detect significant change in symptom burden that correlated with changes in functional impairment in relation to antibiotic therapy, but rigorous assessments have not yet been reported for two other symptom questionnaires (Aucott et al., 2022; Citera et al., 2017). However, given the current uncertainty in knowledge of disease mechanism, risk factors, and defined sets of symptoms, symptom questionnaires and clinical evaluation scales cannot be used as standalone diagnostic tools, and these publications were not further examined.

Four publications reported on the direct detection of B. burgdorferi by identifying live cells from blood samples or through xenodiagnosis (Phillips et al., 1998; Marques et al., 2014), by amplification of bacterial DNA in urine samples (Bayer et al., 1996), or by immunohistochemical imaging of intact cells and bacterial-derived exopolysaccharide in tissue samples (Sapi et al., 2019). While the last study was not conducted as diagnostic research, as it was conducted on autopsy samples of organ tissues, it does shed light on the types of samples that may be considered for development of future Lyme IACI diagnosis if the goal is to detect persisting pathogens. Xenodiagnosis is a unique method that, though unlikely to be widely adopted for routine clinical use, may be a useful tool in research studies to assess treatment response and shed light on pathogenesis mechanisms. A second clinical trial is underway, but its results have not yet been reported (NIAID, 2024).

Fourteen studies explored indirect detection methods which examined a variety of biomarkers. The majority of these were immune markers, including autoimmune antibodies (Greco et al., 2011; Jacek et al., 2013; Miller et al., 2024), antibodies specific to B. burgdorferi (Coyle et al., 1994; Fleming et al., 2004; Jacek et al., 2013), and other indicators of inflammation or immune activation (Dattwyler et al., 1988; Jacek et al., 2013; Stricker et al., 2002, 2009; Uhde et al., 2016). With the exception of three publications focused on anti-borrelial antibodies, there was no overlap in the potential diagnostic targets (i.e., no two independent studies reported on the same target). Three studies used single-photon emission computed tomography, functional magnetic resonance imaging, and diffusion tensor imaging to assess structural and functional differences in the brain of those with Lyme IACI (Donta et al., 2012; Marvel et al., 2022; Plutchok et al., 1999).[9] One study used positron emission tomography with radiotracer to reveal higher level of the mitochondrial translocator protein (TSPO), a

---

[9] See Box 3-2 in Chapter 3 for additional comments related to neuroimaging and Lyme IACI.

marker for in vivo immune activation in the central nervous system, in specific brain regions of patients experiencing persistent symptoms compared with a set of historical healthy controls (Coughlin et al., 2018). The last two studies of indirect detection methods sought to identify changes in the gut microbiome or serum metabolites that are unique in those with Lyme IACI compared with control groups (healthy volunteers, individuals who recovered from Lyme disease without long-term symptoms, intensive care unit patients) and could be used as a diagnostic signature (Fitzgerald et al., 2021; Morrissette et al., 2020). Despite the breadth of potential biomarkers explored, most of the published research were one-off reports of promising but exploratory approaches.

Biomarkers for diagnosis should be universally present in individuals with Lyme IACI and absent or distinguishable in individuals without Lyme IACI. These disease indicators are often connected with the pathophysiologic processes of the illness. Given the heterogeneity of this condition and implications that there may be distinct subgroups of the Lyme IACI population defined by different disease mechanistic pathways, as well as the potential for interactions between these pathways, it is unknown whether there can be a single biomarker or one group of biomarkers that will be applicable for the entire Lyme IACI population. Consider, for example, the strength of the evidence for attributing persistent symptoms to a Borrelial infection may vary among different individuals even if that is the true root cause of their illness. These variables, such as factors that influence the host immune response (see Chapter 1) or other aspects of disease pathogenesis stemming from the original infection to cause these symptoms, likely also affect the production and level of these biomarkers. It is possible that there are different biomarkers that, together with detailed clinical characteristics, can identify and differentiate subgroups of Lyme IACI. Future research to build on the existing findings or explore new approaches for diagnostics need to consider stratification of study participants or defining the enrollment criteria for a more granular focus to examine potential subgroup-specific criteria.

A significant challenge to diagnostics development, from exploratory research to assay validation, is the limited availability of biological sample material. Such samples would ideally be derived directly from study participants, but the number of necessary samples and the development process may lead to repeat procedures that place an undue burden on study participants and potentially diminish enrollment. Stewardship and the reuse of previously collected samples from another research study could ease this challenge. Biobanks with detailed samples from well-characterized donors with Lyme IACI represent a similar, more systematic approach, with the additional benefit of facilitating validation across studies. These resources appear under-used, however; out of the 15 publications that used human samples (i.e., excluding those that described symptom questionnaires, clinical evaluation scales, and functional neuroimaging), just two made use of established biobanks (Morrissette et al., 2020; Uhde et al., 2016), while three other publications used investigator-collected samples from a previous study (Fitzgerald et al., 2021; Fleming et al., 2004; Jacek et al., 2013) See Chapter 4 for more detailed discussion on the use of biobanks.

The scoping review revealed that research on diagnosis of Lyme IACI remains in the early stages of discovery. No single candidate stands out among the current diverse landscape of potential biomarkers as the most promising diagnostic or prognostic indicator of Lyme IACI, especially given the possibility of subgroups within this condition that are each characterized by a distinct biomarker. Newer technologies with the capacity for multiplex analysis will be valuable when applied to the complexity of Lyme IACI. The ability to obtain many answers at the same time, on the same clinical specimen, under the same conditions of time, temperature, and analyst is both invaluable with respect to data quality and able to lower costs significantly. Going forward, the ideal diagnostic tool to complement new treatment trials is likely to be an in vitro diagnostic that uses easily obtained specimens, has high sensitivity and specificity, and is FDA-approved, regardless of the biomarker that is measured. These biomarker tests must also complement the use of validated instruments (e.g., clinical scales, symptom questionnaires) that document and other clinical characteristics. Additional basic research will be necessary to identify lead candidates and provide data that encourage industry actors to undergo the detailed and costly process of development and approval of in vitro diagnostic tests for Lyme IACI.

Conclusion 2-8: There are no objective, validated biomarkers that are able to guide the diagnosis of Lyme IACI or to help distinguish distinct Lyme IACI subgroups.

KEY QUESTIONS FOR FUTURE RESEARCH

The scoping review underscored several key knowledge gaps in the current understanding of Lyme IACI that are critical to developing effective treatments. An underlying challenge across the existing evidence base for elucidating disease mechanisms and treatment effectiveness is the dearth of sufficiently powered, rigorously designed studies that can illuminate promising pathways for future research. Therefore, the committee offers four key questions that can guide how future research is carried out to identify safe and effective treatments for Lyme IACI.

How Should Lyme IACI and Relevant Lyme IACI Subgroups Be Defined?

As demonstrated in the scoping review, no commonly accepted definition for Lyme IACI exists in the literature. There must be agreement on the population that encompasses Lyme IACI to develop a broadly acceptable definition of the condition and constructively move this research forward. Multiple terms are used to describe the same population or the same subgroups of a broader population. The lack of Lyme IACI definition or common terms hinders the ability to compare results between studies. However, multiple definitions for the Lyme IACI population may be needed for specific purposes. For example, a clinical definition and a research definition are likely to serve different purposes, and both may therefore need to be developed.

People with Lyme IACI exhibit a high degree of diversity in the type and severity of symptoms they experience. To address the heterogeneity of Lyme IACI, research is needed to develop a better understanding of the potential subgroups that make up the Lyme IACI population. First, research must identify which differences in patient phenotypes represent meaningful differences in the cause, pathogenesis, prognosis, or treatment of Lyme IACI. Second, there needs to be consideration for how these differences can be accurately and consistently measured to construct relevant Lyme IACI subgroups. One example that may be relevant to explore is whether previous co-infections alter Lyme IACI prognosis or treatment, suggesting these infections may help define a specific subgroup.

The Potential Role of Objective Biomarkers for Lyme IACI

No biomarkers that can predict disease course or treatment response have been identified for Lyme IACI. To accurately diagnose Lyme IACI, clinicians must know what factors to look for that can distinguish someone with Lyme IACI from someone without the condition. A clinical diagnosis—based on an individual's symptoms—is currently the only available approach to diagnose Lyme IACI. However, this diagnostic approach is imperfect given the lack of a consensus definition for Lyme IACI, the heterogeneity in symptoms, the overlap with symptoms of other IACI, and the potential for missed diagnosis of acute Lyme disease. An observable biomarker or set of biomarkers that are consistently present or altered in individuals with Lyme IACI would provide momentum to diagnosis research. Whether these biomarkers exist for Lyme IACI remains an open question.

It is not clear if there are any differences in biomarker profiles between different types of IACI that can help distinguish an individual with Lyme IACI from another individual with a different IACI. As Chapter 3 will discuss, there are many similarities in symptoms between Lyme IACI and other IACI, and some research has posited that different IACI may share common mechanistic pathways. Given these similarities, understanding how biomarkers do and do not differ between different types of IACI, such as Lyme IACI and Long COVID, will facilitate developing specific diagnostic tools, as well as to guiding treatment research. It is important to acknowledge that distinguishing biomarkers may never be discovered. While biomarkers are a useful tool, researchers and clinicians will need to continue using clinical profiles—such as symptom presentation and severity—to guide syndromic diagnosis and treatment.

What Is the Pathogenesis behind Lyme IACI?

Research has so far been unable to determine the mechanistic pathways leading to Lyme IACI. As noted previously, many of the studies on mechanisms have been narrowly focused on observing a single or small set of characteristics (e.g., identifying a simple set of biomarkers). Ideally, researchers would know where to look when investigating the pathogenesis of a disease. But due to the complexity of Lyme IACI and multiple proposed mechanisms, it is important to ask whether different approaches to generating data may be more fruitful. Prospective studies that capture data longitudinally across a wide range of domains that might be relevant to Lyme IACI mechanisms could be a transformative approach that would accelerate discoveries. However, such an approach will generate massive amounts of data, posing the question of how to organize and analyze those data in a timely and meaningful manner.

Factors Beyond Borrelia spp. *Infection*

Given the insufficient research on Lyme IACI, little is known about the underlying mechanisms that cause individuals with this condition to experience symptoms. One of the primary open questions that demands research is the degree to which prior Lyme disease is responsible for Lyme IACI symptoms. While there is a clear association between an exposure to *B. burgdorferi* and developing chronic nonspecific symptoms (Aucott et al., 2022), the potential for other factors to contribute to the development of Lyme IACI symptoms is poorly understood. Even when Lyme disease is clearly documented and treated before the initiation of Lyme IACI symptoms, there may be other factors that contribute in addition to infection by *Borrelia spp.* that have not been sufficiently explored. For example, the potential contribution of environmental factors has been described in other IACI, including ME/CFS (Crawley and Smith, 2007), Long COVID (Zhang et al., 2023b), and Gulf War illness (IOM, 2005), but it has received little attention in Lyme IACI. Similarly, there is little research on the differences between individuals with documented Lyme disease who develop Lyme IACI, and those who return to health. Such research could illuminate predictors of Lyme IACI symptom development as well as point to potential mechanisms and potential prevention strategies.

How Should Lyme IACI Be Treated Prior to a Full Understanding of its Pathogenesis?

Treatments for Lyme IACI would ideally be tailored to address a defined problem, whether it is the underlying disease mechanisms or the resultant symptoms. Given the poor understanding of Lyme IACI's pathogenic mechanisms, focusing research on the discovery of curative treatments that act on disease mechanisms will likely prolong the wait for effective Lyme IACI treatments. While a survey of individuals with persistent symptoms following Lyme disease showed that a majority of respondents viewed symptom relief alone as less important than a cure, 96% reported that reducing symptom severity was very or critically important (Johnson, 2020). Near-term research into treatments that address Lyme IACI symptoms can be responsive to the immediate priorities of people with Lyme IACI, with mechanistic research occurring in parallel to generate evidence that could lead to the development of a cure.

As discussed earlier in this chapter, it may be difficult to distinguish individuals with Lyme IACI from others who may have been exposed to any number of pathogens that are capable of leading to similar symptoms, particularly in light of the near-ubiquitous exposure to SARS-CoV-2. Given these shared symptoms (discussed in detail in Chapter 3), it is worth considering whether treatment trials need to be specific to Lyme IACI or if individuals with similar conditions can be enrolled within a single trial. On the other hand, results of clinical trials for one disease area may be applicable for treatment of similar symptoms associated with other IACI. The answer to this question may hinge on the specific symptoms that the intervention aims to address as well as emerging evidence on the potential for common mechanistic pathways between different IACI. Moreover, if multiple IACI can be evaluated simultaneously in a trial, researchers will need to consider how these studies can be designed to generate informative results. This will also require inquiry into how outcomes can be consistently measured in these trials. For example, research will need to address whether there are biomarkers shared between IACI that are reliably responsive to treatment or if other measures such as patient-reported outcomes are more reliable.

There are many different, and at times opposing, viewpoints to consider in determining which potential Lyme IACI treatments are a priority for future research. But determining priorities is important. Due to the limited resources, a trial cannot be conducted for every potential treatment. A fundamental question is how to systematically identify the interventions that are the most promising, while acknowledging that different individuals and organizations will likely have their own priorities that reflect their own unique value systems.

Which Outcomes Should Be Used to Evaluate Whether Lyme IACI Treatments Work?

There is no agreed-upon method for measuring disease severity or symptom improvement in Lyme IACI research. Although three symptom scales or questionnaires have been developed for Lyme IACI, only one has reported rigorously designed validation measures (Fallon et al., 2019). In the absence of objective measures of disease, PRO measures or clinician evaluations are often used to measure treatment outcomes. Given their widespread use, it is necessary to consider whether these approaches to measurement are accurately and consistently measuring what they are intended to measure. For example, the question of whether general PROs capture relevant changes in the symptoms experienced in Lyme IACI has never been thoroughly evaluated. Moving forward, it will be necessary to identify the most meaningful, valid outcome measures to people living with Lyme IACI, clinicians, and regulators for use in clinical trials.

Conclusion 2-9: The heterogeneity of patient-reported symptoms and characteristics, in the absence of objective diagnostic findings specific to Lyme IACI, likely obscures important patient subgroups in treatment studies and hinders confirmation of new findings. PTLDS is one defined group that is part of the heterogeneous Lyme IACI patient population.

Conclusion 2-10: The lack of a consensus definition for Lyme IACI is a critical barrier for advancing research to understand disease mechanism and develop new treatments by preventing data aggregation, meta-analyses, or replication for confirmatory studies.

REFERENCES

Aaron, D. G., E. Y. Adashi, and I. G. Cohen. 2024. The U.S. FDA's new rule for regulating laboratory-developed tests. *JAMA Health Forum* 5(10):e242917.

Adjemian, J., I. B. Weber, J. McQuiston, K. S. Griffith, P. S. Mead, W. Nicholson, A. Roche, M. Schriefer, M. Fischer, O. Kosoy, J. J. Laven, R. A. Stoddard, A. R. Hoffmaster, T. Smith, D. Bui, P. P. Wilkins, J. L. Jones, P. N. Gupton, C. P. Quinn, N. Messonnier, C. Higgins, and D. Wong. 2012. Zoonotic infections among employees from Great Smoky Mountains and Rocky Mountain national parks, 2008–2009. *Vector Borne Zoonotic Diseases* 12(11):922–931.

American College of Rheumatology. 2023. *Fibromyalgia.* https://rheumatology.org/patients/fibromyalgia (accessed January 27, 2025).

Asch, E. S., D. I. Bujak, M. Weiss, M. G. Peterson, and A. Weinstein. 1994. Lyme disease: An infectious and postinfectious syndrome. *Journal of Rheumatology* 21(3):454–461.

Asprusten, T. T., L. Sletner, and V. B. B. Wyller. 2021. Are there subgroups of chronic fatigue syndrome? An exploratory cluster analysis of biological markers. *Journal of Translational Medicine* 19(1):48.

Aucott, J. N., L. A. Crowder, and K. B. Kortte. 2013. Development of a foundation for a case definition of post-treatment Lyme disease syndrome. *International Journal of Infectious Diseases* 17(6):e443–e449.

Aucott, J. N., M. J. Soloski, A. W. Rebman, L. A. Crowder, L. J. Lahey, C. A. Wagner, W. H. Robinson, and K. T. Bechtold. 2016. CCL19 as a chemokine risk factor for posttreatment Lyme disease syndrome: A prospective clinical cohort study. *Clinical and Vaccine Immunology* 23(9):757–766.

Aucott, J. N., T. Yang, I. Yoon, D. Powell, S. A. Geller, and A. W. Rebman. 2022. Risk of post-treatment Lyme disease in patients with ideally-treated early Lyme disease: A prospective cohort study. *International Journal of Infectious Diseases* 116:230–237.

Bauchner, H., R. M. Golub, and P. B. Fontanarosa. 2019. Reporting and interpretation of randomized clinical trials. *JAMA* 322(8):732–735.

Bayer, M. E., L. Zhang, and M. H. Bayer. 1996. Borrelia burgdorferi DNA in the urine of treated patients with chronic Lyme disease symptoms. A PCR study of 97 cases. *Infection* 24(5):347–353.

Bouquet, J., M. J. Soloski, A. Swei, C. Cheadle, S. Federman, J.-N. Billaud, A. W. Rebman, B. Kabre, R. Halpert, M. Boorgula, J. N. Aucott, and C. Y. Chiu. 2016. Longitudinal transcriptome analysis reveals a sustained differential gene expression signature in patients treated for acute Lyme disease. *mBio* 7(1):10.1128/mbio.00100-00116.

Bransfield, R. C., D. M. Aidlen, M. J. Cook, and S. Javia. 2020. A clinical diagnostic system for late-stage neuropsychiatric Lyme borreliosis based upon an analysis of 100 patients. *Healthcare (Basel)* 8(1):13.

Bretherick, A. D., S. J. McGrath, A. Devereux-Cooke, S. Leary, E. Northwood, A. Redshaw, P. Stacey, C. Tripp, J. Wilson, S. Chowdhury, I. Lewis, Ø. Almelid, S. V. Baby, T. Baker, H. Becher, T. Boutin, M. Clyde, D. Garcia, J. Ireland, S. M. Kerr, E. McDowall, D. Perry, G. L. Samms, V. Vitart, J. C. Wolfe, and C. P. Ponting. 2023. Typing myalgic encephalomyelitis by infection at onset: A decodeme study. *NIHR Open Research* 3:20.

Brisson, D., D. E. Dykhuizen, and R. S. Ostfeld. 2008. Conspicuous impacts of inconspicuous hosts on the Lyme disease epidemic. *Proceedings: Biological Sciences* 275(1631):227–235.

Califf, R. M. 2018. Biomarker definitions and their applications. *Experimental Biology and Medicine (Maywood)* 243(3):213–221.

Cameron, D. 2008. Severity of Lyme disease with persistent symptoms. Insights from a double-blind placebo-controlled clinical trial. *Minerva Medical* 99(5):489–496.

Choutka, J., V. Jansari, M. Hornig, and A. Iwasaki. 2022. Unexplained post-acute infection syndromes. *Nature Medicine* 28(5):911–923.

Chung, M. K., M. Caboni, P. Strandwitz, A. D'Onofrio, K. Lewis, and C. J. Patel. 2023. Systematic comparisons between Lyme disease and post-treatment Lyme disease syndrome in the U.S. with administrative claims data. *eBioMedicine* 90:104524.

Citera, M., P. R. Freeman, and R. I. Horowitz. 2017. Empirical validation of the Horowitz Multiple Systemic Infectious Disease Syndrome Questionnaire for suspected Lyme disease. *International Journal of General Medicine* 10:249–273.

Clarke, D. J. B., A. W. Rebman, A. Bailey, M. L. Wojciechowicz, S. L. Jenkins, J. E. Evangelista, M. Danieletto, J. Fan, M. W. Eshoo, M. R. Mosel, W. Robinson, N. Ramadoss, J. Bobe, M. J. Soloski, J. N. Aucott, and A. Ma'ayan. 2021. Predicting Lyme disease from patients' peripheral blood mononuclear cells profiled with RNA sequencing. *Frontiers in Immunology* 12:636289.

Coughlin, J. M., T. Yang, A. W. Rebman, K. T. Bechtold, Y. Du, W. B. Mathews, W. G. Lesniak, E. A. Mihm, S. M. Frey, E. S. Marshall, H. B. Rosenthal, T. A. Reekie, M. Kassiou, R. F. Dannals, M. J. Soloski, J. N. Aucott, and M. G. Pomper. 2018. Imaging glial activation in patients with post-treatment Lyme disease symptoms: A pilot study using [11C]DPA-713 PET. *J Neuroinflammation* 19;15(1):346.

Coyle, P. K., L. B. Krupp, C. Doscher, and K. Amin. 1994. *Borrelia burgdorferi* reactivity in patients with severe persistent fatigue who are from a region in which Lyme disease is endemic. *Clinical Infectious Diseases* 18(Suppl 1):S24–S27.

Crawley, E., and G. Davey Smith. 2007. Is chronic fatigue syndrome (CFS/ME) heritable in children, and if so, why does it matter? *Archives of Disease in Childhood* 92(12):1058–1061.

Crossland, N. A., X. Alvarez, and M. E. Embers. 2018. Late disseminated Lyme disease: Associated pathology and spirochete persistence posttreatment in rhesus macaques. *American Journal of Pathology* 188(3):672–682.

D'Adamo, C. R., C. R. McMillin, K. W. Chen, E. K. Lucas, and B. M. Berman. 2015. Supervised resistance exercise for patients with persistent symptoms of Lyme disease. *Medicine & Science in Sports & Exercise* 47(11):2291-2298.

Dattwyler, R. J., D. J. Volkman, B. J. Luft, J. J. Halperin, J. Thomas, and M. G. Golightly. 1988. Seronegative Lyme disease. *New England Journal of Medicine* 319(22):1441–1446.

DeLong, A. K., B. Blossom, E. L. Maloncy, and S. E. Phillips. 2012. Antibiotic retreatment of Lyme disease in patients with persistent symptoms: A biostatistical review of randomized, placebo-controlled, clinical trials. Contemporary Clinical Trials 33(6):1132-1142.

DeLong, A., M. Hsu, and H. Kotsoris. 2019. Estimation of cumulative number of post-treatment Lyme disease cases in the U.S., 2016 and 2020. *BMC Public Health* 19(1):352.

Derderian, G. P., and N. Otenbaker. 2024. A prospective study of patients with post treatment Lyme disease syndrome treated with modified VFEM energy. *Journal of Cosmetic Dermatology* 23(6):2044–2048.

Donta, S. T. 1997. Tetracycline therapy for chronic Lyme disease. *Clinical Infectious Diseases* 25(Supplement_1):S52–S56.

Donta, S. T. 2003. Macrolide therapy of chronic Lyme disease. *Medical Science Monit* 9(11):PI136–PI142.

Donta, S. T., R. B. Noto, and J. A. Vento. 2012. SPECT brain imaging in chronic Lyme disease. *Clinical Nuclear Medicine* 37(9):e219–e222.

Elhaj, R., and J. M. Reynolds. 2023. Chemical exposures and suspected impact on Gulf War veterans. *Military Medical Research* 10(1):11.

Fallon, J., D. I. Bujak, S. Guardino, and A. Weinstein. 1999. The Fibromyalgia Impact Questionnaire: A useful tool in evaluating patients with post–Lyme disease syndrome. *Arthritis Care & Research* 12(1):42–47.

Fallon, B. A., F. A. Tager, J. G. Keilp, N. Weiss, L. Fein, and K. B. Liegner. 1999. Repeated antibiotic treatment in chronic Lyme disease. *Journal of Spirochetal and Tick-Borne Diseases* 6.

Fallon, B. A., J. G. Keilp, K. M. Corbera, E. Petkova, C. B. Britton, E. Dwyer, I. Slavov, J. Cheng, J. Dobkin, D. R. Nelson, and H. A. Sackeim. 2008. A randomized, placebo-controlled trial of repeated IV antibiotic therapy for Lyme encephalopathy. *Neurology* 70(13):992–1003.

Fallon, B. A., E. Petkova, J. G. Keilp, and C. B. Britton. 2012. A reappraisal of the U.S. clinical trials of post-treatment Lyme disease syndrome. *Open Neurology Journal* 6:79-87.

Fallon, B. A., N. Zubcevik, C. Bennett, S. Doshi, A. W. Rebman, R. Kishon, J. R. Moeller, N. R. Octavien, and J. N. Aucott. 2019. The General Symptom Questionnaire-30 (GSQ-30): A brief measure of multi-system symptom burden in Lyme disease. *Frontiers in Medicine (Lausanne)* 6:283.

Fallon, B. A., M. Kuvaldina, N. Zubcevik, R. DeBiasi, S. B. Mulkey, C. Chiu, F. Chow, K. Paolino, R. Lai, D. Putrino, A. Proal, M. Pavlicova, and J. Aucott. 2025. Proposed research classification criteria for Lyme disease in infection associated chronic illness studies. *Frontiers in Medicine* 12.

Faro, M., N. Sàez-Francás, J. Castro-Marrero, L. Aliste, T. Fernández de Sevilla, and J. Alegre. 2016. Gender differences in chronic fatigue syndrome. *Rheumatologíca Clínica* 12(2):72–77.

Fitzgerald, B. L., B. Graham, M. J. Delorey, A. Pegalajar-Jurado, M. N. Islam, G. P. Wormser, J. N. Aucott, A. W. Rebman, M. J. Soloski, J. T. Belisle, and C. R. Molins. 2021. Metabolic response in patients with post-treatment Lyme disease symptoms/syndrome. *Clinical Infectious Diseases* 73(7):e2342–e2349.

Fleming, R. V., A. R. Marques, M. S. Klempner, C. H. Schmid, L. G. Dally, D. S. Martin, and M. T. Philipp. 2004. Pre-treatment and post-treatment assessment of the C(6) test in patients with persistent symptoms and a history of Lyme borreliosis. *European Journal of Clinical Microbiology & Infectious Diseases* 23(8):615–618.

Glatz, M., M. Golestani, H. Kerl, and R. R. Müllegger. 2006. Clinical relevance of different IgG and IgM serum antibody responses to *Borrelia burgdorferi* after antibiotic therapy for erythema migrans: Long-term follow-up study of 113 patients. *Archives of Dermatology* 142(7):862–868.

Gluckman, S. J., A. L. Komaroff, and K. Law. 2025. *Patient education: Myalgic encephalomyelitis/chronic fatigue syndrome (beyond the basics)*. https://www.uptodate.com/contents/myalgic-encephalomyelitis-chronic-fatigue-syndrome-beyond-the-basics/print (accessed March 20, 2025).

Gould, L. H., A. Fathalla, J. C. Moïsi, and J. H. Stark. 2024. Racial and ethnic disparities in Lyme disease in the United States. *Zoonoses and Public Health* 71(5):469–479.

Greco, T. P., Jr., A. M. Conti-Kelly, and T. P. Greco. 2011. Antiphospholipid antibodies in patients with purported "chronic Lyme disease." *Lupus* 20(13):1372–1377.

Haley, R. W., G. Kramer, J. Xiao, J. A. Dever, and J. F. Teiber. 2022. Evaluation of a gene–environment interaction of PON1 and low-level nerve agent exposure with Gulf War illness: A prevalence case-control study drawn from the U.S. Military Health Survey's national population sample. *Environmental Health Perspectives* 130(5):057001.

HHS (Department of Health and Human Services), FDA (Food and Drug Administration), CDER (Center for Drug Evaluation and Research), CBER (Center for Biologics Evaluation and Research), and CDRH (Center for Devices and Radiological Health). 2009. *Guidance for industry—Patient-reported outcome measures: Use in medical product development to support labeling claims*. https://www.fda.gov/media/77832/download (accessed January 27, 2025).

Hodzic, E., D. Imai, S. Feng, and S. W. Barthold. 2014. Resurgence of persisting non-cultivable *Borrelia burgdorferi* following antibiotic treatment in mice. *PLOS One* 9(1):e86907.

Horowitz, R., and P. R. Freeman. 2016. The use of dapsone as a novel "persister" drug in the treatment of chronic Lyme disease/post treatment Lyme disease syndrome. *Journal of Clinical and Experimental Dermatology Research* 07.

Horowitz, R. I., and P. R. Freeman. 2018. Precision medicine: The role of the MSIDS model in defining, diagnosing, and treating chronic Lyme disease/post treatment Lyme disease syndrome and other chronic illness: Part 2. *Healthcare (Basel)* 6(4):129.

Horowitz, R. I., and P. R. Freeman. 2019. Precision medicine: Retrospective chart review and data analysis of 200 patients on dapsone combination therapy for chronic Lyme disease/post-treatment Lyme disease syndrome: Part 1. *International Journal of General Medicine* 12:101–119.

Horowitz, R. I., J. Fallon, and P. R. Freeman. 2023. Comparison of the efficacy of longer versus shorter pulsed high dose dapsone combination therapy in the treatment of chronic Lyme disease/post treatment lyme disease syndrome with bartonellosis and associated coinfections. *Microorganisms* 11(9):2301.

Hu, L., A. C. Steere, and K. K. Hall. 2025. *Patient education: Lyme disease symptoms and diagnosis (beyond the basics)*. https://www.uptodate.com/contents/lyme-disease-symptoms-and-diagnosis-beyond-the-basics (accessed March 20, 2025).

IOM (Institute of Medicine). 2005. *Gulf War and health: Volume 3: Fuels, combustion products, and propellants*. Washington, DC: The National Academies Press.

IOM. 2011. *Relieving pain in America: A blueprint for transforming prevention, care, education, and research*. Washington, DC: The National Academies Press.

Jacek, E., B. A. Fallon, A. Chandra, M. K. Crow, G. P. Wormser, and A. Alaedini. 2013. Increased IFNα activity and differential antibody response in patients with a history of Lyme disease and persistent cognitive deficits. *Journal of Neuroimmunology* 255(1–2):85–91.

Jernigan, D. A., M. C. Hart, K. K. Dodd, S. Jameson, and T. Farney. 2021. Induced native phage therapy for the treatment of Lyme disease and relapsing fever: A retrospective review of first 14 months in one clinic. *Cureus* 13(11):e20014.

Johnson, L., M. Shapiro, R. B. Stricker, J. Vendrow, J. Haddock, and D. Needell. 2020. Antibiotic treatment response in chronic Lyme disease: Why do some patients improve while others do not? *Healthcare* 8(4):383.

Johnson, L. 2020. Outcomes Important to Lyme Patients: Results of a Lymedisease.org Patient Survey Conducted in 2015. figshare. https://doi.org/10.6084/m9.figshare.10010534.v1.

Johnson, L., M. Shapiro, S. Janicki, J. Mankoff, and R. B. Stricker. 2023. Does biological sex matter in Lyme disease? The need for sex-disaggregated data in persistent illness. *International Journal of General Medicine* 16:2557–2571.

Kaplan, R. F., R. P. Trevino, G. M. Johnson, L. Levy, R. Dornbush, L. T. Hu, J. Evans, A. Weinstein, C. H. Schmid, and M. S. Klempner. 2003. Cognitive function in post-treatment Lyme disease: Do additional antibiotics help? *Neurology* 60(12):1916–1922.

Klein, S. L., and K. L. Flanagan. 2016. Sex differences in immune responses. *Nature Reviews Immunology* 16(10):626–638.

Klempner, M. S., L. T. Hu, J. Evans, C. H. Schmid, G. M. Johnson, R. P. Trevino, D. Norton, L. Levy, D. Wall, J. McCall, M. Kosinski, and A. Weinstein. 2001. Two controlled trials of antibiotic treatment in patients with persistent symptoms and a history of Lyme disease. *New England Journal of Medicine* 345(2):85–92.

Klempner, M. S., P. J. Baker, E. D. Shapiro, A. Marques, R. J. Dattwyler, J. J. Halperin, and G. P. Wormser. 2013. Treatment trials for post-Lyme disease symptoms revisited. *American Journal of Medicine* 126(8):665–669.

Krupp, L. B., L. G. Hyman, R. Grimson, P. K. Coyle, P. Melville, S. Ahnn, R. Dattwyler, and B. Chandler. 2003. Study and treatment of post Lyme disease (STOP-LD): A randomized double masked clinical trial. *Neurology* 60(12):1923–1930.

Lemieux, J. E., W. Huang, N. Hill, T. Cerar, L. Freimark, S. Hernandez, M. Luban, V. Maraspin, P. Bogovic, K. Ogrinc, E. Ruzic-Sabljic, P. Lapierre, E. Lasek-Nesselquist, N. Singh, R. Iyer, D. Liveris, K. D. Reed, J. M. Leong, J. A. Branda, A. C. Steere, G. P. Wormser, F. Strle, P. C. Sabeti, I. Schwartz, and K. Strle. 2023. Whole genome sequencing of *Borrelia burgdorferi* isolates reveals linked clusters of plasmid-borne accessory genome elements associated with virulence. *bioRxiv* [Preprint]. Feb 27:2023.02.26.530159. Update in: *PLOS Pathogens*, 2023, 19(8):e1011243.

Logigian, E. L., R. F. Kaplan, and A. C. Steere. 1990. Chronic neurologic manifestations of Lyme disease. *New England Journal of Medicine* 323(21):1438–1444.

Marques, A. 2008. Chronic Lyme disease: A review. *Infectious Disease Clinics of North America* 22(2):341–360, vii–viii.

Marques, A. 2022. Persistent symptoms after treatment of Lyme disease. *Infectious Disease Clinics of North America* 36(3):621–638.

Marques, A., S. R. Telford, 3rd, S. P. Turk, E. Chung, C. Williams, K. Dardick, P. J. Krause, C. Brandeburg, C. D. Crowder, H. E. Carolan, M. W. Eshoo, P. A. Shaw, and L. T. Hu. 2014. Xenodiagnosis to detect *Borrelia burgdorferi* infection: A first-in-human study. *Clinical Infectious Diseases* 58(7):937–945.

Marvel, C. L., K. H. Alm, D. Bhattacharya, W. Rebman Alison, A. Bakker, O. P. Morgan, J. A. Creighton, E. A. Kozero, A. Venkatesan, P. A. Nadkarni, and J. N. Aucott. 2022. A multimodal neuroimaging study of brain abnormalities and clinical correlates in post treatment Lyme disease. *PLOS One* 10(17):e0271425.

Mauvais-Jarvis, F., N. Bairey Merz, P. J. Barnes, R. D. Brinton, J. J. Carrero, D. L. DeMeo, G. J. De Vries, C. N. Epperson, R. Govindan, S. L. Klein, A. Lonardo, P. M. Maki, L. D. McCullough, V. Regitz-Zagrosek, J. G. Regensteiner, J. B. Rubin, K. Sandberg, and A. Suzuki. 2020. Sex and gender: Modifiers of health, disease, and medicine. *The Lancet* 396(10250):565–582.

Mayo-Wilson, E., N. Fusco, T. Li, H. Hong, J. K. Canner, and K. Dickersin. 2017. Multiple outcomes and analyses in clinical trials create challenges for interpretation and research synthesis. *Journal of Clinical Epidemiology* 86:39–50.

Miller, J. B., A. W. Rebman, M. D. V. de Flores, H. Wang, E. Darrah, and J. N. Aucott. 2024. Annexin A2 antibodies in post-treatment Lyme disease. *Therapeutic Advances in Infectious Disease* 11:20499361241242971.

Monaghan, M., S. Norman, M. Gierdalski, A. Marques, J. E. Bost, and R. L. DeBiasi. 2024. Pediatric Lyme disease: Systematic assessment of post-treatment symptoms and quality of life. *Pediatric Research* 95(1):174–181.

Morrissette, M., N. Pitt, A. González, P. Strandwitz, M. Caboni, A. W. Rebman, R. Knight, A. D'Onofrio, J. N. Aucott, M. J. Soloski, and K. Lewis. 2020. A distinct microbiome signature in posttreatment Lyme disease patients. *mBio* 11(5):e02310-20.

Murray, L., C. Alexander, C. Bennett, M. Kuvaldina, G. Khalsa, and B. Fallon. 2022. Kundalini yoga for post-treatment Lyme disease: A preliminary randomized study. *Healthcare (Basel)* 10(7):1314.

Mustafiz, F., J. Moeller, M. Kuvaldina, C. Bennett, and B. A. Fallon. 2022. Persistent symptoms, Lyme disease, and prior trauma. *Journal of Nervous and Mental Disorders* 210(5):359–364.

MyLymeData. 2019. *2019 chart book—MyLymeData registry*. https://www.lymedisease.org/2019-mylymedata-highlights.pdf (accessed January 28, 2025).

NCFH (National Center for Farmworker Health). 2023. *Tickborne disease risk and perceptions among outdoor workers in Hunterdon and Morris counties, New Jersey*. https://www.ncfh.org/uploads/3/8/6/8/38685499/final_ncfh_tiksnow_report_6.28.23.pdf (accessed November 27, 2024).

NIAID (National Institute of Allergy and Infectious Diseases. 2024. *Xenodiagnosis after antibiotic treatment for Lyme disease*. https://www.clinicaltrials.gov/study/NCT02446626 (accessed January 27, 2025).

Nicolson, G., R. Settineri, and R. Ellithorpe. 2012. Glycophospholipid formulation with NADH and CoQ10 significantly reduces intractable fatigue in western blot-positive 'chronic Lyme disease' patients: Preliminary report. *Functional Foods in Health and Disease* 2:35–47.

NIH (National Institute of Health). 2025. *Patient-Reported Outcomes Measurement Information System (PROMIS)*. https://commonfund.nih.gov/promis/index (accessed January 27, 2025).

NIH Reporter. 2025. *A prospective study of persistent symptoms of Lyme disease*. https://reporter.nih.gov/search/OzWUFp3Ng0GcgLPybQbQkQ/project-details/10862287 (accessed January 27, 2025).

Pavia, C. S., and G. P. Wormser. 2014. Culture of the entire mouse to determine whether cultivable *Borrelia burgdorferi* persists in infected mice treated with a five-day course of ceftriaxone. *Antimicrobial Agents and Chemotherapy* 58(11):6701–6703.

Phillips, S. E., L. H. Mattman, D. Hulínská, and H. Moayad. 1998. A proposal for the reliable culture of *Borrelia burgdorferi* from patients with chronic Lyme disease, even from those previously aggressively treated. *Infection* 26(6):364–367.

Piacentino, J. D., and B. S. Schwartz. 2002. Occupational risk of Lyme disease: An epidemiological review. *Occupational and Environmental Medicine* 59(2):75–84.

Plutchok, J. J., R. S. Tikofsky, K. B. Liegner, J. M. Kochevan, B. A. Fallon, and R. L. Van Heertum. Tc-99m HMPAO brain SPECT imaging in chronic Lyme disease. 1999. *Journal of Spirochetal and Tick-Borne Diseases* 6:117–122.

Rebman, A. W., K. T. Bechtold, T. Yang, E. A. Mihm, M. J. Soloski, C. B. Novak, and J. N. Aucott. 2017. The clinical, symptom, and quality-of-life characterization of a well-defined group of patients with posttreatment Lyme disease syndrome. *Frontiers in Medicine* 4.

Rebman, A. W., and J. N. Aucott. 2020. Post-treatment Lyme disease as a model for persistent symptoms in Lyme disease. *Frontiers in Medicine* 7:57.

Sapi, E., R. S. Kasliwala, H. Ismail, J. P. Torres, M. Oldakowski, S. Markland, G. Gaur, A. Melillo, K. Eisendle, K. B. Liegner, J. Libien, and J. E. Goldman. 2019. The long-term persistence of *Borrelia burgdorferi* antigens and DNA in the tissues of a patient with Lyme disease. *Antibiotics (Basel)* 8(4):183.

Shadick, N. A., C. B. Phillips, E. L. Logigian, A. C. Steere, R. F. Kaplan, V. P. Berardi, P. H. Duray, M. G. Larson, E. A. Wright, K. S. Ginsburg, J. N. Katz, and M. H. Liang. 1994. The long-term clinical outcomes of Lyme disease. A population-based retrospective cohort study. *Annals of Internal Medicine* 121(8):560–567.

Shere-Wolfe, K. D., N. George, G. M. Al Kibria, R. Silk, and C. S. Alexander. 2024. A multimodal Ayurveda and mind–body therapeutic intervention for chronic symptoms attributed to a postinfectious syndrome: A pilot study. *Journal of Integrative and Complementary Medicine* 30(5):450–458.

Solomon, S. P., E. Hilton, B. S. Weinschel, S. Pollack, and E. Grolnick. 1998. Psychological factors in the prediction of Lyme disease course. *Arthritis & Rheumatism* 11(5):419–426.

Stricker, R. B., J. Burrascano, and E. Winger. 2002. Longterm decrease in the CD57 lymphocyte subset in a patient with chronic Lyme disease. *Annals of Agricultural and Environmental Medicine* 9(1):111–113.

Stricker, R. B., V. R. Savely, N. C. Motanya, and P. C. Giclas. 2009. Complement split products C3a and C4a in chronic Lyme disease. *Scandinavian Journal of Immunology* 69(1):64–69.

Sun, T. Y., J. Hardin, H. R. Nieva, K. Natarajan, R. F. Cheng, P. Ryan, and N. Elhadad. 2023. Large-scale characterization of gender differences in diagnosis prevalence and time to diagnosis. *medRxiv* [Preprint]. Oct 16:2023.10.12.23296976.

TBDWG (Tick-Borne Disease Working Group). 2018. *Tick-Borne Disease Working Group 2018 report to Congress*. https://www.hhs.gov/sites/default/files/tbdwg-report-to-congress-2018.pdf (accessed November 27, 2024).

TBDWG. 2020. *Tick-Borne Disease Working Group 2020 report to Congress*. https://www.hhs.gov/sites/default/files/tbdwg-2020-report_to-ongress-final.pdf (accessed November 27, 2024).

TBDWG. 2022. *Tick-Borne Disease Working Group 2022 report to Congress.* https://www.hhs.gov/sites/default/files/tbdwg-2022-report-to-congress.pdf (accessed November 27, 2024).

Turk, S. P., K. Lumbard, K. Liepshutz, C. Williams, L. Hu, K. Dardick, G. P. Wormser, J. Norville, C. Scavarda, D. McKenna, D. Follmann, and A. Marques. 2019. Post-treatment Lyme disease symptoms score: Developing a new tool for research. *PLOS One* 14(11):e0225012.

Uhde, M., M. Ajamian, X. Li, G. P. Wormser, A. Marques, and A. Alaedini. 2016. Expression of C-reactive protein and serum amyloid a in early to late manifestations of Lyme disease. *Clinical Infectious Diseases* 63(11):1399–1404.

Ursinus, J., H. D. Vrijmoeth, M. G. Harms, A. D. Tulen, H. Knoop, S. A. Gauw, T. P. Zomer, A. Wong, I. H. M. Friesema, Y. M. Vermeeren, L. A. B. Joosten, J. W. Hovius, B. J. Kullberg, and C. C. van den Wijngaard. 2021. Prevalence of persistent symptoms after treatment for Lyme borreliosis: A prospective observational cohort study. *The Lancet Regional Health—Europe* 6:100142.

Vaes, A. W., M. Van Herck, Q. Deng, J. M. Delbressine, L. A. Jason, and M. A. Spruit. 2023. Symptom-based clusters in people with ME/CFS: An illustration of clinical variety in a cross-sectional cohort. *Journal of Translational Medicine* 21(1):112.

Verschoor, Y. L., A. Vrijlandt, R. Spijker, R. M. van Hest, H. Ter Hofstede, K. van Kempen, A. J. Henningsson, and J. W. Hovius. 2022. Persistent *Borrelia burgdorferi* sensu lato infection after antibiotic treatment: Systematic overview and appraisal of the current evidence from experimental animal models. *Clinical Microbiology Reviews* 35(4):e0007422.

Walitt, B., K. Singh, S. R. LaMunion, M. Hallett, S. Jacobson, K. Chen, Y. Enose-Akahata, R. Apps, J. J. Barb, P. Bedard, R. J. Brychta, A. W. Buckley, P. D. Burbelo, B. Calco, B. Cathay, L. Chen, S. Chigurupati, J. Chen, F. Cheung, L. M. K. Chin, B. W. Coleman, A. B. Courville, M. S. Deming, B. Drinkard, L. R. Feng, L. Ferrucci, S. A. Gabel, A. Gavin, D. S. Goldstein, S. Hassanzadeh, S. C. Horan, S. G. Horovitz, K. R. Johnson, A. J. Govan, K. M. Knutson, J. D. Kreskow, M. Levin, J. J. Lyons, N. Madian, N. Malik, A. L. Mammen, J. A. McCulloch, P. M. McGurrin, J. D. Milner, R. Moaddel, G. A. Mueller, A. Mukherjee, S. Muñoz-Braceras, G. Norato, K. Pak, I. Pinal-Fernandez, T. Popa, L. B. Reoma, M. N. Sack, F. Safavi, L. N. Saligan, B. A. Sellers, S. Sinclair, B. Smith, J. Snow, S. Solin, B. J. Stussman, G. Trinchieri, S. A. Turner, C. S. Vetter, F. Vial, C. Vizioli, A. Williams, S. B. Yang, A. Nath, and the Center for Human Immunology, Autoimmunity, and Inflammation Consortium. 2024. Deep phenotyping of post-infectious myalgic encephalomyelitis/chronic fatigue syndrome. *Nature Communications* 15(1):907.

Weitzner, E., D. McKenna, J. Nowakowski, C. Scavarda, R. Dornbush, S. Bittker, D. Cooper, R. B. Nadelman, P. Visintainer, I. Schwartz, and G. P. Wormser. 2015. Long-term assessment of post-treatment symptoms in patients with culture-confirmed early Lyme disease. *Clinical Infectious Diseases* 61(12):1800–1806.

Wormser, G. P., R. J. Dattwyler, E. D. Shapiro, J. J. Halperin, A. C. Steere, M. S. Klempner, P. J. Krause, J. S. Bakken, F. Strle, G. Stanek, L. Bockenstedt, D. Fish, J. S. Dumler, and R. B. Nadelman. 2006. The clinical assessment, treatment, and prevention of Lyme disease, human granulocytic anaplasmosis, and babesiosis: Clinical practice guidelines by the Infectious Diseases Society of America. *Clinical Infectious Diseases* 43(9):1089–1134.

Wormser, G. P., E. Weitzner, D. McKenna, R. B. Nadelman, C. Scavarda, and J. Nowakowski. 2015. Long-term assessment of fatigue in patients with culture-confirmed Lyme disease. *American Journal of Medicine* 128(2):181–184.

Wormser, G. P., D. McKenna, C. L. Karmen, K. D. Shaffer, J. H. Silverman, J. Nowakowski, C. Scavarda, E. D. Shapiro, and P. Visintainer. 2020. Prospective evaluation of the frequency and severity of symptoms in Lyme disease patients with erythema migrans compared with matched controls at baseline, 6 months, and 12 months. *Clinical Infectious Diseases* 71(12):3118–3124.

Wormser, G. P., D. McKenna, K. D. Shaffer, J. H. Silverman, C. Scavarda, and P. Visintainer. 2021. Evaluation of selected variables to determine if any had predictive value for, or correlated with, residual symptoms at approximately 12 months after diagnosis and treatment of early Lyme disease. *Diagnostic Microbiology and Infectious Disease* 100(3):115348.

Zhang, H., C. Zang, Z. Xu, Y. Zhang, J. Xu, J. Bian, D. Morozyuk, D. Khullar, Y. Zhang, A. S. Nordvig, E. J. Schenck, E. A. Shenkman, R. L. Rothman, J. P. Block, K. Lyman, M. G. Weiner, T. W. Carton, F. Wang, and R. Kaushal. 2023a. Data-driven identification of post-acute SARS-CoV-2 infection subphenotypes. *Nature Medicine* 29(1):226–235.

Zhang, Y., H. Hu, V. Fokaidis, C. L. V, J. Xu, C. Zang, Z. Xu, F. Wang, M. Koropsak, J. Bian, J. Hall, R. L. Rothman, E. A. Shenkman, W. Q. Wei, M. G. Weiner, T. W. Carton, and R. Kaushal. 2023b. Identifying environmental risk factors for post-acute sequelae of SARS-CoV-2 infection: An EHR-based cohort study from the recover program. *Environmental Advances* 11:100352.

3

Building on Research from Other Infection-Associated Chronic Illnesses

Lyme infection-associated chronic illnesses (IACI) are among the many chronic illnesses that are potentially triggered by an infectious agent. Also called "post-acute infectious syndromes," such other conditions with similar subjective symptoms of unclear etiology have been described following viral, bacterial, and parasitic infections (Choutka et al., 2022).[1] These may be related to a specific pathogen, such as Long COVID and post-polio syndrome, or may not have a clear connection to specific pathogens, such as with as myalgic encephalomyelitis/chronic fatigue syndrome (ME/CFS). However, while several potential disease mechanisms have been hypothesized, including the possibility of overlap or interactions between more than one process, the pathogenesis of Lyme IACI and other IACI remains unknown (Arron et al. 2024; Bai and Richardson 2023; Choutka et al., 2022; Davis et al. 2023; Komaroff and Lipkin, 2023).

The potential link to infectious agents and parallels in symptoms contribute to the hypothesis that there may be common mechanisms among Lyme IACI and other IACI that lead to these chronic symptoms (NASEM, 2024b). Thus, there may be treatment approaches or therapeutic agents that act on common causative pathways to alleviate symptoms across more than one of these similar diseases. For example, dysautonomia symptoms have been reported in Lyme IACI, Long COVID, and ME/CFS, which would

---

[1] Collectively these are referred to as "infection-associated chronic illnesses" (IACI) in this report while acknowledging that no single infectious agent has been linked to ME/CFS and that whether there is a definitive infectious origin for the condition as a whole remains debated and uncertain.

suggest therapeutic agents for autonomic nervous system dysfunction as an avenue for exploration (Adler et al., 2024). Existing knowledge and ongoing research from ME/CFS have already helped shape treatment strategies to ameliorate Long COVID symptoms (Bonilla et al., 2023; Petracek et al., 2023). Similar opportunities exist for knowledge sharing to inform Lyme IACI research and address the unmet need for new treatments.

Stigmatization and dismissal or minimization of their symptoms in social spheres and in seeking health care are common experiences shared by those living with chronic symptoms from IACI, even as objectively measurable pathology affirms the severity of their symptoms (Ali et al., 2014; IOM, 2015; NASEM, 2024a). People living with IACI have shared how these debilitating symptoms have reverberated throughout their daily lives and the profound impact on their social, economic, mental, and physical well-being. The debilitating impact that these symptoms have on people's health and quality of life must be matched by an equal urgency to provide high-quality scientific evidence for clinical decision-making.

In this chapter, the committee explores research conducted concerning IACI other than Lyme IACI, with a focus on how findings from such research may be drawn upon to advance Lyme IACI treatment. A full understanding of disease etiology and mechanisms remain elusive in IACI, though these likely involve a complex combination of pathogen, host, and environmental factors (Peluso et al., 2024). The generally insufficient understanding of the causes of IACI impedes evaluation and prioritization of candidate treatments that target disease etiology and pathogenesis, which may be further complicated by the possibility that multiple causes or risk factors may be responsible for developing IACI. In the absence of robust data to inform mechanism-based disease targets and treatments, the committee examined findings on treatments aimed at alleviating symptoms and the associated evidence base to any available knowledge on disease mechanisms.

Surveying Potential Treatments with Focus on ME/CFS and Long COVID

Of the many chronic illnesses potentially associated with an infectious trigger, ME/CFS and Long COVID have emerged as two with the most robust evidence bases—one built over decades of research, the other driven by the sudden and immense disease burden stemming from the global pandemic. Based on the significant overlap in symptoms among Lyme IACI, Long COVID, and ME/CFS (Table 3-1) as well as potential insights from the research infrastructure that have been established around ME/CFS and Long COVID, the committee centered this evidence review around these two conditions.

TABLE 3-1 Symptoms Commonly Reported for IACI

Symptoms	Lyme IACI	Long COVID	ME/CFS
Neurocognitive function (memory loss, brain fog)	x	x	x
Fatigue	x	x	x
Musculoskeletal pain (myalgia, arthralgia)	x	x	x
Sleep impairment (difficulty with sleep, unrefreshing sleep)	x	x	x
Mental health symptoms (depression, anxiety)	x	x	x
Headache	x	x	x
Dysautonomia symptoms	x	x	x
Gastrointestinal symptoms	x	x	x
Paresthesia	x	x	
Stiff neck	x		
Tremors/twitching	x		
Change in taste/smell		x	
Rash and hair loss		x	
Post-exertional malaise[1]		x	x
Food/chemical sensitivities			x
Lymphadenopathy			x
Increased susceptibility to viruses			x

[1] Post-exertional malaise has not been evaluated separately from measures of fatigue in studies on Lyme IACI.
NOTE: IACI = infection-associated chronic illnesses; ME/CFS = myalgic encephalomyelitis/chronic fatigue syndrome.

The committee surveyed systematic reviews and meta-analyses published since 2020 that described randomized trials evaluating pharmacological and nonpharmacological treatments for the two conditions. While the committee's search focused on ME/CFS and Long COVID, the initial literature search was broadly conducted to incorporate reviews on other IACI, if available. A descriptive summary of the results of randomized trials that have been assessed in review articles is offered in this section. There were three reviews that evaluated studies assessing treatments for other IACI based on mechanistic pathways: one summarized studies on the effects of plasmapheresis on amyloid fibrin(ogen) particles in people with Long

COVID (Fox et al., 2023), the second examined studies that evaluated the efficacy of nutraceutical interventions to target mitochondrial dysfunction in individuals living with ME/CFS (Maksoud et al., 2021), and the third summarized ongoing clinical trials that target proposed disease mechanisms in Long COVID (Chee et al., 2023). The rest of the systematic reviews evaluated studies of treatments to alleviate persistent symptoms without specifically targeting a particular disease mechanism or etiology. There was also a notable lack of studies focused on the pediatric population. As more knowledge is generated on disease mechanisms from other IACI and on promising therapeutic interventions for children and adolescents, it will be important to examine the possible applicability to Lyme IACI research for this subpopulation as well.

Conclusion 3-1: There is an insufficient understanding of the underlying mechanisms that cause Lyme IACI and of how Lyme IACI is similar to and distinct from other IACI.

CLINICAL EVIDENCE ON SYMPTOM-BASED APPROACHES TO TREATMENTS FOR IACI

There is overlap in many of the symptoms ascribed to Lyme IACI, ME/CFS, Long COVID, and other chronic conditions suspected of having an infectious trigger. Table 3-1 provides an overview of the most commonly noted symptoms in the literature for Lyme IACI, Long COVID, and ME/CFS, drawn from reviews on similarities and differences among the conditions (Bai and Richardson, 2023; Choutka et al., 2022; Komaroff and Lipkin, 2023). It should be noted, however, that these lists of symptoms are not intended to provide a case definition or diagnostic criteria for the associated illnesses or conditions. Heterogeneity in symptoms among people living with IACI is a central feature of these conditions. While there can be a subset of core or characteristic symptoms, or subsets of symptom clusters associated with each condition, individual experiences with the disease may differ from one person to the next. Research on different IACIs, such as Long COVID, has generally not prioritized patient-reported symptoms or lived experience into the study's goals, approach, or outcome measures as standard practice (Zeraatkar et al., 2024).

In Lyme IACI, an analysis of self-reported information in a patient-led registry found that the three most commonly reported symptoms were neurologic—cognitive impairment or neuropathy (84 percent), fatigue (64 percent), and musculoskeletal pain (57 percent) (Johnson et al., 2018). These symptoms were reported by many individuals as severe, with symptoms related to pain, mental health, physical health, and general poor health affecting quality of life on a majority of days within a 30-day period (Johnson et al., 2014). Additional observational studies have also found that fatigue, pain, and cognitive impairment were among the most frequent symptoms exhibited by individuals living with Lyme IACI (Aucott et al., 2013; Rebman et al., 2017). These three symptoms are also extremely common in both adults and children living with Long COVID and ME/CFS (Komaroff and Lipkin, 2023; Rao et al., 2024; Rowe et al., 2017). Given these findings, the committee organized their assessment of current evidence for the effectiveness of treatments of other IACI around the core symptoms of fatigue, pain, and cognitive dysfunction, while remaining inclusive of the literature that addresses other common symptoms as well as approaches that may mitigate more than one symptom.

This section summarizes current evidence from randomized trials on the treatment of other IACI, with a focus on ME/CFS and Long COVID. The summary is organized by the major symptoms described in Lyme IACI. The evidence presented in this section is not intended to be a comprehensive review of treatments for other IACI. The committee prioritized scientific findings that are supported by a compilation of evidence and systematically reviewed over new claims whose results have not yet been reviewed or replicated. The literature search was thus limited to meta-analyses and systematic reviews published since 2020, and the outcomes of individual randomized trials within those reviews are summarized below. An important limitation of relying on published reviews to identify current evidence is the potential exclusion of well-designed, high-quality, or promising late-breaker studies that were not captured in review articles due to temporal or scope parameters. Another key limitation in this method is the reliance on reporting effectiveness of interventions based on the outcome cutoff defined in individual studies. However, this approach is intended to provide a broad overview of the evidence on treatments for other IACI and enable the committee to examine evidence that has been replicated in multiple studies, when available. While studies differed in the use of outcome measurements and analyses to determine effectiveness, on balance, none of the interventions described in this section have consistent, compelling evidence suggesting effectiveness.

Fatigue

While fatigue may be perceived by the public as a general, transient experience, the fatigue experienced by people with IACI is often severe and intractable and may or may not be worsened by physical activity. Fatigue may be caused by inadequate signaling from the central nervous system to the rest of the body to initiate or sustain a task (i.e., central fatigue), by inadequate signaling or responses from muscle receptors (i.e., peripheral fatigue), or by a combination of the two. Yet the specific pathogenic pathways that lead to these alterations in neuromuscular signaling and responses remain poorly understood (Staud, 2012). This complexity suggests that effective treatment of fatigue will likely require a better understanding of its pathogenesis in different individuals and circumstances in which pharmacological or nonpharmacological strategies that exert change on multiple pathways may be more likely to succeed in symptom management.

Evidence in Adults

Both medications and nonpharmacologic interventions have been evaluated using randomized trials for their effects on fatigue in adults. Overall, for ME/CFS there were more reports of beneficial effects among studies on nonpharmacologic interventions than among studies on medications or complementary and alternative medicine (Kim et al., 2020). Similarly, a systematic review of randomized trials for Long COVID (inclusive of publications up until December 2023) did not identify any pharmaceutical interventions that improved fatigue in this population (Zeraatkar et al., 2024). Single studies of individuals with ME/CFS have suggested potential benefit for methylphenidate (a central nervous system stimulant) or coenzyme Q10 with nicotinamide adenine dinucleotide in its reduced form (NADH, a hypothesized mitochondrial modulator) (hypothesized mitochondrial modulator) to alleviate fatigue (Blockmans et al., 2006; Castro-Marrero et al., 2015); although these studies were randomized and controlled, both were small trials with fewer than 50 participants in their treatment arms. Evidence from medium-to-larger trials for ME/CFS on the potential effect on fatigue of hydro- or fludrocortisone at various dose ranges remain conflicted, with benefit reported in one randomized crossover study including 32 patients (Cleare et al., 1999), but not in four other randomized trials (Blockmans et al., 2003; McKenzie et al., 1998; Peterson et al., 1998; Rowe et al., 2001). These findings alone are not sufficient to justify immediate adoption of these interventions in randomized trials for the treatment of fatigue in Lyme IACI. Further research into the abovementioned products for the treatment of fatigue in other IACI, including Lyme IACI, must be supported by reasonable biological plausibility and any additional preclinical or clinical data that supports the treatments' effects. Many trials described in the available literature have small sample sizes (<100), the results have not been replicated, and understanding of the therapeutic mechanisms—which would bolster confidence in any observed effects—may be lacking.

Cognitive behavioral therapy (CBT) and graded exercise therapy have been studied as nonpharmaceutical interventions to improve fatigue for ME/CFS and, more recently, for Long COVID. However, several important caveats must be kept in mind when considering the trial outcomes related to these two approaches. CBT is an established psychological intervention with roots in treating mental health conditions that has also been found to be effective in managing aspects of many chronic diseases (Halford and Brown, 2009; Taylor, 2006). CBT can alleviate mental health–related comorbidities (e.g., depression, anxiety) and help develop coping strategies for individuals living with chronic illnesses. Whether CBT may improve other aspects of IACI through additional mechanistic pathways remains to be determined.

Graded exercise therapy was initially explored as an intervention for ME/CFS based on the hypothesis that deconditioning is a main cause of post-exertional malaise in ME/CFS. However, exercise therapy may in fact exacerbate symptoms of ME/CFS for some individuals and can lead individuals to adopt coping behaviors to be able to complete the exercise regimen, which does not reflect symptom improvement. Furthermore, there are criticisms surrounding analyses and outcome reporting of a major trial involving these interventions (Geraghty, 2017; White et al., 2017). Within this context, clinical trial design and outcome interpretations need to consider whether the trial endpoints reflect a temporary remission, masking, or actual sustained recovery of symptoms such that accurate conclusions can be drawn and reported. As discussed below, there is currently insufficient evidence to consider CBT and graded exercise therapy as preferred therapeutic options for ME/CFS or Long COVID (Sanal-Hayes et al., 2023; Wilshire et al., 2018).

A high-level overview of trials involving CBT found mixed results in trials in individuals with ME/CFS and Long COVID. One complication in the interpretation of trial results or of an aggregated analysis is the variation in the CBT protocols used across different studies. In one systematic review, improvement in fatigue was reported in six out of 10 randomized trials of CBT that enrolled at least 45 participants with ME/CFS (or at least 23 participants for randomized crossover trials) (Deale et al., 1997; Janse et al., 2018; Kim et al., 2020; Prins et al., 2001; Sharpe et al., 1996; White et al., 2011; Wiborg et al., 2015), and other trials reported similar potential benefits in reduction of fatigue in ME/CFS (O'Dowd et al., 2006; Stubhaug et al., 2008). Similarly, CBT may be beneficial for managing fatigue associated with Long COVID, but these findings were based on low-certainty evidence and require additional study (Kuut et al., 2023; Zeraatkar et al., 2024). Two randomized trials reported that less intense self-guided instruction based on CBT for people with ME/CFS led to improvement in fatigue and physical function (Knoop et al., 2008), though the improvement in physical function was restricted to a subgroup of participants with physical disabilities at baseline in one of the studies (Tummers et al., 2012). While individuals with ME/CFS reported some improvement in fatigue in studies of CBT, this was not always associated with increased activity level and can be interpreted as an adaptation instead of improvement in the underlying disease (Toogood et al., 2021). CBT has also been evaluated for other post-infectious fatigue, with positive outcomes reported in a study of Q fever fatigue syndrome compared with an oral medication placebo group, though comparison between groups receiving CBT and oral antibiotics was not performed (Keijmel et al., 2017).

Graded exercise therapy has in the past been suggested as a therapy that could address post-exertional malaise, a symptom that has been described for ME/CFS and Long COVID but has not been differentiated from general fatigue in Lyme IACI research. It is important to note that exercise regimens that address respiratory, cardiovascular, and musculoskeletal deconditioning as sources of physical fatigue are contraindicated for a subset of individuals with ME/CFS. Post-exertional malaise has been linked with distinct pathological changes in muscles, including mitochondrial dysfunction and abnormal lactic acid accumulation (Appelman et al., 2024), but such changes have yet to be evaluated in Lyme IACI. Overall, current evidence suggests that a patient-led, self-paced approach to physical activity is more likely to be beneficial than pre-set therapy regimens (Fowler-Davis, 2021). Graded exercise therapy was found to have some benefit in two studies of ME/CFS (Wearden et al., 1998; White et al., 2011), and self-managed graded exercise or other self-paced physical activity reported reduction in the severity of fatigue in ME/CFS (Clark et al., 2017; Marques et al., 2015). A meta-analysis of randomized trials studying graded exercise therapy for individuals with Long COVID found overall improvement in fatigue from structured physical activities, including aerobic, multimodal, breathing, and tai chi exercises. However, the majority of these studies were assessed to have high risk of bias, and additional rigorously designed studies are needed to confirm efficacy (Cheng et al., 2024). A critical context for these findings is the lack of a reliable method to distinguish individuals who may benefit with exercise therapy from others for whom it is detrimental.

Complementary and alternative medicine or health strategies have also been explored for the management of fatigue in ME/CFS and Long COVID. Acupuncture or therapeutic abdominal massages have been suggested to improve fatigue symptoms in people with ME/CFS and Long COVID (Huanan et al., 2017; Kim et al., 2015; Lam et al., 2024; Ng and Yiu, 2013). Isometric yoga, alone or in combination with pharmacotherapy, was reported to have some benefits for ME/CFS (Oka et al., 2014). Other complementary and alternative interventions that suggest potential benefit to an individual's health are based on data considered to be low confidence and would require well-designed, adequately powered studies to determine whether there are meaningful benefits. These include a variety of Chinese herbal medicines used alone or co-administered with conventional pharmaceuticals; integrative medicine approaches, including muscle relaxation and meditation; nutrient supplements, such as probiotic microbes and enzymes; aromatherapy; and traditional Chinese medicine (Chen et al., 2024; Hawkins et al., 2022; Pang et al., 2022; Rathi et al., 2021).

Evidence in Pediatrics

Of the literature described in the review papers the committee assessed, only two studies of ME/CFS measured outcomes in the pediatric population. These found improvement in fatigue and general physical scoring in children following CBT interventions (Kim et al., 2020; Nijhof et al., 2012; Stulemeijer et al., 2005).

Pain

Current research generally categorizes pain into three types based on its source and pathophysiology (Cao et al., 2024). Nociceptive pain stems from inflammation and tissue damage and is usually treatable with analgesics. Neuropathic pain results from nerve damage and responds poorly to analgesics. Nociplastic pain is a relatively new concept that describes pain not associated with detectable involvement of nociceptive or neuropathic pathways (i.e., pain in the absence of tissue or nerve damage). The etiology for nociplastic pain remains poorly understood, though enhanced pain and sensory processing in the central nervous system or altered pain modulation have been proposed as possibilities (Kaplan et al., 2024). While such overall categorization based on a mechanistic understanding of pain can be informative for the development and application of treatments, different types of pain may occur simultaneously in individual people.

Pain can decrease the quality of life, and chronic pain in particular is associated with serious comorbidities, including depression, anxiety, fatigue, and cognitive impairment (Cao et al., 2024; Fitzcharles et al., 2021). Pharmacological options for pain relief largely work on cellular targets for inflammation or various signaling receptors in the neurosensory pathway. In addition, nonpharmaceutical interventions such as cognitive behavioral therapy, exercise, acupuncture, and others have demonstrated effectiveness in general pain management.

Evidence in Adults

Clinical trials targeting pain in Long COVID and ME/CFS populations have been limited. Analgesics, including opiates and naloxone were found to have minimal effects in ME/CFS by a small study with 41 participants (Hermans et al., 2018). A randomized trial of 54 participants assessing psycho-spiritual mental health education in ME/CFS found that the intervention improved well-being, with a decrease in daily interference from pain. (El-Mokadem et al., 2023).

Chronic pain symptoms have been reported following other infections beyond COVID. For example, people recovering from chikungunya fever, a mosquito-transmitted viral disease characterized by severe debilitating joint pain, often experience ongoing musculoskeletal and neuropathic pain for months to years (WHO, 2025). A systematic review identified two small randomized trials that suggested some benefit from physical therapy or exercise in improving physical function and reducing pain in those individuals (de Oliveira et al., 2019; Neumann et al., 2021). A third randomized trial identified in the systematic review found transcranial direct current stimulation to significantly improve pain in this patient population, but it had no effect on physical function or the quality of life (Silva-Filho et al., 2018).

Post-polio syndrome is another disorder for which a systematic review and meta-analysis of randomized, controlled trials of treatment was available. This review examined evidence on intravenous immunoglobulin therapy and concluded that it was unlikely to improve pain, fatigue, or muscle strength. However, these trials had small sample sizes, and further study would be needed to determine whether certain patient subgroups might respond to the therapy (Huang et al., 2015).

Evidence in Pediatrics

A review found that despite the prevalence and impact of pain, very few pediatric studies had measured it, and no studies were found on pain management in children. The treatments studied focused primarily on the overall management of ME/CFS for pediatric populations. As more research is conducted to identify effective therapeutic options for pain associated with ME/CFS and other IACI in adults, additional safety, efficacy, and dosing studies will need to be conducted in pediatric populations to determine if these treatments are also appropriate for children (Ascough et el., 2020).

Cognitive Dysfunction

People living with IACI have described "brain fog" that may include attention deficits (e.g., an inability to concentrate or maintain focus), mental fatigue (e.g., reduced task processing speed), language loss (e.g., difficulties finding words), and other impairments in memory, reasoning, and executive functions (IOM, 2015; NASEM 2024a; Touradji et al., 2019). While many reported symptoms have subjective qualities, there are established methods and tools to measure neurologic and cognitive function that can be used to connect patient-reported outcomes to objectively characterize neurocognitive decline. The causes of these types of cognitive symptoms remain elusive. Available data in Long COVID suggest two potential mechanisms that may occur alone or in combination: inflammation involving the central nervous system and vascular dysfunction from SARS-CoV-2 infection (Spudich and Nath, 2022). Reductions in gray matter thickness and global brain size have also been noted in some individuals with Long COVID in comparisons of MRI scans before and after COVID-19 infection, suggesting damage to the central nervous system (Komaroff and Lipkin, 2023). Markers of neuroinflammation and other physiological changes in brain structure have similarly been measured for ME/CFS (Lee et al., 2024; Walitt et al., 2024). People living with IACI may simultaneously experience pain, depression, and anxiety, which are each known from other conditions to affect different aspects of cognition (James and Ferguson, 2020; Robinson et al., 2013), complicating efforts to dissect cause and effect.

Evidence in Adults

Pathogen persistence is a possible cause of ongoing inflammation or structural changes in IACI that may lead to cognitive impairment, and anti-infectives have been explored as treatment options. In a subset of individuals with ME/CFS who had elevated Epstein-Barr viral and human herpesvirus 6 titers, treatment with valganciclovir, an RNA polymerase inhibitor antiviral drug, was associated with minor improvement in cognitive symptoms when given for 6 months (Montoya et al., 2013). The Toll-like receptor 3 agonist polyI:polyC12U (also known as rintatolimod or Ampligen) has antiviral and immunomodulatory properties and yielded mild improvements to cognitive deficit in a small, randomized trial for ME/CFS (Strayer et al., 1994). It has been approved for use in severe cases of ME/CFS in Argentina but not in the United States and is being tested for efficacy in Long COVID with mixed read-outs from a recent phase II trial (AIM ImmunoTech, 2024).

Various other pharmaceutical treatments have been evaluated for their potential to improve cognition in Long COVID. Two medications with known neurological applications, donepezil chlorhydrate (a cholinesterase inhibitor approved for Alzheimer's disease) and an investigational endocannabinoid treatment for neurodegenerative diseases, were not found to improve cognitive function (Pooladgar et al., 2023; Versace et al., 2023). The serotonergic antidepressant drug vortioxetine may have potential to improve depression and general health-related quality of life, but no effects on cognitive function were detected (McIntyre et al., 2024). Famotidine, a selective histamine 2 (H2) receptor antagonist, was reported to lead to some improvement in cognitive function (Momtazmanesh et al., 2023). While the evidence assessed above was all drawn from randomized, controlled trials, the sample sizes examined were small and the findings need to be confirmed by larger trials.

Nonpharmaceutical approaches have also been evaluated for improvement of cognitive functioning in Long COVID and have also yielded mixed results. A meditation program was shown to improve processing speed in a small cohort (Hausswirth et al., 2023), but breathing training and a mobile app guide to motivational and rehabilitation activities in a randomized controlled trial of 100 people with Long COVID were not found to affect cognitive function (Philip et al., 2022, Samper-Pardo et al., 2023). As described above, a meta-analysis of randomized, controlled trials evaluating exercise therapies suggested improvement in fatigue but did not find effects on cognitive impairment (Cheng et al., 2024). No improvement in executive function and processing speed was found after transcranial direct current stimulation (Oliver-Mas et al., 2023). Some improvement in cognitive function from hyperbaric oxygen was reported in a randomized trial of 73 participants; approximately 10 percent of participants in both the treatment and control arms experienced trauma resulting from pressure changes in the hyperbaric chamber where participants received the intervention or sham treatment (Zilberman-Itskovich et al., 2022).

Available findings from three small randomized trials of alternative medicine approaches to treat cognitive dysfunction are inconclusive, given the variety of supplements evaluated and the inconsistency in the effects on cognitive symptoms. A randomized trial with 31 participants with Long COVID found that a cannabidiol-rich hemp-derived product did not improve cognition compared with baseline (Young et al., 2024). A randomized trial of 100 participants evaluating an adaptogen mixture in people with Long COVID showed improvement in cognitive performance, anxiety, and depression in both the treatment and placebo groups compared with baseline, but no difference in the three symptoms between the treatment and placebo groups. This finding suggests the intervention was no different than a placebo in addressing cognition, anxiety, or depression (Karosanidze et al., 2022). A nutritional supplement consisting of a combination of ethylmethylhydroxypyridine succinate and meldonium, tested in a randomized trial of 30 participants with Long COVID, led to a small improvement in cognitive function compared with a placebo control (Tanashyan et al., 2023).

Evidence in Pediatrics

No randomized trials included in systematic reviews or meta-analyses on ME/CFS or Long COVID interventions specifically address cognitive dysfunction in the pediatric or adolescent population.

OPPORTUNITIES FOR TRANSLATING PROMISING APPROACHES TO LYME IACI

Through the survey of systematic reviews and meta-analyses of ME/CFS and Long COVID clinical research summarized above, the committee did not identify specific treatment approaches with sufficient support of beneficial effects and determined that the available evidence do not support prioritizing development or translation of these interventions to treat Lyme IACI. This should not be interpreted to mean that these treatment approaches do not have merit and should not be pursued as potential treatments for Lyme IACI. Instead, there is an opportunity for future evaluations of potential IACI treatments to be conducted with trials that incorporate—and stratify results according to—different IACI populations, including the Lyme IACI population. Given the similarities in the major symptoms, these future clinical trials can be developed to address a shared symptom and consider enrollment criteria based on a carefully defined syndromic definition that includes people with Lyme IACI along with others with ME/CFS and Long COVID. Likewise, research findings on disease mechanisms in other IACI can be explored to understand if these findings also apply for Lyme IACI.

There may be concerns that treatments to address disease symptoms rather than etiology or a fully known mechanistic pathway may be imprecise and do not address the need for curative treatments. However, therapeutics that aim to alleviate symptoms have been developed and approved for many intractable diseases while research to elucidate the pathogenesis and root cause continue being carried out. Examples range from mental health (e.g., depression) to autonomic disorders that have been reported for IACI (e.g., clinical studies on repurposed drugs for symptoms of POTS) (Cui et al., 2024; Vernino et al. 2021). Notably, the etiology of the three examples are unknown, but a number of pharmaceutical and nonpharmaceutical interventions have been identified to mitigate the disease manifestations and research to develop new treatments remain active. The approach to developing new treatments for IACI through symptom mitigation would focus on any available knowledge of the immediate causes for the symptoms, identify if there are parallels with other known diseases, and design studies such that data and samples can be collected to further understanding of the disease mechanism(s). One example of success in developing new treatments through this research approach is in fibromyalgia, a chronic condition with indeterminate etiology and symptoms similar to those in other IACI, particularly ME/CFS (Box 3-1).

> **BOX 3-1**
> **Developing Effective Treatments to Mitigate Symptoms: Case Study with Fibromyalgia**
>
> Fibromyalgia is a complex chronic condition characterized by diffuse symptoms such as fatigue, sleep impairment, muscle and joint pain and stiffness, and cognitive dysfunction, limiting daily function and quality of life. Like Lyme IACI, it is an invisible illness, without clear diagnostic tests, and has often been met with stigma and a perception of not being a "real" medical condition. The pathophysiology of the disorder is not well understood. Chronic, widespread pain is the main symptom of fibromyalgia. However, standard treatments for nociceptive pain, such as non-steroid anti-inflammatory drugs or opioids, have no or reduced effectiveness. Progress was made in treatment after functional magnetic resonance imaging studies of the brain demonstrated altered pain processing, which provided objective evidence to the condition and patient experience and opened the door for evaluating pain treatments that work through the central nervous system. This line of research subsequently led to three therapeutics receiving approval from the Food and Drug Administration for treatment of fibromyalgia (pregabalin, duloxetine, and milnacipran). Further investigations into disease pathogenesis have built on these successes, including studies of potential new treatments and improved understanding of mechanistic pathways to optimize treatment decisions (e.g., toward identifying individuals who respond better to one medication than other therapeutics).
>
> While these medications are not curative, their development demonstrates the possibility of developing therapeutics that improve the quality of life for many patients despite lacking knowledge of the etiology or a full understanding of the pathogenesis of a disease.
>
> SOURCE: Gracely et al. (2002), Sluka and Clauw (2016), Schmidt-Wilke and Clauw (2011).

Ongoing Lyme IACI Trials Informed by Other Disease Areas

There are few ongoing clinical trials registered on ClinicalTrials.gov for interventions to address Lyme IACI that draw from findings in other disease areas such as Long COVID, ME/CFS, and fibromyalgia.[2] These interventions are briefly discussed below. While these interventions are in

---

[2] This section highlights clinical trials that are listed as active or suspended on ClinicalTrials.gov as of March 17, 2025. It does not include review of trials that have been terminated or withdrawn.

the early stages of evaluation, they demonstrate the potential for translating treatment approaches from disease areas similar to those of Lyme IACI. As of March 2025, there are also a number of other ongoing clinical trials that explore treatments for Long COVID and ME/CFS; however, these experimental interventions have not been applied to Lyme IACI.[3]

Vagus Nerve Stimulation

Vagus nerve stimulation (VNS) is a procedure using a medical device to stimulate the vagus nerve with electrical impulses, which engages both afferent and efferent fibers to alter brain activity and systemic inflammation (Mayo Clinic, 2023). The implanted device has been approved by the Food and Drug Administration (FDA) to treat pharmaco-resistant epilepsy and severe, recurrent depression as well as for use in stroke rehabilitation programs. There are also noninvasive devices that may be held against the skin of the neck to stimulate the cervical branch of the nerve or on the ear to stimulate its auricular branch, which has only afferent fibers. Noninvasive VNS devices haves been used to treat cluster headaches and migraines and have been shown to block pain signals (Mayo Clinic, 2023). In recent years, pilot studies using VNS to treat individuals with Long COVID has demonstrated early but promising effects for symptoms including fatigue, sleep, and mood (Khan et al., 2024; Lladós et al., 2024). There is an ongoing clinical trial investigating transcutaneous auricular VNS in people with persistent symptoms after Lyme disease (NCT05776251) (Columbia University, n.d., 2024).

Transcranial Direct Current Stimulation

Transcranial direct current stimulation (tDCS) is performed using a noninvasive neuromodulation medical device that delivers a low electrical current to the scalp of an individual and modulates brain functions. tDCS does not alter brain structure but instead selectively modulates neuronal activity in regions of the brain to alter brain activity (Thair et al., 2017). The device is not currently FDA-approved for use outside of clinical research. A systematic review and meta-analysis of six randomized trials of tDCS for the treatment of major depressive disorder found that tDCS was superior to placebo and comparable to antidepressant drugs in addressing depression symptoms (Brunoni et al., 2016). A trial of the medical

---

[3] Clinical trials for Long COVID and ME/CFS can be found through searching on ClinicalTrials.gov, CenterWatch (https://www.centerwatch.com/clinical-trials/listings) or on patient organization websites such as the American Myalgic Encephalomyelitis and Chronic Fatigue Syndrome Society (https://ammes.org/clinical-trials/) (accessed March 16, 2025).

device for the treatment of symptoms of Lyme IACI was recently launched (NCT03500770). The Clinical Trials Network for Lyme and Other Tick-Borne Diseases is planning to test tDCS and cognitive retraining for the treatment of brain fog and will plan to examine the feasibility of long-term tDCS for individuals with persistent cognitive symptoms following a Lyme infection (Columbia University, n.d.). tDCS is also being tested by the RECOVER-NEURO clinical trial to assess the devices' impacts on Long COVID symptoms, such as brain fog (RECOVER, 2024).

Sana Device

The Sana Device is a wearable device that uses a combination of audio and visual stimulation to encourage mental relaxation with the goal of reducing chronic pain, among other intended health effects. It does not have FDA approval for treatment of any medical conditions, but it has been tested in clinical trials for relieving symptoms of fibromyalgia, as well as chronic neuropathic pain. Results are not available for the fibromyalgia study, and results from the chronic pain study, which have not yet gone through peer review, suggest the device was effective in reducing pain in the small study sample (Tabacof et al., 2024). There is currently a clinical trial to evaluate the effectiveness of the device on reducing chronic pain associated with PTLDS (NCT06655844).

Psilocybin

Psilocybin is a psychedelic agent that has been tested to treat several neurological and psychiatric conditions. Psilocybin is also being evaluated in a pilot study for the treatment of symptom burden in individuals with post-treatment Lyme disease (PTLD) (Johns Hopkins Medicine, 2024). The study is expected to be completed in April of 2025 (JHU, 2024).

Lumbrokinase

Building on Long COVID research that identified amyloid fibrin(ogen) particles as a potential cause for fatigue and other dysautonomia symptoms, thrombolytic enzymes, including lumbrokinase, have been proposed as potential therapeutic agents for Long COVID (Kell et al., 2024). Lumbrokinase is available as an oral supplement but does not have approved pharmaceutical indications (Mihara et al., 1991). A recent clinical trial has been initiated to test the efficacy of lumbrokinase in treating adults with Long COVID, PTLDS, or ME/CFS (Putrino et al., n.d.) (NCT06511050).

Applying New Research Methods to Lyme IACI

Opportunities for knowledge sharing between Lyme IACI and other conditions are not limited to breakthrough biomedical or clinical findings. Sharing technical knowledge such as methods and pitfalls learned from Long COVID research can facilitate application of new techniques to Lyme IACI studies that may unveil novel findings. A comparison between research into neurological manifestations of Long COVID and Lyme IACI is one example of the imbalance in application of modern research tools between two disease areas that share similar neurocognitive symptoms (Box 3-2). While early findings on potential links between neurological structure and function in Long COVID require further confirmatory research, sharing of techniques, protocols, and study designs can promote uptake of new technologies that have not been previously applied to Lyme IACI and facilitate coordination that enable meta-analyses across disease areas.

Epigenomics are another emerging area of Long COVID research with potential application to Lyme IACI. Infections are capable of triggering epigenetic changes, such as DNA methylation, which alter gene expression and have been known to contribute to disease pathogenesis for multiple conditions including ME/CFS (de Vega and McGowan, 2017). Studies of individuals with Long COVID have also described methylation of genes involved in immune responses and other biological processes that may shed light on the disease mechanism (Calzari et al., 2024; Lee et al., 2024). A genomewide DNA methylation study has been conducted in participants with neuroborreliosis following a *B. burgdorferi* infection (Henningsson et al., 2024), but epigenomic studies, which may contribute to improved understanding of pathogenesis, have yet to be conducted in a population with Lyme IACI.

Conclusion 3-2: Research findings for any single IACI may be informative for other IACI. Coordination to studying these illnesses and conditions can advance research for all IACI, including Lyme IACI.

Lessons from Diagnosis of Other Infection-Associated Chronic Illnesses

There are no specific diagnostic tests for Lyme IACI (see Chapter 2), Long COVID, or ME/CFS due to the incomplete understanding of etiology and lack of objective markers (IOM, 2015; NASEM, 2024a). Biomarker research is ongoing for Long COVID and ME/CFS and, if successful, may be transformative for both the development of potential diagnostic tests (Davis et al., 2023) and advancing our understanding of these conditions. Moreover, research on biomarkers in conditions like Long COVID may

BOX 3-2
Applying New Research Tools to Lyme IACI:
A Case Study on Neuroscience

Involvement of the central nervous system was recognized early on in many people with Long COVID, which has led to considerable exploration into the potential neurological mechanisms and biomarkers of disease. Although additional research is needed to confirm the preliminary findings discussed here, this area of research is one example of how new techniques being used in Long COVID are lacking in Lyme IACI research, and there is an opportunity to translate methodologies and protocols from one IACI to another.

Neuroimaging studies in Long COVID research have developed protocols using modern imaging techniques, such as specific magnetic resonance imaging scan sequences, to characterize brain changes and investigate links between brain structure and function with neurological symptoms. By contrast, neuroimaging studies conducted in Lyme IACI have been few and far between, particularly in the United States. These limited number of studies have reported brain abnormalities associated with long-term sequelae of Lyme disease, but there has been a dearth of follow-up studies to confirm and further characterize such findings. Moreover, exploration of Lyme IACI brain pathophysiology has been outpaced by modern neuroimaging techniques applied to Long COVID research. For instance, decreased cerebral perfusion in Lyme IACI was reported in a small number of studies in the early 2000s. Since then, MRI methods have been developed that provide relatively higher spatial and temporal resolution and are safer to administer (i.e., forgo the need for radioactive agents), which have been applied to the study of Long COVID multiple times. Similarly, studies of white matter integrity in Long COVID quickly outnumbered the only study conducted to date in Lyme IACI. Other state-of-the-art neuroimaging measures that have been applied to the study of Long COVID, but not yet to Lyme IACI, include those that study blood–brain barrier permeability, cortical thickness, and functional connectivity.

SOURCE: Besteher et al. (2024), Fallon et al. (2003), Greene et al. (2024), Marvel et al. (2022), Mohammadi et al. (2024), Nelson et al. (2025), Newberg et al. (2002).

inform the development of diagnostics for Lyme IACI if similar mechanisms exist. For example, several similar psychiatric conditions share the same inflammation-related biomarkers (Yuan et al., 2019).

In the absence of validated diagnostic tests, a syndromic definition has been developed for Long COVID (NASEM, 2024a), and ME/CFS has had a multitude of proposed case definitions and diagnostic criteria (IOM, 2015; Lim and Son, 2020). The 2015 Institute of Medicine (IOM) diagnostic criteria for ME/CFS enabled clinicians to make diagnoses based primarily on the presence of symptoms, as opposed to the lengthy approach that largely relied on a diagnosis by exclusion, which was commonly used before the diagnostic criteria (Bateman et al., 2021). Making a diagnosis of ME/CFS still involves a degree of ruling out other potential causes of an individual's symptoms, but the availability of standardized, evidence-based definitions is critical for making reliable and timely diagnoses. In addition, significant efforts have been made over the years to develop and validate patient-reported outcome measures for use in ME/CFS research that will likely complement the use of biomarkers in clinical diagnosis. These standardized and validated assessments of symptoms include those developed specifically for ME/CFS, such as the DePaul Symptom Questionnaire, and more general research tools such as the Short Form 36-Item Health Survey (Jason & Sunnquist, 2018).[4]

The definitions and criteria for Long COVID and ME/CFS, while imperfect, can be useful in guiding clinical diagnoses and appropriate care. However, it is not known whether there are meaningful differences among different IACI that would affect treatment. Research that compares treatment responses across participants with different IACI diagnoses will be needed to determine if certain interventions are more effective for certain populations. In the absence of such evidence, tailoring treatment to the symptoms of each individual patient will continue to be important to clinical practice.

Notably, disease definitions may have multiple applications. A definition for the purposes of research may need to be more narrowly tailored to ensure that the patient populations in various studies are comparable. A clinical definition used in diagnosis or for disability determinations may be broader to suggest possible treatment approaches or facilitate access to care or benefits. In the example of ME/CFS, the IOM criteria are more commonly used in the clinical care setting, while the Canadian Consensus Criteria are more frequently seen as a definition in clinical research.[5]

Key research findings must be incorporated into disease definitions to maintain relevance and clinical utility. Definitions of ME/CFS have been

---

[4] Common data elements for ME/CFS list many other patient-reported measures of study outcomes and end points, see: NINDS, n.d.

[5] As presented to the committee in open session by Nancy Klimas on July 11, 2024.

revised many times to reflect emerging evidence and the Long COVID definition was developed with the intention to be reviewed at regular intervals for necessary updates (Lim and Son, 2020; NASEM, 2024a). Given the incomplete and evolving understanding of Lyme IACI, it is critical that future efforts to develop research or clinical definitions for Lyme IACI follow a similar approach to allow periodic review and modification to reflect new evidence as it develops.

Other Considerations in Research Strategies for Infection-Associated Chronic Illnesses

In addition to potential directions for clinical research, opportunities to incorporate new techniques, and approaches to developing working definitions in the absence of diagnostic tests for Lyme IACI, there are several strategies that have helped advance research on other IACI. These strategies are, to date, generally absent or underused in the field of Lyme IACI research.

Standardization

A standardized and clear definition for a patient population, and any relevant subgroups, can streamline clinical trial recruitment and guide application of research findings to the appropriate group in clinical practice. The consensus definitions for Long COVID and ME/CFS provide a common reference point for researchers to interpret results from across different studies. For Lyme IACI, PTLDS is used for research purposes and describes a well-defined group within the Lyme IACI population (see Chapter 2; Wormser et al., 2006). While PTLDS has an important role in the research that has been conducted to date, the balance toward its stringency inevitably excludes many individuals with similar symptoms for whom the evidence for prior Lyme disease is uncertain or who have less severe symptoms. Standardized definitions for Lyme IACI would serve as a common reference point to advance research for this disease and could provide a clear pathway for including people who do not fit the PTLDS criteria in future research. To facilitate a coordinated IACI research approach, efforts to develop a Lyme IACI definition could consider how it aligns or differs from the limitations, rationale, and steps for improvement for the proposed Long COVID definition (Ely et al., 2024).

Standardization in scientific research also ensures there are commonly accepted outcome measures that promote a consistent approach to collecting data (e.g., patient characteristics, study endpoints) and allow for meta-analyses and other cross-study comparisons. Data standardization can be particularly important when symptom assessments include subjective measures that may be obtained through a variety of tools which are not always interchangeable or comparable, and may not be validated (Machado et al., 2021). For example, common measurements for fatigue in the IACI literature reviewed in this chapter included a number of tools that differed in their utility, such as the Fatigue Severity Scale (a unidimensional tool with good potential to detect change over disease course), and Fatigue Impact Scale (a multidimensional tool with poor potential to detect change over disease course), and the relevant subscale of the generic short-form 36 (SF-36) (Whitehead, 2009).[6] Efforts to standardize patient-reported outcome measures include NIH-supported development of several robust measurement systems, including the Patient-Reported Outcomes Measurement Information System (PROMIS®) and Neuro-QoL™ (Cella et al., 2012; Health Measures, 2025; NIH OSC, 2025). Research on other IACI has benefited from establishment of core data standards and preferred outcome measurement tools. The National Institute of Neurological Disorders and Stroke, in collaboration with the Centers for Disease Control and Prevention, convened working groups to assemble common data elements (CDEs) for clinical research on ME/CFS (NIH, n.d.b). The publication of these CDEs has helped to orient the research field around reliable and consistent outcome measures which enable researchers to make direct comparisons between studies.[7] Efforts to develop CDEs for standardization in Long COVID research is also in progress (Walters et al., 2024).

Coordination

In 2022, the Department of Health and Human Services released the National Research Action Plan describing the federal government's research agenda for Long COVID and ongoing research efforts across different federal agencies (HHS, 2022). The action plan also serves as a blueprint to guide future investment, identify research priorities, and outline actions to advance those priorities. One such priority is a call to apply the knowledge gained from ME/CFS and other IACI to address Long COVID. The action plan also calls to situate Long COVID research within the broader IACI context and acknowledges that advancement of Long COVID research needs to be built on intersectoral collaborations among people with IACI, and academic and private sector research, as well as interdisciplinary collaborations. Coordination through a similar action plan for people living with Lyme IACI, researchers, and research funders can provide a strategic

---

[6] Unidimensional fatigue measure tool is one that includes measure of just one factor, usually fatigue severity. Multidimensional measure tool capture two or more factors (e.g., fatigue severity, duration, pattern over time, etc.).

[7] As presented to the committee in open session by Nancy Klimas on July 11, 2024.

vision to advance Lyme IACI research within the broader context of other similar conditions. In particular, coordination of research efforts—and standards, where appropriate—across various IACI would facilitate knowledge and resource sharing that could accelerate treatment innovations for people with IACI symptoms regardless of the initial infectious agent. This includes the potential identification of common disease pathways and therapeutic targets, but also the identification of differences between Lyme IACI and other conditions. The HHS Office of Long COVID Research and Practice, though closing, was a vital mechanism to coordinate government initiatives on Long COVID and demonstrates the value of aligning efforts across a complex research ecosystem (HHS, 2025).

One option for aligning research efforts across multiple sites is to establish coordinating centers. There are different ways to structure and run coordinating centers, but core functions include administrative organization and operation of trials or research programs that are often complex, interdisciplinary, and multisite. For example, tasks that coordinating centers generally undertake on behalf of a research network or program can be categorized into the following four themes:

1. structural: coordinating centers may provide input on the organizational structure or governance of a research program;
2. collaboration development: facilitating connections between and synergy within the research program or network, including the prioritization of activities;
3. operational: administrative and technological tasks, with a focus on promoting compatibility; and
4. data: efforts to promote data interoperability between individual research sites (Rolland et al., 2017).

Several coordinating centers have demonstrated the utility of this design as an effective tool that reduces administrative burden for complex trials and improves research efficiency (Rolland et al., 2011, 2017). A coordinating center can also support a network of decentralized clinical trials, which may allow a larger participant pool from different geographic locations, and a convergence of greater expertise than trials that rely on personnel at a single site.

The NIH already supports a data management and coordinating center for the ME/CFS Research Network (MECFS Net, n.d.) and an administrative coordinating center for the Researching COVID to Enhance Recovery (RECOVER) initiative on Long COVID (RTI International, 2021). However, there is not currently a coordinating center dedicated to Lyme IACI research. As Chapter 4 will discuss, there is a Clinical Trials Network Coordinating Center for Lyme and other Tick-borne Diseases, though as the name indicates, the center covers a broad variety of diseases beyond Lyme IACI.

Conclusion 3-3: *The Lyme IACI field needs leadership in promoting and supporting coordination between research sites and investigators to conduct research with minimal redundancy, maximize outcomes from the limited available resources, and enable cross-IACI initiatives.*

Expanded Data Collection

Data are the key to unlocking scientific discoveries. But when conducting research, it is critical to collect and analyze the right data—data that can answer the target research questions. Expanded data collection is only cost-effective when there is a clear benefit, and otherwise may lead to waste in time and unnecessary harm for trial participants, loss of time and effort for research staff and participants, and excess samples that consume precious storage space. Therefore, it is important to have a strategy for collecting the necessary data to answer research questions.

One strategy to expanding data collections could be drawn from the recent deep phenotyping study conducted to elucidate the pathogenesis of post-infectious ME/CFS. This involves measuring a broad array of health markers from participants (e.g., cognition, motor skills, cardiopulmonary health, laboratory testing, imaging results) for comparison between individuals with ME/CFS and health controls (Walitt et al., 2024). In this study, researchers performed "physiological measures, physical and cognitive performance testing, and biochemical, microbiological, and immunological assays of blood, cerebrospinal fluid, muscle, and stool" of the recruited participants, accruing a massive dataset that could be probed to detect unique features of the ME/CFS patients. Despite a small sample size of 17 ME/CFS patients and 21 healthy controls, data from the study led to a hypothesis involving simultaneous immune dysfunction and microbiome dysbiosis that may result in a cascade of symptoms. The data also pointed to several biomarkers that could assist in the diagnosis of ME/CFS, highlighted sex differences, and identified potential treatment targets based on the proposed pathogenesis model.

Another strategy is to broaden, instead of deepen, the data that are collected. To address challenges with the overlapping symptoms and potential infectious origins of different IACI, studies could include participants from a variety of IACI (possibly also people with similar symptoms of uncertain origin). Studies that collect data on multiple IACI provide an opportunity to more rapidly identify commonalities and potential treatments with wide benefit for different diseases. Analysis of these large datasets could also identify treatments for specific subsets of patients, including patient subgroups, or mechanistic understandings may be discernible across a multi-IACI dataset. It can be challenging to design studies that identify and ideally stratify relevant subgroups across these different diseases, which may have different etiology and pathogenesis, including heterogeneity in risk factors such as prior history of trauma, environmental exposures, or genetics. If these strata are not identified and analyzed separately, important findings could be missed among the combined study sample. Additionally, this combined research effort would prove counterproductive if there are significant differences in the etiology, pathogenesis, or risk factor for these diseases. To guard against this possibility, it is important to maintain relevant history and key characteristics of study participants, which can be done through using a standardized core set of common data elements to further facilitate interoperability of the large dataset.

Deepening and broadening the data used in research can be complementary and mutually reinforcing approaches to better understand Lyme IACI. Standardizing outcome measures and definitions are central to successfully collecting and making use of expanded data collections. New approaches to obtaining and analyzing this data are discussed in Chapter 4.

LESSONS LEARNED

Many knowledge gaps remain in understanding the etiology of IACI, impeding the ability to develop treatments and diagnostics for these diseases. This is the case for the recently emerged condition of Long COVID as well as for other chronic syndromes that have been known for decades, including ME/CFS and Lyme IACI. The limiting factor to progress in the basic understanding of IACI does not appear to be exhaustion of scientific or technological exploration. Instead, the interdisciplinary, comprehensive approach that is necessary to address these complex illnesses and conditions requires significant and sustained investment in high quality basic and clinical research.

Widespread acknowledgment of the public health burden from COVID-19 and Long COVID among policymakers and research funders has led to significant support for Long COVID research that was essential to yielding the substantial body of evidence for this condition. The RECOVER Initiative, established in 2021 as a nationwide research program to fully understand, diagnose, and treat Long COVID, received $1.7 billion in funding through a combination of Congressional appropriations and repurposed NIH funding (NIH, 2024). In contrast, Lyme disease research, which encompasses research on Lyme IACI, has received a total of $475 million in NIH funding over 15 years between 2008 and 2023 (Figure 3-1) (NIH, n.d.a). The limited funding for Lyme IACI research has been attributed to varied factors, including a historic lack of recognition of the disease, poor understanding of the pathophysiology,[8] shifting priorities in the absence of a national research strategy, and challenges with alignment and coordination among different research partners—such as people with lived experience and funding organizations.[9] Increased funding has a direct impact on the quantity and quality of studies that can be conducted. While an imperfect count, a search of for active trials on "Long COVID" through ClinicalTrials.gov yields 299 results, whereas the same search for "post-treatment Lyme disease" returns 9 studies.[10] More broadly speaking, while NIH-funded programs and initiatives are crucial to advancing biomedical research and scientific knowledge, adjunctive research often led through the expertise of other agencies are also important for addressing a wide-reaching public health problem like Lyme IACI. For example, the Agency for Health Research and Quality supports expansion of comprehensive, multidisciplinary clinics for Long COVID, which can play a key role as community trial sites (AHRQ, 2025). While the Centers for Disease Control and Prevention is largely involved in surveillance and prevention of vector-borne diseases, they can be key partners in conducting necessary epidemiological studies (see Chapter 2), participating in development of new diagnostics and evaluate their use in case surveillance, and educating clinicians to disseminate use of research and clinical definitions for Lyme IACI.

Conclusion 3-4: Lyme IACI research is conducted with limited resources without a centralized body and with no formal standardized definition of patient population, outcomes, or mechanisms to promote collaboration among investigators, transparency of existing resources, and data sharing.

Support for long-term, sustainable clinical research infrastructure and initiatives, including adjunctive research, may be costly as they will likely be years-long endeavors involving investigators across multiple locations and disciplines. But long-term engagement also builds a collaborative ecosystem among researchers and patient participants that can provide return on the initial investment by enabling more rapid mobilization for future work and streamlined dissemination of study outcomes.

Although the available evidence does not support the immediate translation of any particular intervention from ME/CFS and Long COVID research to Lyme IACI, the adoption of the research approaches from these conditions is supported by available evidence. Common standards for research definitions and metrics would greatly improve the capacity to draw

---

[8] As presented to the committee in open session by Wendy Adams on July 11, 2024.
[9] As presented to the committee in open session by Leith States on July 11, 2024.
[10] Search performed at https://clinicaltrials.gov/ on January 15, 2025.

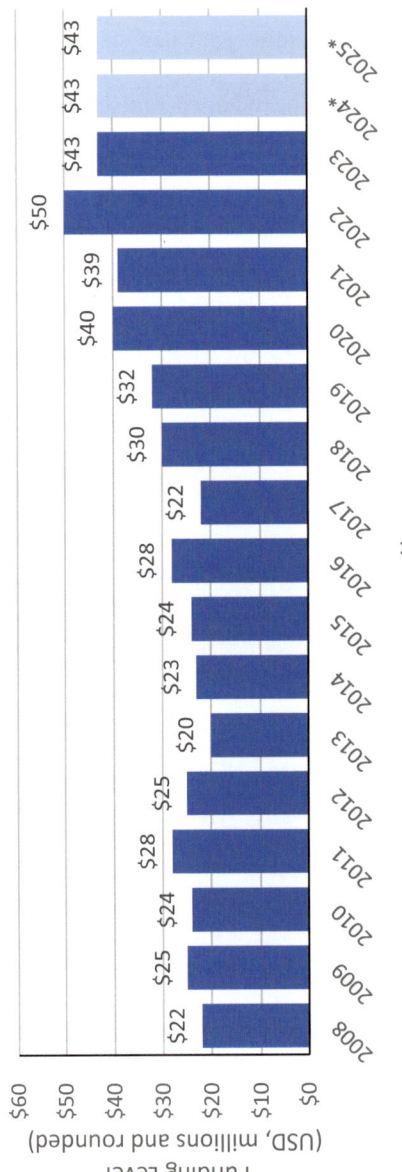

FIGURE 3-1 NIH funding for Lyme disease research, 2008–2025.
NOTES: Asterisks indicate that funding levels for 2024 and 2025 are estimates provided by NIH and have not been finalized as of March 2025. Research for persistent symptoms related to Lyme disease is part of this overall funding. NIH = National Institutes of Health.

comparisons between individual studies on Lyme IACI. Centralized coordination will be particularly important for streamlining Lyme IACI research efforts—and IACI research broadly, and would help increase efficiency and avoid duplicative studies and efforts. Research coordination within Lyme IACI and among different IACI would also promote the sharing of data and limited resources among researchers. Applying these lessons in Lyme IACI research will be important to advance the pace of discoveries.

REFERENCES

Adler, B. L., T. Chung, P. C. Rowe, and J. Aucott. 2024. Dysautonomia following Lyme disease: A key component of post-treatment lyme disease syndrome? *Front Neurology* 15:1344862.

AIM ImmunoTech. 2024. *AIM ImmunoTech announces that analysis of AMP-518 complete clinical patient data underscores Ampligen's potential to improve the post-covid condition of fatigue.* https://aimimmuno.com/aim-immunotech-announces-that-analysis-of-amp-518-complete-clinical-patient-data-underscores-ampligens-potential-to-improve-the-post-covid-condition-of-fatigue/ (accessed January 27, 2025).

Ali, A., L. Vitulano, R. Lee, T. R. Weiss, and E. R. Colson. 2014. Experiences of patients identifying with chronic Lyme disease in the healthcare system: A qualitative study. *BMC Family Practice* 15(1):79.

Appelman, B., B. T. Charlton, R. P. Goulding, T. J. Kerkhoff, E. A. Breedveld, W. Noort, C. Offringa, F. W. Bloemers, M. van Weeghel, B. V. Schomakers, P. Coelho, J. J. Posthuma, E. Aronica, W. Joost Wiersinga, M. van Vugt, and R. C. I. Wüst. 2024. Muscle abnormalities worsen after post-exertional malaise in Long COVID. *Nature Communications* 15(1):17.

AHRQ (Agency for Healthcare Research and Quality). 2025. *AHRQ efforts to address Long COVID.* https://www.ahrq.gov/coronavirus/long-covid.html (accessed March 16, 2025).

Arron, H. E., B. D. Marsh, D. B. Kell, M. A. Khan, B. R. Jaeger, and E. Pretorius. 2024. Myalgic encephalomyelitis/chronic fatigue syndrome: The biology of a neglected disease. *Frontiers in Immunology* 15:1386607.

Ascough, C., H. King, T. Serafimova, L. Beasant, S. Jackson, L. Baldock, A. E. Pickering, J. Brooks, and E. Crawley. 2020. Interventions to treat pain in paediatric CFS/ME: A systematic review. *BMJ Paediatrics Open* 4(1):e000617.

Aucott, J. N., A. W. Rebman, L. A. Crowder, and K. B. Kortte. 2013. Post-treatment Lyme disease syndrome symptomatology and the impact on life functioning: Is there something here? *Quality of Life Research* 22(1):75–84.

Bai, N. A., and C. S. Richardson. 2023. Posttreatment Lyme disease syndrome and myalgic encephalomyelitis/chronic fatigue syndrome: A systematic review and comparison of pathogenesis. *Chronic Diseases and Translational Medicine* 9(3):183–190.

Bateman, L., A. C. Bested, H. F. Bonilla, B. V. Chheda, L. Chu, J. M. Curtin, T. T. Dempsey, M. E. Dimmock, T. G. Dowell, D. Felsenstein, D. L. Kaufman, N. G. Klimas, A. L. Komaroff, C. W. Lapp, S. M. Levine, J. G. Montoya, B. H. Natelson, D. L. Peterson, R. N. Podell, I. R. Rey, I. S. Ruhoy, M. A. Vera-Nunez, and B. P. Yellman. 2021. Myalgic encephalomyelitis/chronic fatigue syndrome: Essentials of diagnosis and management. *Mayo Clinic Proceedings* 96(11):2861–2878.

Besteher, B., T. Rocktäschel, A. P. Garza, M. Machnik, J. Ballez, D.-L. Helbing, K. Finke, P. Reuken, D. Güllmar, C. Gaser, M. Walter, N. Opel, and I. Rita Dunay. 2024. Cortical thickness alterations and systemic inflammation define Long COVID patients with cognitive impairment. *Brain, Behavior, and Immunity* 116:175–184.

Blockmans, D., P. Persoons, B. Van Houdenhove, M. Lejeune, and H. Bobbaers. 2003. Combination therapy with hydrocortisone and fludrocortisone does not improve symptoms in chronic fatigue syndrome: A randomized, placebo-controlled, double-blind, crossover study. *American Journal of Medicine* 114(9):736–741.

Blockmans, D., P. Persoons, B. Van Houdenhove, and H. Bobbaers. 2006. Does methylphenidate reduce the symptoms of chronic fatigue syndrome? *American Journal of Medicine* 119(2):167.E23–167.E30.

Bonilla, H., M. J. Peluso, K. Rodgers, J. A. Aberg, T. F. Patterson, R. Tamburro, L. Baizer, J. D. Goldman, N. Rouphael, A. Deitchman, J. Fine, P. Fontelo, A. Y. Kim, G. Shaw, J. Stratford, P. Ceger, M. M. Costantine, L. Fisher, L. O'Brien, C. Maughan, J. G. Quigley, V. Gabbay, S. Mohandas, D. Williams, and G. A. McComsey. 2023. Therapeutic trials for Long COVID-19: A call to action from the interventions taskforce of the RECOVER initiative. *Frontiers in Immunology* 14:1129459.

Brunoni, A. R., A. H. Moffa, F. Fregni, U. Palm, F. Padberg, D. M. Blumberger, Z. J. Daskalakis, D. Bennabi, E. Haffen, A. Alonzo, and C. K. Loo. 2016. Transcranial direct current stimulation for acute major depressive episodes: Meta-analysis of individual patient data. *British Journal of Psychiatry* 208(6):522–531.

Calzari, L., D. F. Dragani, L. Zanotti, E. Inglese, R. Danesi, R. Cavagnola, A. Brusati, F. Ranucci, A. M. Di Blasio, L. Persani, I. Campi, S. De Martino, A. Farsetti, V. Barbi, M. Gottardi Zamperla, G. N. Baldrighi, C. Gaetano, G. Parati, and D. Gentilini. 2024. Epigenetic patterns, accelerated biological aging, and enhanced epigenetic drift detected 6 months following COVID-19 infection: Insights from a genome-wide DNA methylation study. *Clinical Epigenetics* 16(1):112.

Cao, B., Q. Xu, Y. Shi, R. Zhao, H. Li, J. Zheng, F. Liu, Y. Wan, and B. Wei. 2024. Pathology of pain and its implications for therapeutic interventions. *Signal Transduction and Targeted Therapy* 9(1):155.

Castro-Marrero, J., M. D. Cordero, M. J. Segundo, N. Sáez-Francàs, N. Calvo, L. Román-Malo, L. Aliste, T. Fernández de Sevilla, and J. Alegre. 2015. Does oral coenzyme Q10 plus NADH supplementation improve fatigue and biochemical parameters in chronic fatigue syndrome? *Antioxidants & Redox Signaling* 22(8):679–685.

Cella, D., J. S. Lai, C. J. Nowinski, D. Victorson, A. Peterman, D. Miller, F. Bethoux, A. Heinemann, S. Rubin, J. E. Cavazos, A. T. Reder, R. Sufit, T. Simuni, G. L. Holmes, A. Siderowf, V. Wojna, R. Bode, N. McKinney, T. Podrabsky, K. Wortman, S. Choi, R. Gershon, N. Rothrock, and C. Moy. 2012. Neuro-QoL: Brief measures of health-related quality of life for clinical research in neurology. *Neurology* 78(23):1860-1867.

Chee, Y. J., B. E. Fan, B. E. Young, R. Dalan, and D. C. Lye. 2023. Clinical trials on the pharmacological treatment of Long COVID: A systematic review. *Journal of Medical Virology* 95(1):e28289.

Chen, X. Y., C. L. Lu, Q. Y. Wang, X. R. Pan, Y. Y. Zhang, J. L. Wang, J. Y. Liao, N. C. Hu, C. Y. Wang, B. J. Duan, X. H. Liu, X. Y. Jin, J. Hunter, and J. P. Liu. 2024. Traditional, complementary and integrative medicine for fatigue post COVID-19 infection: A systematic review of randomized controlled trials. *Integrative Medicine Research* 13(2):101039.

Cheng, X., M. Cao, W.-F. Yeung, and D. S. T. Cheung. 2024. The effectiveness of exercise in alleviating Long COVID symptoms: A systematic review and meta-analysis. *Worldviews on Evidence-Based Nursing* 21(5):561–574.

Choutka, J., V. Jansari, M. Hornig, and A. Iwasaki. 2022. Unexplained post-acute infection syndromes. *Nature Medicine* 28(5):911–923.

Cui, L., S. Li, S. Wang, X. Wu, Y. Liu, W. Yu, Y. Wang, Y. Tang, M. Xia, and B. Li. 2024. Major depressive disorder: Hypothesis, mechanism, prevention and treatment. *Signal Transduction and Targeted Therapy* 9(1):30.

Clark, L. V., F. Pesola, J. M. Thomas, M. Vergara-Williamson, M. Beynon, and P. D. White. 2017. Guided graded exercise self-help plus specialist medical care versus specialist medical care alone for chronic fatigue syndrome (GETSET): A pragmatic randomised controlled trial. *Lancet* 390(10092):363–373.

Cleare, A. J., E. Heap, G. S. Malhi, S. Wessely, V. O'Keane, and J. Miell. 1999. Low-dose hydrocortisone in chronic fatigue syndrome: A randomised crossover trial. *The Lancet* 353(9151):455–458.

Columbia University. n.d. *Clinical Trials Network for Lyme and Other Tick-Borne Diseases: Active clinical studies.* https://www.lymectn.org/Studies.aspx (accessed January 15, 2025).

Davis, H. E., L. McCorkell, J. M. Vogel, and E. J. Topol. 2023. Long COVID: Major findings, mechanisms and recommendations. *Nature Reviews Microbiology* 21(3):133–146.

Deale, A., T. Chalder, I. Marks, and S. Wessely. 1997. Cognitive behavior therapy for chronic fatigue syndrome: A randomized controlled trial. *American Journal of Psychiatry* 154(3):408–414.

de Oliveira, B. F. A., P. R. C. Carvalho, A. S. de Souza Holanda, R. Dos Santos, F. A. X. da Silva, G. W. P. Barros, E. C. de Albuquerque, A. T. Dantas, N. G. Cavalcanti, A. Ranzolin, A. Duarte, and C. D. L. Marques. 2019. Pilates method in the treatment of patients with chikungunya fever: A randomized controlled trial. *Clinical Rehabilitation* 33(10):1614–1624.

de Vega, W. C., and P. O. McGowan. 2017. The epigenetic landscape of myalgic encephalomyelitis/chronic fatigue syndrome: Deciphering complex phenotypes. *Epigenomics* 9(11):1337–1340.

El-Mokadem, J. F. K., K. DiMarco, T. M. Kelley, and L. Duffield. 2023. Three principles/innate health: The efficacy of psycho-spiritual mental health education for people with chronic fatigue syndrome. *Spirituality in Clinical Practice* 10(4):289–303.

Ely, E. W., L. M. Brown, and H. V. Fineberg. 2024. Long COVID defined. *New England Journal of Medicine* 391(18):1746–1753.

Fallon, B. A., J. Keilp, I. Prohovnik, R. V. Heertum, and J. J. Mann. 2003. Regional cerebral blood flow and cognitive deficits in chronic Lyme disease. *The Journal of Neuropsychiatry Clinical Neuroscience* 15(3):326–332.

Fitzcharles, M. A., S. P. Cohen, D. J. Clauw, G. Littlejohn, C. Usui, and W. Häuser. 2021. Nociplastic pain: Towards an understanding of prevalent pain conditions. *The Lancet* 397(10289):2098–2110.

Fowler-Davis, S., R. Young, T. Maden-Wilkinson, W. Hameed, E. Dracas, E. Hurrell, R. Bahl, E. Kilcourse, R. Robinson, and R. Copeland. 2021. Assessing the acceptability of a co-produced Long COVID intervention in an underserved community in the UK. *International Journal of Environmental Research and Public Health* 18(24):13191.

Fox, T., B. J. Hunt, R. A. Ariens, G. J. Towers, R. Lever, P. Garner, and R. Kuehn. 2023. Plasmapheresis to remove amyloid fibrin(ogen) particles for treating the post-COVID-19 condition. *Cochrane Database of Systematic Reviews* 7(7):CD015775.

Geraghty, K. J. 2017. 'Pace-gate': When clinical trial evidence meets open data access. *Journal of Health Psychology* 22(9):1106–1112.

Gracely, R. H., F. Petzke, J. M. Wolf, and D. J. Clauw. 2002. Functional magnetic resonance imaging evidence of augmented pain processing in fibromyalgia. *Arthritis & Rheumatology* 46(5):1333–1343.

Greene, C., R. Connolly, D. Brennan, A. Laffan, E. O'Keeffe, L. Zaporojan, J. O'Callaghan, B. Thomson, E. Connolly, R. Argue, J. F. M. Meaney, I. Martin-Loeches, A. Long, C. N. Cheallaigh, N. Conlon, C. P. Doherty, and M. Campbell. 2024. Blood–brain barrier disruption and sustained systemic inflammation in individuals with Long COVID-associated cognitive impairment. *Nature Neuroscience* 27(3):421–432.

Halford, J., and T. Brown. 2009. Cognitive–behavioural therapy as an adjunctive treatment in chronic physical illness. *Advances in Psychiatric Treatment* 15(4):306–317.

Hausswirth, C., C. Schmit, Y. Rougier, and A. Coste. 2023. Positive impacts of a four-week neuro-meditation program on cognitive function in post-acute sequelae of COVID-19 patients: A randomized controlled trial. *International Journal of Environmental Research and Public Health* 20(2):1361.

Hawkins, J., C. Hires, L. Keenan, and E. Dunne. 2022. Aromatherapy blend of thyme, orange, clove bud, and frankincense boosts energy levels in post-COVID-19 female patients: A randomized, double-blinded, placebo controlled clinical trial. *Complementary Therapies in Medicine* 67:102823.

HHS (Department of Health and Human Services). 2022. *National research action plan on Long COVID*. https://www.covid.gov/sites/default/files/documents/National-Research-Action-Plan-on-Long-COVID-08012022.pdf (accessed November 27, 2024).

HHS. 2025. *The office of Long COVID research and practice OLC*. https://www.hhs.gov/longcovid/index.html (accessed March 27, 2025).

Health Measures. 2025. *Search & view measures*. https://www.healthmeasures.net/search-view-measures?task=Search.search (accessed March 15, 2025).

Henningsson, A. J., S. Hellberg, M. Lerm, and S. Sayyab. 2024. Genome-wide DNA methylation profiling in Lyme neuroborreliosis reveals altered methylation patterns of HLA genes. *Journal of Infectious Diseases* 229(4):1209–1214.

Hermans, L., J. Nijs, P. Calders, L. De Clerck, G. Moorkens, G. Hans, S. Grosemans, T. Roman De Mettelinge, J. Tuynman, and M. Meeus. 2018. Influence of morphine and naloxone on pain modulation in rheumatoid arthritis, chronic fatigue syndrome/fibromyalgia, and controls: A double-blind, randomized, placebo-controlled, cross-over study. *Pain Practice* 18(4):418–430.

Huanan, L., W. Jingui, Z. Wei, Z. Na, H. Xinhua, S. Shiquan, S. Qing, H. Yihao, Z. Runchen, and M. Fei. 2017. Chronic fatigue syndrome treated by the traditional Chinese procedure abdominal tuina: A randomized controlled clinical trial. *Journal of Traditional Chinese Medicine* 37(6):819–826.

Huang, Y. H., H. C. Chen, K. W. Huang, P. C. Chen, C. J. Hu, C. P. Tsai, K. W. Tam, and Y. C. Kuan. 2015. Intravenous immunoglobulin for postpolio syndrome: A systematic review and meta-analysis. *BMC Neurology* 15:39.

IOM (Institute of Medicine). 2015. *Beyond myalgic encephalomyelitis/chronic fatigue syndrome: Redefining an illness*. Washington, DC: The National Academies Press.

James, R. J. E., and E. Ferguson. 2020. The dynamic relationship between pain, depression and cognitive function in a sample of newly diagnosed arthritic adults: A cross-lagged panel model. *Psychological Medicine* 50(10):1663–1671.

Janse, A., M. Worm-Smeitink, G. Bleijenberg, R. Donders, and H. Knoop. 2018. Efficacy of web-based cognitive–behavioural therapy for chronic fatigue syndrome: Randomised controlled trial. *British Journal of Psychiatry* 212(2):112–118.

Jason, L. A., and M. Sunnquist. 2018. The development of the DePaul Symptom Questionnaire: Original, expanded, brief, and pediatric versions. *Front Pediatr* 6:330.

JHU (Johns Hopkins University). 2024. Effects of psilocybin in post-treatment lyme disease. In: ClinicalTrials.gov. Available from https://clinicaltrials.gov/study/NCT05305105?cond=Post-Treatment%20Lyme%20Disease&rank=5 (accessed November 27, 2025).

Johns Hopkins Medicine. 2024. *Psychiatry and behavioral sciences*. https://www.hopkinsmedicine.org/psychiatry/research/psychedelics-research (accessed January 15, 2025).

Johnson, L., S. Wilcox, J. Mankoff, and R. B. Stricker. 2014. Severity of chronic Lyme disease compared to other chronic conditions: A quality of life survey. *PeerJ* 2:e322.

Johnson, L., M. Shapiro, and J. Mankoff. 2018. Removing the mask of average treatment effects in chronic Lyme disease research using big data and subgroup analysis. *Healthcare (Basel)* 6(4):124.

Kaplan, C. M., E. Kelleher, A. Irani, A. Schrepf, D. J. Clauw, and S. E. Harte. 2024. Deciphering nociplastic pain: Clinical features, risk factors and potential mechanisms. *Nature Reviews Neurology* 20(6):347–363.

Karosanidze, I., U. Kiladze, N. Kirtadze, M. Giorgadze, N. Amashukeli, N. Parulava, N. Iluridze, N. Kikabidze, N. Gudavadze, L. Gelashvili, V. Koberidze, E. Gigashvili, N. Jajanidze, N. Latsabidze, N. Mamageishvili, R. Shengelia, A. Hovhannisyan, and A. Panossian. 2022. Efficacy of adaptogens in patients with long COVID-19: A randomized, quadruple-blind, placebo-controlled trial. *Pharmaceuticals* 15(3):345.

Keijmel, S. P., C. E. Delsing, G. Bleijenberg, J. W. M. van der Meer, R. T. Donders, M. Leclercq, L. M. Kampschreur, M. van den Berg, T. Sprong, M. H. Nabuurs-Franssen, H. Knoop, and C. P. Bleeker-Rovers. 2017. Effectiveness of long-term doxycycline treatment and cognitive-behavioral therapy on fatigue severity in patients with Q fever fatigue syndrome (Qure study): A randomized controlled trial. *Clinical Infectious Diseases* 64(8):998–1005.

Kell, D. B., M. A. Khan, B. Kane, G. Y. H. Lip, and E. Pretorius. 2024. Possible role of fibrinaloid microclots in postural orthostatic tachycardia syndrome (POTS): Focus on Long COVID. *Journal of Personalized Medicine* 14(2):170.

Khan, M. W. Z., M. Ahmad, S. Qudrat, F. Afridi, N. A. Khan, Z. Afridi, Fahad, T. Azeem, and J. Ikram. 2024. Vagal nerve stimulation for the management of long COVID symptoms. *Infectious Medicine* 3(4):100149.

Kim, J. E., B. K. Seo, J. B. Choi, H. J. Kim, T. H. Kim, M. H. Lee, K. W. Kang, J. H. Kim, K. M. Shin, S. Lee, S. Y. Jung, A. R. Kim, M. S. Shin, H. J. Jung, H. J. Park, S. P. Kim, Y. H. Baek, K. E. Hong, and S. M. Choi. 2015. Acupuncture for chronic fatigue syndrome and idiopathic chronic fatigue: A multicenter, nonblinded, randomized controlled trial. *Trials* 16:314.

Kim, D. Y., J. S. Lee, S. Y. Park, S. J. Kim, and C. G. Son. 2020. Systematic review of randomized controlled trials for chronic fatigue syndrome/myalgic encephalomyelitis (CFS/ME). *Journal of Translational Medicine* 18(1):7.

Knoop, H., J. W. van der Meer, and G. Bleijenberg. 2008. Guided self-instructions for people with chronic fatigue syndrome: Randomised controlled trial. *British Journal of Psychiatry* 193(4):340–341.

Komaroff, A. L., and W. I. Lipkin. 2023. ME/CFS and long COVID share similar symptoms and biological abnormalities: Road map to the literature. *Frontiers in Medicine (Lausanne)* 10:1187163.

Kuut, T. A., F. Müller, I. Csorba, A. Braamse, A. Aldenkamp, B. Appelman, E. Assmann-Schuilwerve, S. E. Geerlings, K. B. Gibney, R. A. A. Kanaan, K. Mooij-Kalverda, T. C. Olde Hartman, D. Pauëlsen, M. Prins, K. Slieker, M. van Vugt, S. P. Keijmel, P. Nieuwkerk, C. P. Rovers, and H. Knoop. 2023. Efficacy of cognitive–behavioral therapy targeting severe fatigue following coronavirus disease 2019: Results of a randomized controlled trial. *Clinical Infectious Diseases* 77(5):687–695.

Lam, W. C., D. Wei, H. Li, L. Yao, S. Zhang, M. X. Y. Lai, Y. Zheng, J. W. F. Yeung, A. Y. L. Lau, A. Lyu, Z. Bian, A. M. Cheung, and L. L. D. Zhong. 2024. The use of acupuncture for addressing neurological and neuropsychiatric symptoms in patients with long COVID: A systematic review and meta-analysis. *Frontiers in Neurology* 15:1406475.

Lee, J.-S., W. Sato, and C.-G. Son. 2024. Brain-regional characteristics and neuroinflammation in ME/CFS patients from neuroimaging: A systematic review and meta-analysis. *Autoimmunity Reviews* 23(2):103484.

Lim, E.-J., and C.-G. Son. 2020. Review of case definitions for myalgic encephalomyelitis/chronic fatigue syndrome (ME/CFS). *Journal of Translational Medicine* 18(1):289.

Lladós, G., M. Massanella, R. Coll-Fernández, R. Rodríguez, E. Hernández, G. Lucente, C. López, C. Loste, J. R. Santos, S. España-Cueto, M. Nevot, F. Muñoz-López, S. Silva-Arrieta, C. Brander, M. J. Durà, P. Cuadras, J. Bechini, M. Tenesa, A. Martinez-Piñeiro, C. Herrero, A. Chamorro, A. Garcia, E. Grau, B. Clotet, R. Paredes, L. Mateu, M.-M. José, R.-F. Carmina, P. Anna, E. Carla, V. Nuria, V. Roger, A. Julia, M. Toni, M. Julia, and C. Ivette. 2024. Vagus nerve dysfunction in the post-COVID-19 condition: A pilot cross-sectional study. *Clinical Microbiology and Infection* 30(4):515–521.

Machado, M. O., N.-Y. C. Kang, F. Tai, R. D. S. Sambhi, M. Berk, A. F. Carvalho, L. P. Chada, J. F. Merola, V. Piguet, and A. Alavi. 2021. Measuring fatigue: A meta-review. *International Journal of Dermatology* 60(9):1053–1069.

Maksoud, R., C. Balinas, S. Holden, H. Cabanas, D. Staines, and S. Marshall-Gradisnik. 2021. A systematic review of nutraceutical interventions for mitochondrial dysfunctions in myalgic encephalomyelitis/chronic fatigue syndrome. *Journal of Translational Medicine* 19(1):81.

Marques, M., V. De Gucht, I. Leal, and S. Maes. 2015. Effects of a self-regulation based physical activity program (the "4-steps") for unexplained chronic fatigue: A randomized controlled trial. *International Journal of Behavioral Medicine* 22(2):187–196.

Marvel, C. L., K. H. Alm, D. Bhattacharya, W. Rebman Alison, A. Bakker, O. P. Morgan, J. A. Creighton, E. A. Kozero, A. Venkatesan, P. A. Nadkarni, and J. N. Aucott. 2022. A multimodal neuroimaging study of brain abnormalities and clinical correlates in post treatment Lyme disease. *PLOS One* 10(17).

Mayo Clinic. 2023. *Vagus nerve stimulation.* https://www.mayoclinic.org/tests-procedures/vagus-nerve-stimulation/about/pac-20384565 (accessed January 15, 2025).

McIntyre, R. S., L. Phan, A. T. H. Kwan, R. B. Mansur, J. D. Rosenblat, Z. Guo, G. H. Le, L. M. W. Lui, K. M. Teopiz, F. Ceban, Y. Lee, J. Bailey, R. Ramachandra, J. Di Vincenzo, S. Badulescu, H. Gill, P. Drzadzewski, and M. Subramaniapillai. 2024. Vortioxetine for the treatment of post-COVID-19 condition: A randomized controlled trial. *Brain* 147(3):849–857.

McKenzie, R., A. O'Fallon, J. Dale, M. Demitrack, G. Sharma, M. Deloria, D. Garcia-Borreguero, W. Blackwelder, and S. E. Straus. 1998. Low-dose hydrocortisone for treatment of chronic fatigue syndrome: A randomized controlled trial. *JAMA* 280(12):1061–1066.

Mihara, H., H. Sumi, T. Yoneta, H. Mizumoto, R. Ikeda, M. Seiki, and M. Maruyama. 1991. A novel fibrinolytic enzyme extracted from the earthworm, lumbricus rubellus. *Japanese Journal of Physiology* 41(3):461–472.

MECFS Net (Myalgic Encephalomyelitis/Chronic Fatigue Syndrome Research Network). n.d. *Research centers.* https://mecfs.rti.org/centers/ (accessed February 5, 2025).

Mohammadi, S., S. Ghaderi, and F. Fatehi. 2024. Brain perfusion alterations in patients and survivors of COVID-19 infection using arterial spin labeling: A systematic review. *Brain-X* 2(3):e70007.

Momtazmanesh, S., S. Ansari, Z. Izadi, P. Shobeiri, V. Vatankhah, A. Seifi, F. Ghiasvand, M. Bahrami, M. Salehi, A. A. Noorbala, and S. Akhondzadeh. 2023. Effect of famotidine on cognitive and behavioral dysfunctions induced in post-COVID-19 infection: A randomized, double-blind, and placebo-controlled study. *Journal of Psychosomatic Research* 172:111389.

Montoya, J. G., A. M. Kogelnik, M. Bhangoo, M. R. Lunn, L. Flamand, L. E. Merrihew, T. Watt, J. T. Kubo, J. Paik, and M. Desai. 2013. Randomized clinical trial to evaluate the efficacy and safety of valganciclovir in a subset of patients with chronic fatigue syndrome. *Journal of Medical Virology* 85(12):2101–2109.

NASEM (National Academies of Sciences, Engineering, and Medicine). 2024a. *A Long COVID definition: A chronic, systemic disease state with profound consequences.* Washington, DC: The National Academies Press.

NASEM. 2024b. *Toward a common research agenda in infection-associated chronic illnesses: Proceedings of a workshop.* Washington, DC: The National Academies Press.

Nelson, B. K., L. N. Farah, S. A. Saint, C. Song, T. S. Field, V. Sossi, A. J. Stoessl, C. Wellington, W. G. Honer, D. Lang, N. D. Silverberg, and W. J. Panenka. 2025. Diffusion tensor imaging after COVID-19 infection: A systematic review. *NeuroImage* 310:121150.

Neumann, I. L., D. A. de Oliveira, E. L. de Barros, S. S. G. da, L. S. de Oliveira, A. L. Duarte, C. D. Marques, A. T. Dantas, D. Dantas, G. R. de Siqueira, and A. da Silva Tenório. 2021. Resistance exercises improve physical function in chronic chikungunya fever patients: A randomized controlled trial. *European Journal of Physical and Rehabilitation Medicine* 57(4):620–629.

Newberg, A., A. Hassan, and A. Alavi. 2002. Cerebral metabolic changes associated with Lyme disease. *Nuclear Medicine Communication* 23(8):773–777.

Ng, S. M., and Y. M. Yiu. 2013. Acupuncture for chronic fatigue syndrome: A randomized, sham-controlled trial with single-blinded design. *Alternative Therapies in Health and Medicine* 19(4):21–26.

NIH (National Institutes of Health). n.d.a. *Estimates of funding for various research, condition, and disease categories (RCDC).* https://report.nih.gov/funding/categorical-spending#/ (accessed January 28, 2025).

NIH. n.d.b. *Myalgic encephalomyelitis/chronic fatigue syndrome.* https://www.commondataelements.ninds.nih.gov/Myalgic%20Encephalomyelitis/Chronic%20Fatigue%20Syndrome#pane-89 (accessed January 27, 2025).

NIH. 2024. *NIH adds funds to long COVID-19 research, advances work on new clinical trials.* https://www.nih.gov/about-nih/who-we-are/nih-director/statements/nih-adds-funds-long-covid-19-research-advances-work-new-clinical-trials (accessed January 28, 2025).

NINDS (National Institute of Neurological Disorders and Stroke). n.d. *Myalgic encephalomyelitis/chronic fatigue syndrome.* https://www.commondataelements.ninds.nih.gov/Myalgic%20Encephalomyelitis/Chronic%20Fatigue%20Syndrome (accessed March 15, 2025).

NIH OSC (National Institute of Health Office of Strategic Coordination – The Common Fund). 2025. *Patient-reported outcomes measurement information system (PROMIS).* https://commonfund.nih.gov/patient-reported-outcomes-measurement-information-system-promis (accessed March 15, 2025).

Nijhof, S. L., G. Bleijenberg, C. S. Uiterwaal, J. L. Kimpen, and E. M. van de Putte. 2012. Effectiveness of internet-based cognitive behavioural treatment for adolescents with chronic fatigue syndrome (FITNET): A randomised controlled trial. *The Lancet* 379(9824):1412–1418.

O'Dowd, H., P. Gladwell, C. A. Rogers, S. Hollinghurst, and A. Gregory. 2006. Cognitive behavioural therapy in chronic fatigue syndrome: A randomised controlled trial of an outpatient group programme. *Health Technology Assessment* 10(37):iii–iv, ix–x, 1–121.

Oka, T., T. Tanahashi, T. Chijiwa, B. Lkhagvasuren, N. Sudo, and K. Oka. 2014. Isometric yoga improves the fatigue and pain of patients with chronic fatigue syndrome who are resistant to conventional therapy: A randomized, controlled trial. *Biopsychosocial Medicine* 8(1):27.

Oliver-Mas, S., C. Delgado-Alonso, A. Delgado-Álvarez, M. Díez-Cirarda, C. Cuevas, L. Fernández-Romero, A. Matias-Guiu, M. Valles-Salgado, L. Gil-Martínez, M. J. Gil-Moreno, M. Yus, J. Matias-Guiu, and J. A. Matias-Guiu. 2023. Transcranial direct current stimulation for post-COVID fatigue: A randomized, double-blind, controlled pilot study. *Brain Communications* 5(2):fcad117.

Pang, W., F. Yang, Y. Zhao, E. Dai, J. Feng, Y. Huang, Y. Guo, S. Zhou, M. Huang, W. Zheng, J. Ma, H. Li, Q. Li, L. Hou, S. Zhang, H. Wang, Q. Liu, B. Zhang, and J. Zhang. 2022. Qingjin yiqi granules for post-COVID-19 condition: A randomized clinical trial. *Journal of Evidence-Based Medicine* 15(1):30–38.

Peluso, M. J., M. R. Hanson, and S. G. Deeks. 2024. Infection-associated chronic conditions: Why long COVID is our best chance to untangle Osler's web. *Science Translational Medicine* 16(773):eado2101.

Peterson, P. K., A. Pheley, J. Schroeppel, C. Schenck, P. Marshall, A. Kind, J. M. Haugland, L. J. Lambrecht, S. Swan, and S. Goldsmith. 1998. A preliminary placebo-controlled crossover trial of fludrocortisone for chronic fatigue syndrome. *Archives of Internal Medicine* 158(8):908–914.

Petracek, L. S., C. A. Broussard, R. L. Swope, and P. C. Rowe. 2023. A case study of successful application of the principles of ME/CFS care to an individual with long COVID. *Healthcare* 11(6):865. https://www.mdpi.com/2227-9032/11/6/865 (accessed February 4, 2025).

Philip, K. E. J., H. Owles, S. McVey, T. Pagnuco, K. Bruce, H. Brunjes, W. Banya, J. Mollica, A. Lound, S. Zumpe, A. M. Abrahams, V. Padmanaban, T. H. Hardy, A. Lewis, A. Lalvani, S. Elkin, and N. S. Hopkinson. 2022. An online breathing and wellbeing programme (ENO Breathe) for people with persistent symptoms following COVID-19: A parallel-group, single-blind, randomised controlled trial. *The Lancet Respiratory Medicine* 10(9):851–862.

Pooladgar, P., M. Sakhabakhsh, S. Soleiman-Meigooni, A. Taghva, M. Nasiri, and I. A. Darazam. 2023. The effect of donepezil hydrochloride on post-COVID memory impairment: A randomized controlled trial. *Journal of Clinical Neuroscience* 118:168–174.

Prins, J. B., G. Bleijenberg, E. Bazelmans, L. D. Elving, T. M. de Boo, J. L. Severens, G. J. van der Wilt, P. Spinhoven, and J. W. van der Meer. 2001. Cognitive behaviour therapy for chronic fatigue syndrome: A multicentre randomised controlled trial. *The Lancet* 357(9259):841–847.

Putrino, D., A. Proal, and M. Doerstling. n.d. *Lumbrokinase long COVID & ME/CFS clinical trial.* https://polybio.org/projects/lumbrokinase-longcovid-me-cfs-clinical-trial/ (accessed February 4, 2025).

Rao, S., R. S. Gross, S. Mohandas, C. R. Stein, A. Case, B. Dreyer, N. M. Pajor, H. T. Bunnell, D. Warburton, E. Berg, J. B. Overdevest, M. Gorelik, J. Milner, S. Saxena, R. Jhaveri, J. C. Wood, K. E. Rhee, R. Letts, C. Maughan, N. Guthe, L. Castro-Baucom, and M. S. Stockwell. 2024. Postacute sequelae of SARS-COV-2 in children. *Pediatrics* 153(3).

Rathi, A., S. B. Jadhav, and N. Shah. 2021. A randomized controlled trial of the efficacy of systemic enzymes and probiotics in the resolution of post-COVID fatigue. *Medicines (Basel)* 8(9):47.

Rebman, A. W., K. T. Bechtold, T. Yang, E. A. Mihm, M. J. Soloski, C. B. Novak, and J. N. Aucott. 2017. The clinical, symptom, and quality-of-life characterization of a well-defined group of patients with posttreatment Lyme disease syndrome. *Frontiers in Medicine* 4:224.

RECOVER (Researching COVID to Enhance Recovery). 2024. *RECOVER-NEURO clinical trial.* https://recovercovid.org/neuro (accessed November 27, 2024).

Robinson, O. J., K. Vytal, B. R. Cornwell, and C. Grillon. 2013. The impact of anxiety upon cognition: Perspectives from human threat of shock studies. *Frontiers in Human Neuroscience* 7:203.

Rolland, B., B. R. Smith, and J. D. Potter. 2011. Coordinating centers in cancer epidemiology research: The Asia Cohort Consortium coordinating center. *Cancer Epidemiology, Biomarkers & Prevention* 20(10):2115–2119.

Rolland, B., C. P. Lee, and J. D. Potter. 2017. Greater than the sum of its parts: A qualitative study of the role of the coordinating center in facilitating coordinated collaborative science. *Journal of Research Administration* 48(1):65–85.

Rowe, P. C., H. Calkins, K. DeBusk, R. McKenzie, R. Anand, G. Sharma, B. A. Cuccherini, N. Soto, P. Hohman, S. Snader, K. E. Lucas, M. Wolff, and S. E. Straus. 2001. Fludrocortisone acetate to treat neurally mediated hypotension in chronic fatigue syndrome: A randomized controlled trial. *JAMA* 285(1):52–59.

Rowe, P. C., R. A. Underhill, K. J. Friedman, A. Gurwitt, M. S. Medow, M. S. Schwartz, N. Speight, J. M. Stewart, R. Vallings, and K. S. Rowe. 2017. Myalgic encephalomyelitis/chronic fatigue syndrome diagnosis and management in young people: A primer. *Frontiers in Pediatrics* 5.

RTI International. 2021. RTI International is supporting NIH initiative to study "long COVID." https://www.rti.org/announcements/rti-international-supporting-nih-initiative-study-long-covid (accessed February 5, 2025).

Samper-Pardo, M., S. León-Herrera, B. Oliván-Blázquez, F. Méndez-López, M. Domínguez-García, and R. Sánchez-Recio. 2023. Effectiveness of a telerehabilitation intervention using recovery app of long COVID patients: A randomized, 3-month follow-up clinical trial. *Science Reports* 13(1):7943.

Sanal-Hayes, N. E. M., M. McLaughlin, L. D. Hayes, J. L. Mair, J. Ormerod, D. Carless, N. Hilliard, R. Meach, J. Ingram, and N. F. Sculthorpe. 2023. A scoping review of "pacing" for management of myalgic encephalomyelitis/chronic fatigue syndrome (ME/CFS): Lessons learned for the long COVID pandemic. *Journal of Translational Medicine* 21(1):720.

Schmidt-Wilcke, T., and D. J. Clauw. 2011. Fibromyalgia: From pathophysiology to therapy. *Nature Reviews Rheumatology* 7(9):518–527.

Sharpe, M., K. Hawton, S. Simkin, C. Surawy, A. Hackmann, I. Klimes, T. Peto, D. Warrell, and V. Seagroatt. 1996. Cognitive behaviour therapy for the chronic fatigue syndrome: A randomized controlled trial. *BMJ* 312(7022):22–26.

Silva-Filho, E., A. H. Okano, E. Morya, J. Albuquerque, E. Cacho, G. Unal, M. Bikson, and R. Pegado. 2018. Neuromodulation treats chikungunya arthralgia: A randomized controlled trial. *Science Reports* 8(1):16010.

Sluka, K. A., and D. J. Clauw. 2016. Neurobiology of fibromyalgia and chronic widespread pain. *Neuroscience* 338:114–129.

Spudich, S., and A. Nath. 2022. Nervous system consequences of COVID-19. *Science* 375(6578):267–269.

Staud, R. 2012. Peripheral and central mechanisms of fatigue in inflammatory and noninflammatory rheumatic diseases. *Current Rheumatology Reports* 14(6):539–548.

Strayer, D. R., W. A. Carter, I. Brodsky, P. Cheney, D. Peterson, P. Salvato, C. Thompson, M. Loveless, D. E. Shapiro, W. Elsasser, D. H. Gillespie, and C. Z. Thompson. 1994. A controlled clinical trial with a specifically configured RNA drug, poly(I).poly(C12U), in chronic fatigue syndrome. *Clinical Infectious Diseases* 18(Suppl 1):S88–S95.

Stubhaug, B., S. A. Lie, H. Ursin, and H. R. Eriksen. 2008. Cognitive–behavioural therapy v. mirtazapine for chronic fatigue and neurasthenia: Randomised placebo-controlled trial. *British Journal of Psychiatry* 192(3):217–223.

Stulemeijer, M., L. W. de Jong, T. J. Fiselier, S. W. Hoogveld, and G. Bleijenberg. 2005. Cognitive behaviour therapy for adolescents with chronic fatigue syndrome: Randomised controlled trial. *BMJ* 330(7481):14.

Tabacof, L., R. Howard, J. Bower, E. Breyman, S. Dewil, J. Tosto-Mancuso, R. Hanbury, B. Carmouche, M. Robberson, A. Fry, and D. Putrino. 2024. Audio-visual stimulation therapy for chronic neuropathic pain: A sham-controlled randomized clinical trial. *medRxiv*:2024.2008.2012.24311569.

Tanashyan, M., S. Morozova, A. Raskurazhev, and P. Kuznetsova. 2023. A prospective randomized, double-blind placebo-controlled study to evaluate the effectiveness of neuroprotective therapy using functional brain MRI in patients with post-COVID chronic fatigue syndrome. *Biomed & Pharmacotherapy* 168:115723.

Taylor, R. R. 2006. *Cognitive behavioral therapy for chronic illness and disability*, Cognitive behavioral therapy for chronic illness and disability. New York, NY: Springer Science + Business Media.

Thair, H., A. L. Holloway, R. Newport, and A. D. Smith. 2017. Transcranial direct current stimulation (tDCS): A beginner's guide for design and implementation. *Frontiers in Neuroscience* 11:641.

Toogood, P. L., D. J. Clauw, S. Phadke, and D. Hoffman. 2021. Myalgic encephalomyelitis/chronic fatigue syndrome (ME/CFS): Where will the drugs come from? *Pharmacological Research* 165:105465.

Touradji, P., J. N. Aucott, T. Yang, A. W. Rebman, and K. T. Bechtold. 2019. Cognitive decline in post-treatment Lyme disease syndrome. *Archives of Clinical Neuropsychology* 34(4):455–465.

Tummers, M., H. Knoop, A. van Dam, and G. Bleijenberg. 2012. Implementing a minimal intervention for chronic fatigue syndrome in a mental health centre: A randomized controlled trial. *Psychological Medicine* 42(10):2205–2215.

Vernino, S., K. M. Bourne, L. E. Stiles, B. P. Grubb, A. Fedorowski, J. M. Stewart, A. C. Arnold, L. A. Pace, J. Axelsson, J. R. Boris, J. P. Moak, B. P. Goodman, K. R. Chémali, T. H. Chung, D. S. Goldstein, A. Diedrich, M. G. Miglis, M. M. Cortez, A. J. Miller, R. Freeman, I. Biaggioni, P. C. Rowe, R. S. Sheldon, C. A. Shibao, D. M. Systrom, G. A. Cook, T. A. Doherty, H. I. Abdallah, A. Darbari, and S. R. Raj. 2021. Postural orthostatic tachycardia syndrome (POTS): State of the science and clinical care from a 2019 National Institutes of Health expert consensus meeting - part 1. *Autonomic Neuroscience: basic & clinical* 235:102828.

Versace, V., P. Ortelli, S. Dezi, D. Ferrazzoli, A. Alibardi, I. Bonini, M. Engl, R. Maestri, M. Assogna, V. Ajello, E. Pucks-Faes, L. Saltuari, L. Sebastianelli, M. Kofler, and G. Koch. 2023. Co-ultramicronized palmitoylethanolamide/luteolin normalizes $GABA_B$-ergic activity and cortical plasticity in long COVID-19 syndrome. *Clinical Neurophysiology* 145:81–88.

Walitt, B., K. Singh, S. R. LaMunion, M. Hallett, S. Jacobson, K. Chen, Y. Enose-Akahata, R. Apps, J. J. Barb, P. Bedard, R. J. Brychta, A. W. Buckley, P. D. Burbelo, B. Calco, B. Cathay, L. Chen, S. Chigurupati, J. Chen, F. Cheung, L. M. K. Chin, B. W. Coleman, A. B. Courville, M. S. Deming, B. Drinkard, L. R. Feng, L. Ferrucci, S. A. Gabel, A. Gavin, D. S. Goldstein, S. Hassanzadeh, S. C. Horan, S. G. Horovitz, K. R. Johnson, A. J. Govan, K. M. Knutson, J. D. Kreskow, J. Levin, J. J. Lyons, N. Madian, N. Malik, A. L. Mammen, J. A. McCulloch, P. M. McGurrin, J. D. Milner, R. Moaddel, G. A. Mueller, A. Mukherjee, S. Muñoz-Braceras, G. Norato, K. Pak, I. Pinal-Fernandez, T. Popa, L. B. Reoma, M. N. Sack, F. Safavi, L. N. Saligan, B. A. Sellers, S. Sinclair, B. Smith, J. Snow, S. Solin, B. J. Stussman, G. Trinchieri, S. A. Turner, C. S. Vetter, F. Vial, C. Vizioli, A. Williams, S. B. Yang, A. Nath, and the Center for Human Immunology, Autoimmunity, and Inflammation Consortium. 2024. Deep phenotyping of post-infectious myalgic encephalomyelitis/chronic fatigue syndrome. *Nature Communications* 15(1):907.

Walters, K. M., M. Clark, S. Dard, S. S. Hong, E. Kelly, K. Kostka, A. M. Lee, R. T. Miller, M. Morris, M. B. Palchuk, E. R. Pfaff, N3C and RECOVER Consortia. 2024. National COVID cohort collaborative data enhancements: A path for expanding common data models. *Journal of the American Medical Informatics Association* 32(2):391–397.

Wearden, A. J., R. K. Morriss, R. Mullis, P. L. Strickland, D. J. Pearson, L. Appleby, I. T. Campbell, and J. A. Morris. 1998. Randomised, double-blind, placebo-controlled treatment trial of fluoxetine and graded exercise for chronic fatigue syndrome. *British Journal of Psychiatry* 172:485–490.

White, P. D., K. A. Goldsmith, A. L. Johnson, L. Potts, R. Walwyn, J. C. DeCesare, H. L. Baber, M. Burgess, L. V. Clark, D. L. Cox, J. Bavinton, B. J. Angus, G. Murphy, M. Murphy, H. O'Dowd, D. Wilks, P. McCrone, T. Chalder, and M. Sharpe. 2011. Comparison of adaptive pacing therapy, cognitive behaviour therapy, graded exercise therapy, and specialist medical care for chronic fatigue syndrome (PACE): A randomised trial. *The Lancet* 377(9768):823–836.

White, P. D., T. Chalder, M. Sharpe, B. J. Angus, H. L. Baber, J. Bavinton, M. Burgess, L. V. Clark, D. L. Cox, J. C. DeCesare, K. A. Goldsmith, A. L. Johnson, P. McCrone, G. Murphy, M. Murphy, H. O'Dowd, L. Potts, R. Walwyn, and D. Wilks. 2017. Response to the editorial by Dr Geraghty. *Journal of Health Psychology* 22(9):1113–1117.

Whitehead, L. 2009. The measurement of fatigue in chronic illness: A systematic review of unidimensional and multidimensional fatigue measures. *Journal of Pain and Symptom Management* 37(1):107–128.

WHO (World Health Organization). 2025. Chikungunya. https://www.who.int/news-room/fact-sheets/detail/chikungunya (accessed May 10, 2025).

Wiborg, J. F., J. van Bussel, A. van Dijk, G. Bleijenberg, and H. Knoop. 2015. Randomised controlled trial of cognitive behaviour therapy delivered in groups of patients with chronic fatigue syndrome. *Psychotherapy and Psychosomatics* 84(6):368–376.

Wilshire, C. E., T. Kindlon, R. Courtney, A. Matthees, D. Tuller, K. Geraghty, and B. Levin. 2018. Rethinking the treatment of chronic fatigue syndrome—A reanalysis and evaluation of findings from a recent major trial of graded exercise and CBT. *BMC Psychology* 6(1):6.

Wormser, G. P., R. J. Dattwyler, E. D. Shapiro, J. J. Halperin, A. C. Steere, M. S. Klempner, P. J. Krause, J. S. Bakken, F. Strle, G. Stanek, L. Bockenstedt, D. Fish, J. S. Dumler, and R. B. Nadelman. 2006. The clinical assessment, treatment, and prevention of Lyme disease, human granulocytic anaplasmosis, and babesiosis: Clinical practice guidelines by the Infectious Diseases Society of America. *Clinical Infectious Diseases* 43(9):1089–1134.

Young, T. P., J. S. Erickson, S. L. Hattan, S. Guzy, F. Hershkowitz, and M. D. Steward. 2024. A single-blind, randomized, placebo controlled study to evaluate the benefits and safety of endourage targeted wellness formula C sublingual +drops in people with post-acute coronavirus disease 2019 syndrome. *Cannabis and Cannabinoid Research* 9(1):282–292.

Yuan, N., Y. Chen, Y. Xia, J. Dai, and C. Liu. 2019. Inflammation-related biomarkers in major psychiatric disorders: A cross-disorder assessment of reproducibility and specificity in 43 meta-analyses. *Translational Psychiatry* 9(1):233.

Zeraatkar, D., M. Ling, S. Kirsh, T. Jassal, M. Shahab, H. Movahed, J. R. Talukdar, A. Walch, S. Chakraborty, T. Turner, L. Turkstra, R. S. McIntyre, A. Izcovich, L. Mbuagbaw, T. Agoritsas, S. A. Flottorp, P. Garner, T. Pitre, R. J. Couban, and J. W. Busse. 2024. Interventions for the management of long COVID (post-COVID condition): Living systematic review. *BMJ* 387:e081318.

Zilberman-Itskovich, S., M. Catalogna, E. Sasson, K. Elman-Shina, A. Hadanny, E. Lang, S. Finci, N. Polak, G. Fishlev, C. Korin, R. Shorer, Y. Parag, M. Sova, and S. Efrati. 2022. Hyperbaric oxygen therapy improves neurocognitive functions and symptoms of post-COVID condition: Randomized controlled trial. *Scientific Reports* 12(1):11252.

4

Innovative Approaches to Accelerating Lyme IACI Research

Many people living with Lyme infection-associated chronic illnesses (IACI) suffer from debilitating symptoms. There is an urgent need for effective treatments to improve symptoms, function, and quality of life for those affected. Innovative research approaches can accelerate progress toward safe and effective treatments and address the key research questions outlined at the end of Chapter 2. Many of the approaches discussed in this chapter are already being used in Lyme IACI research, but their implementation has been limited thus far. Greater coordination can increase the likelihood that these approaches will be used without duplicated or competing efforts and can also maximize the efficiency of financial resources. To promote such coordination, this chapter offers a common framework for the numerous funder, research, and patient organizations to identify shared research priorities for Lyme IACI treatment studies.

A COMMON FRAMEWORK TO PRIORITIZE LYME IACI RESEARCH

Clinical case reports, small or uncontrolled trials, and anecdotal evidence from people living with Lyme IACI and their care providers have identified therapeutic interventions that may be worthy of further investigation in the effort to understand these interventions' safety, efficacy, and potential for development into approved treatments. The finite nature of funding and other resource constraints generally necessitates prioritization of the areas of research with the greatest potential to improve symptoms, daily function, and quality of life.

Many factors may contribute to or influence what evidence is assessed, how the evidence is weighed, and how these considerations translate into research or funding decisions. Various priorities may be pursued by different research groups or funders in parallel; nonetheless, it is helpful for the field to agree on a general approach to identify research priorities to pursue and to understand the rationale in arriving at these decisions. The committee proposes a framework for research prioritization that outlines a systematic approach to evaluating the available evidence and making decisions (Figure 4-1).

Specifically, this proposed framework is intended to provide a balanced strategy to identify and evaluate potential therapeutic agents to inform prioritization decisions for continued or new research and build toward a portfolio approach to optimally allocate available resources. (1) **Source candidates** may be identified from established or emerging science documented in published or unpublished (e.g., proprietary) data as well as from lived experience or clinical anecdotes (Figure 4-1A). From these sources, these potential therapeutic agents may be grouped into broad (2) **intervention categories** based on their mode of action (e.g., acting on pathogen, host, symptoms, or other processes). This can then inform the relevant criteria for evaluating efficacy, clinical readiness, and safety, as well as other considerations for success in development in a systematic series of (3) **prioritization activities** to assess how a candidate fits into a coordinated portfolio of clinical research.

The series of prioritization activities can include a triage process to rule out candidate agents if they are already being investigated in other robust clinical trials for Lyme IACI, if no preclinical or clinical data on safety exist yet, or if there are insufficient preclinical or clinical data that support treatment effects. This triage reduces redundancies in the research portfolio and redirects research efforts to obtain the necessary data on safety and preliminary indications of efficacy to support consideration in the research portfolio (Figure 4-1B). Therapeutic candidates need to be screened to ensure sufficient toxicology and human data are available to guarantee that they can safely be tested in larger human clinical studies. In some instances, the safety profile of candidates may be well known, such as with approved antimicrobials, but there may be differences between the labeled and proposed use that need to be considered in clinical trials for Lyme IACI (e.g., duration of use). In other cases, the candidate may be a new molecular entity for which comprehensive preclinical development is needed prior to human studies, including toxicology.

Candidates that have been triaged may be evaluated based on four major domains: biological plausibility, availability of supportive preclinical and clinical data, and potential impact (individual and population level), as well as other considerations for the feasibility of clinical development

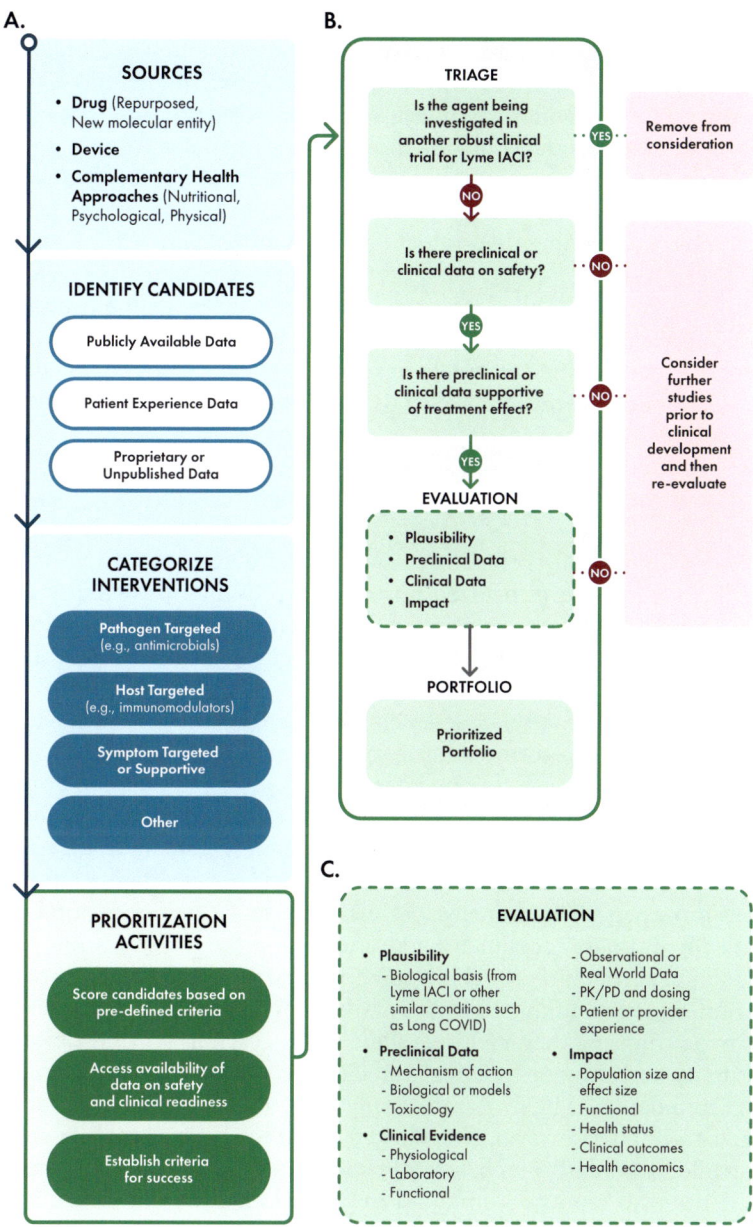

FIGURE 4-1 Framework for research prioritization of Lyme IACI treatment interventions. (A) Overall process for identification and prioritization of Lyme IACI treatment intervention candidates. (B) Decision framework for evaluating identified candidates. (C) Domains for evaluation of triaged candidates. Adapted from Buchman et al. (2021).
NOTES: IACI = infection-associated chronic illness; IND = investigational new drug; PK/PD = pharmacokinetics and pharmacodynamics.

(Figure 4-1C). For each domain, the evaluation considers whether sufficient data exist, whether the data are from rigorously conducted studies, and whether any elements listed within the domain are not required for the assessment of a particular candidate (e.g., real-world data may be applicable to repurposed products but are generally not available for new entities). In addition to a close examination of the available data, prioritization decisions may also consider factors for a viable clinical development pathway of the potential therapeutic product. Some factors include:

- Are the available data sufficient for an investigational new drug application (IND)?[1]
- Are there sufficient supply or manufacturing logistics to enable testing in large-scale clinical trials (and market access if the therapeutic agent is approved)?
- Is it supported or likely to be supported by adequate capital throughout the clinical development pathway?

Overall, potential therapeutic candidates are evaluated to ensure that those included in the prioritized portfolio have a high probability of success, while balancing the inherent risks of failure in clinical development with the envisioned benefit (e.g., high-risk–high-reward candidates may be included in the portfolio).

It is important for the assessment criteria to be clearly defined at the start of this prioritization exercise as part of a rational and systematic review of potential new treatments to avoid post hoc decisions or other sources of bias, even if the specific criteria for each of these domains may differ among the candidate types (e.g., preclinical data may derive from observational studies with human participants for some and from animal models for others). This framework thus serves as a common ground to systematically evaluate, document, and understand the prioritization process for funding, particularly for challenging situations where different researchers or funders may ultimately arrive at different decisions. For instance, consider two promising therapeutic candidates that each have robust biological plausibility and strong preclinical and clinical data that are sufficient for an IND: Candidate A is likely to affect only a subset of patients (e.g., targeting a specific symptom or symptom cluster) and thus have a small population size, while Candidate B is believed to be broadly applicable to a majority of patients who report a common symptom. However, Candidate A has a

---

[1] An investigational new drug application (IND) is "a request for authorization from the Food and Drug Administration (FDA) to administer an investigational drug or biological product to humans." It is a necessary authorization for new potential therapeutic products or uses that have not been previously approved for humans. See: NIH CC (n.d.).

more favorable clinical development pathway (e.g., clear product supply, logistics, and clinical studies design), while the many components in the clinical development pathway for Candidate B are unclear (Table 4-1). One funder may decide to prioritize Candidate A if the targeted symptom does not have any other promising treatment options and the funder perceives this as a high-need area. Given the same analysis, another funder might prioritize Candidate B if they value the larger population size for the potential treatment more, and the decisions align with the funder's "high-risk/high-reward" ethos in supporting new research. Given the dynamic nature of biomedical research, a landscape review of potential therapeutic agents, including those recently reported and those already in the portfolio, must be conducted regularly, rather than being a one-time assessment exercise. This is particularly important in light of the opportunities for applying modern technologies and methods and drawing from similar health conditions to investigate the pathogenesis and treatment of Lyme IACI that may reveal significant findings (see Box 3-2).

TABLE 4-1 Example of Applying Prioritization Assessment of Lyme IACI Treatment Interventions

Evaluation Domain	Hypothetical Candidate A	Hypothetical Candidate B
Plausibility	Established with strong evidence	
Preclinical Data	Sufficient evidence on mechanism of action (in vivo or from relevant model) and toxicology	
Clinical Data	Sufficient evidence supportive of potential clinical efficacy (e.g., physiological or laboratory measurements, functional data, patient or provider experience), favorable PK/PD, etc.	
Impact	Positive function, health status, clinical outcomes reported by patients	Positive function, health status, clinical outcomes reported by patients
	Population size: subset of patient population (estimate ≤25%) with a specific symptom or symptoms cluster	Population size: broadly applicable to patient population (estimate ≥75%) with a commonly reported symptom
	Effect size: An 8-point increase in global SF-36 score	Effect size: An 8-point increase in global SF-36 score
Clinical Development Pathways	Sufficient data for IND Capital/funding not yet secure Supply and logistics pathways are clear Clinical development pathway (phases 1–3) feasible	Sufficient data for IND Capital/funding not yet secure Supply and logistics pathways currently unclear Clinical development pathway (phases 1–3) uncertain

NOTE: IACI = infection-associated chronic illness; IND = investigational new drug; PD = pharmacodynamics; PK = pharmacokinetics.

Prioritization among potential treatments inevitably means some candidates will be excluded from the prioritized portfolio. However, a lower-priority ranking from one round of assessments does not imply that the particular research direction or proposed candidate will not produce results that lead to substantial discoveries and treatments in the future. It is important that the prioritization process be designed to incorporate new evidence as it is generated and allow for ongoing refinement of research priorities.

Given the heterogeneity in people living with Lyme IACI, the committee recognizes the need to consider a variety of interventions, sometimes in combinations, potentially including nonpharmaceutical interventions. Combination therapies have been successfully developed to treat conditions such as cancer (Jin et al., 2023), cardiovascular disease (Agarwal et al., 2024), and immune conditions (Colombel et al., 2010); but there are several challenges in evaluating them through clinical research. These challenges include identifying patients likely to benefit from combination therapy, determining the correct dosing, and designing studies that can provide informative results on the safety and efficacy of the combination. Importantly, enhanced toxicity is a major concern when multiple drugs with varying safety profiles are combined (IOM, 2012).

Ultimately, the committee decided not to apply this framework to propose a specific portfolio of priority candidates for additional study for several reasons. First, the committee acknowledges that individual funders and research organizations may have different perspectives on prioritization. Second, input from people living with Lyme IACI is built into the framework, but the robust community engagement needed to faithfully implement this framework was beyond the capabilities of this committee, given its task and timeline. Finally, the committee did not have all of the relevant expertise or time to evaluate the diversity of potential candidates that are likely to be identified for such an approach.

RESEARCH INFRASTRUCTURE

Careful consideration of needed research infrastructure is important to ensure that studies can answer their proposed research questions. Insufficient or inappropriate research infrastructure can make it challenging, if not impossible, to achieve the goals of a study, delaying treatment discovery and adoption. In this section, the committee evaluated factors related to research infrastructure that may challenge or enable effective research and how these factors can be addressed.

Participant Recruitment and Retention

Recruiting interested individuals who are willing to participate in clinical research is a challenge that is not unique to Lyme IACI research (Houghton et al., 2020). In particular, clinical researchers often fail to recruit representative samples of the intended patient population, commonly underrepresenting racial and ethnic minority groups, children, pregnant and lactating women, and members of rural communities, among others (NASEM, 2022b). The factors that impede people from participating in research are multiple, including mistrust of health care professionals or institutions and the burden of participating in research (Natale et al., 2021).

Mistrust and stigmatization as barriers to research participant recruitment are particularly relevant for Lyme IACI research. Many people with Lyme IACI symptoms have encountered stigmatization and delegitimization when seeking care from medical providers (Dumes, 2020). As a result, they may be suspicious of clinical researchers and the institutions that they represent; conversely, receiving information about clinical research from someone who is perceived as trustworthy by patients is a key facilitator to participant recruitment (Houghton et al., 2020). It will, therefore, be incumbent upon Lyme IACI researchers and clinicians to build trusting relationships with their patients and the Lyme IACI patient community. To improve recruitment, it is also important for researchers to develop relationships with the broad range of health care providers who treat people living with Lyme IACI, since many receive care from primary care physicians, specialized clinics, and complementary and alternative medicine providers (e.g., naturopaths, chiropractors, herbalists) (Ali et al., 2014).

Given the geographic distribution of Lyme IACI without nearby specialized centers for everyone, decentralized clinical trials may be a useful method to allow broader participation. Decentralized trials may be particularly helpful for those with severe symptoms, who may find participating in standard, site-based trials with frequent visits a difficult burden. Decentralized trials also provide an opportunity for community-based clinicians to engage in the conduct of research (Goodson et al., 2022).

Another barrier to participant recruitment in Lyme IACI research is the strict inclusion criteria required in some studies.[2] On the one hand, using strict inclusion criteria promotes a homogeneous study population and ensures that research participants are comparable to one another and facilitates validity the interpretation of study results. On the other hand, certain criteria may prevent many people who want to enroll in a clinical study from doing so and can slow study enrollment, complicate subgroup analyses, and limit the generalizability of research findings to a relatively

---

[2] As presented to the committee in open session by John Aucott on July 11, 2024.

small subset of the overall patient population. Expanding the study population to be more representative of the broader Lyme IACI population can improve access to trials and help produce more generalizable results but will likely require clear definition and analysis of distinct subgroups, increasing the size and costs of trials. For example, designing studies to recruit participants with and without two-tier test confirmation would enable researchers to capture a greater heterogeneity of people with Lyme IACI. Stratifying data collection and analysis based on these or other relevant patient characteristics might help researchers identify subpopulations who respond to treatment.

Ultimately, improving trial recruitment and retention will depend on people living with Lyme IACI being able to see the value in participating in clinical research. To ensure that participation is meaningful, individuals with lived experience need to be involved in the planning and design of Lyme IACI research (NASEM, 2022a). Similarly, providing mechanisms for clinicians to inform research priorities can assist recruitment, given their role in referring patients to research studies.

Study Designs

The design of a study determines the research infrastructure required. Study designs can be divided into two broad categories: interventional, in which study participants are assigned to a new intervention and typically compared with controls, and observational, in which study participants receive no research intervention and instead are observed. Interventional studies are particularly well suited to evaluate the safety and efficacy of treatments. Observational studies can be useful for understanding the natural history and outcomes of a disease, the risk factors for developing a disease or disease progression, and the long-term safety of treatments. While biomedical research has often focused on randomized controlled trials or prospective observational trials as the preferred methods to generate data in clinical research, there is robust literature on how other experimental designs can be relevant in answering some research questions or navigating limitations to the available resources (Brown et al., 2023).

Ultimately, the most appropriate study design will depend on the research question. While many different interventional and observational study designs exist, this section highlights two examples of efficient designs that are well suited to answer pressing research questions for Lyme IACI and that provide long-term value despite high start-up costs.

Interventional Adaptive Platform Trials

Traditional clinical trials are often slow and costly and do not achieve economies of scale. When multiple trials are needed for a given disease area, as is likely the case for Lyme IACI, then the serial or parallel process of setting up and conducting trials grows redundant and offers limited flexibility in adapting as learning unfolds. In contrast, platform trials, which operate off a single master protocol (Woodcock and LaVange, 2017), and adaptive trial designs, which enable flexibility in how the study is conducted by responding to evidence as it is generated (Pallmann et al., 2018), offer a learning system that can accelerate evidence generation and adapt to the most important priorities for the development of effective treatments.

Adaptive platform trials can change over time in response to emerging data, allowing new treatments to be added as they become available and ineffective treatments to be dropped in order to optimize the use of resources and time. For example, if a specific subset of participants, such as individuals with a particular condition or several subpopulations across different conditions, respond more favorably to the intervention, the randomization could be adapted to increase the number of participants within that subset who are assigned to that intervention. Master protocols used within platform trials may allow the study of multiple interventions and populations, increasing the efficiency of evidence generation. By using a common placebo or control group and shared infrastructure, the time and resources required to test new treatments can be reduced. Moreover, having a single overarching trial structure synchronizes administrative, operational, and analytical approaches to efficiently test multiple drugs or devices simultaneously or in an accelerated, semi-sequential process.

Although more resources may be needed up front to establish a flexible platform, once it is operational the potential benefits can exceed the marginal costs for each additional intervention tested when the adaptive trial is thoughtfully designed and executed. Alternatively, the serial process of one trial at a time generates operational delays and opportunity costs that could be avoided (Mahlich et al., 2021). Examples of well-designed, successful platform trial platforms include the RECOVERY (RECOVERY Collaborative Group, 2021), REMAP-CAP (REMAP-CAP Investigators, 2021), and ACTIV-6 platforms (Naggie et al., 2022). All of these were performed in the setting of acute COVID-19 in which multiple interventions needed to be tested efficiently with common data collection and endpoints.

The advantages of adaptive platform trials may be particularly relevant for Lyme IACI research, since it is complex condition likely involving multiple subpopulations of interest and mechanisms to target. However, it should be noted that adaptive designs often rely on interim analyses that depend on surrogate markers to assess benefit. In many disease areas, such surrogates do not necessarily correlate with outcomes and may not allow for a full evaluation of safety if the trials are shortened. Notably, there are no known biomarkers for Lyme IACI that correlate to treatment response, though several have been suggested in the literature (see Chapter 2).

Observational Prospective Studies

Prospective longitudinal studies are important for developing a fundamental understanding of the characteristics and mechanisms of Lyme IACI. Longitudinal study designs permit researchers to observe change over time. When longitudinal studies are conducted prospectively, research participants are observed starting before the outcome of interest occurs (e.g., disease development or symptom resolution). As described in Chapter 2, between 5 and 36 percent of people diagnosed with Lyme disease experience persistent symptoms 6 months or more after antibiotic treatment, but the causes and pathogenesis of these persistent symptoms remain unknown. A major benefit of obtaining prospective longitudinal data is that it enables researchers to study the development and progression of Lyme IACI in a group of individuals starting from the time they receive a Lyme disease diagnosis. Understanding how Lyme IACI develops and progresses can inform the design of targeted treatments. Several prospective, longitudinal studies designed to provide insights on Lyme IACI mechanisms and disease progression are in progress at the time of this report's publication (Box 4-1).

For the evidence generated by prospective observational studies to be informative, the studies must be well designed. Ideally, participants would be enrolled soon after *Borrelia spp.* infection and followed regularly for several years. Timely enrollment requires early detection of Lyme disease, which is often complicated by the inconsistent display of symptoms following infection and imperfect diagnostics (Branda and Steere, 2021; Schwartz et al., 2017). Notwithstanding, this study design would enable examination of the disease course and help identify factors that predict which individuals will return to health versus those who will develop Lyme IACI. Moreover, such studies could be designed to incorporate comparison groups, such as individuals with IACI symptoms of unknown origin, or people without *Borrelia spp.* infection, to evaluate how the comparison groups change over time relative to the participants with *Borrelia spp.* infection, given the similarities between Lyme IACI and other IACI, and the high prevalence of IACI-like symptoms in the general population (Wormser et al., 2020). Recruiting and following sufficiently large cohorts of study participants is important for several reasons. First, Lyme IACI is highly heterogeneous, and studies must have large enough sample sizes to capture that heterogeneity and help to understand its relevance to disease progression and treatment. Furthermore, large cohorts whose exposures have been well characterized over time provide greater opportunities to identify risk factors and novel therapeutic targets. For example, sex differences that are influenced by reproductive stage could be masked in a small study.

Because prospective longitudinal studies are expensive and time-intensive, they often are designed to gather data on many different exposures

> **BOX 4-1**
> **Ongoing Longitudinal Observational Studies in Lyme IACI in the U.S.**
>
> The Study of Lyme Disease Immunology and Clinical Events (SLICE) is a longstanding research study conducted by the Johns Hopkins University Lyme Disease Research Center. SLICE enrolls individuals who have recently acquired Lyme disease as well as healthy controls to better understand the disease course and outcomes of individuals diagnosed with Lyme disease. The study examines several aspects of Lyme IACI, including symptom characterization, molecular biomarkers, and the risk of developing Lyme IACI after *B. burgdorferi* infection.
>
> The Mucosal and Systemic Signatures Triggered by Responses to Infectious Organisms (MAESTRO) study at the Massachusetts Institute of Technology is another longitudinal study designed to understand how IACI symptoms develop. The MAESTRO study explores IACI broadly and includes study arms of people with Lyme disease, Lyme IACI, and Long COVID, as well as healthy controls. Researchers collect biological samples from participants to conduct antibody and metagenomic analyses. Ultimately, the study is designed to analyze why some individuals who acquire an infectious disease develop chronic symptoms after the acute infection is treated and what mechanisms contribute to the development of those chronic symptoms.
>
> A newly established prospective longitudinal study coordinated out of Tufts University—in collaboration with Northwestern University, MaineHealth, and Massachusetts General Hospital—will examine the outcomes of enrolled participants after the diagnosis of Lyme disease. The aim of the study is to explore potential mechanisms of Lyme IACI by following participants over time after Lyme disease diagnosis and treatment. Researchers also plan to establish a biobank with specimens collected during the study that can be used by other researchers.
>
> SOURCE: Aucott et al. (2016, 2022), LaPoint (2024), Rebman et al. (2017), SLICE Study (n.d.), Tufts University (2024).

that may be of interest. Collecting and storing well-characterized biological samples (e.g., serum, cells, tissues) during a prospective longitudinal study can increase the study's value and potential for use in future research as new knowledge and assays are developed. Furthermore, the application of machine learning (ML), which is discussed in more detail later in this chapter, to large datasets generated through these types of studies may help detect new and relevant factors, including genetics, co-infections, or prior infections that may result in a confluence of events that lead to Lyme IACI. The complexity of these contributions may be masked in the results of smaller studies, which is why large-scale, prospective longitudinal studies are critical to understanding the etiology and pathogenesis of Lyme IACI.

Trial Networks

Multicenter trials are a feasible approach to conducting studies that are intended to enroll large numbers of participants. Such projects are harmonized for study participant recruitment and data-collection methods and can help speed enrollment, allowing large datasets to be acquired in a relatively short time frame. However, multicenter trials require centralized oversight (e.g., a principal investigator or oversight committee), with significant administrative burden, and are expensive to execute. Trial networks can help facilitate multicenter trials, coordinate or facilitate single-center studies, and can help address the costliness of multicenter studies by reducing the administrative costs incurred by each site. One such network already operates in the Lyme disease area, the Clinical Trials Network (CTN) for Lyme and Other Tickborne Diseases, based at Columbia University. The CTN model provides a means of collaboration and general research support to Lyme studies at other sites within the network.

As explained in Chapter 3, coordinating centers can help promote harmonization and decrease administrative burden on individual sites within a trial network. For example, coordinating centers can facilitate the development or selection of uniform data content and formats used by the sites participating in the network. Moreover, the use of common data elements (CDEs) can improve data interoperability among sites by aligning common case definitions, metrics, outcomes, and data formats. Data interoperability is critical within a trial network, especially when the network is conducting a multisite trial, to allow data generated from distinct sites to be aggregated and analyzed together.

The use of a single institutional review board (sIRB) can also help ease administrative burden within a multisite trial by streamlining the IRB process through a single institution (Wolinetz and Collins, 2017). In fact, certain National Institutes of Health (NIH)–funded research that is conducted at multiple sites may require use of a sIRB (NIH, 2016).[3] A platform protocol, a type of master protocol, is another tool that trial networks can use to reduce the burden on individual sites and promote coordination within the network. Similar to platform trials, platform protocols enable the study of multiple interventions for a specific disease over time (Woodcock and LaVange, 2017). A platform protocol offers the benefit of allowing all sites within the network to operate off the same protocol while conducting research on different interventions. Ideally, the existing trial network infrastructure could be used to launch large-scale multi-site clinical trials with identical protocols across study sites. Each site could, in addition, include specialized research arms to explore additional avenues of research.

Conclusion 4-1: Clinical trial networks can foster collaboration across disparate sites that conduct Lyme IACI research.

Data Sources

Advancing Lyme IACI research will require the integration and gathering of diverse data sources to address scientific questions accurately and efficiently. The previously mentioned study designs highlight the importance of tailoring research infrastructure to the specific types of data needed to address issues. In addition to different study designs, it will also be necessary to use data sources whose contents extend beyond what clinical trials traditionally collect. The sections below explore these data sources and provide an overview of their unique benefits, limitations, and background for their use in research.

Real-World Data

The Food and Drug Administration defines real-world data (RWD) as "data relating to patient health status and/or the delivery of health care routinely collected from a variety of sources" (FDA, 2024). Real-world evidence is "the clinical evidence about the usage and potential benefits or risks of a medical product derived from analysis of RWD" (FDA, 2024). Sources of RWD are diverse and can include electronic health records, health insurance claims, product and disease registries, and wearable and other mobile technology. Accordingly, some sources of RWD are also sources of patient-generated data. In addition to the heterogeneity in data sources used to generate RWD, the fact that the data are captured in real-world environments increases the variability within and among the individuals from whom data are collected compared with the carefully defined subjects included in

---

[3] *Cooperative Research*, 45 CFR Part 46.114 (July 19, 2018).

clinical trials. For example, patients may have more variable adherence to the intervention in a study using RWD, compared with a randomized trial. Despite these limitations, RWD can be useful for a number of applications in clinical research and may in some instances, typically through including patients more fully reflective of the heterogeneity of the actual treated population, be better suited than randomized trials to draw conclusions regarding real-world safety, compliance, and effectiveness and to efficiently produce informative results (Simon et al., 2022).

There are a multitude of ways in which RWD can be used in research and decision making, including identifying potential research hypotheses and priorities, conducting long-term safety monitoring, and even making causal inferences about an intervention's effectiveness (Duke-Margolis Center for Health Policy, 2024). Regardless of the application, RWD must be fit for use, meaning that the data can address the relevant research or regulatory questions. Multiple sources of RWD—or a combination of RWD and research data—may ultimately be necessary to improve the fitness of the data (Duke-Margolis Center for Health Policy, 2019).

Assessing the quality of data obtained from an RWD source is fundamental to predicting its likely utility in generating evidence. RWD is generally not produced with future research applications in mind and is often unstructured and heterogeneous and includes errors and missing information (Liu and Panagiotakos, 2022). To address these challenges, it is important to validate that the data meet defined minimum quality principles. While the data-quality principles for RWD may vary across organizations, principles include:

- Conformance: Do the structure and format of the data conform with prespecified standards?
- Completeness: Are data values reported frequently enough for variables of interest (i.e., what is the rate of missingness in the data)?
- Plausibility: Are the data believable and conform with expectations for potential values and relationships? (Duke-Margolis Center for Health Policy, 2019)

ML also presents an opportunity to derive useful information from unstructured RWD, though researchers and clinicians must exercise caution in interpreting results from ML software (Liu and Panagiotakos, 2022).

A particular challenge to the broader adoption of RWD in Lyme IACI is the lack of both generally accepted diagnostic criteria for Lyme IACI and an *International Classification of Diseases* (ICD) code for the disorder. ICD codes provide a standardized approach to tracking a patient's diagnosis, and are therefore ubiquitous in electronic health records and billing claims often used in research employing RWD. However, without clear diagnostic criteria or an ICD code for Lyme IACI, it is challenging to define or identify individuals with Lyme IACI within these RWD sources. However, CDEs may help to identify people with possible Lyme IACI within certain sources of RWD. For example, a Lyme IACI symptom and disease history questionnaire that can both identify potential individuals with Lyme IACI and distinguish patient subgroups based on the likelihood that symptoms are related to Lyme disease would be a useful tool to adopt as a CDE. While it would be infeasible to adopt such a questionnaire as a CDE throughout the entire health system, clinics and registries that frequently encounter patients with Lyme disease and Lyme IACI could increase the research value of the data they collect by incorporating a similar tool into their routine processes. And even clinics without routine Lyme patient encounters could improve the utility of their records for RWD purposes by clearly reporting the method and date of Lyme disease diagnosis and documenting any symptoms that develop after diagnosis.

Patient-Generated Data

One type of real-world data that has been incorporated into existing Lyme IACI research is patient-generated data. Patient-generated data can come in many different forms, such as outcome data collected through a validated self-reporting instrument, data from wearable technologies, and data entered by individuals in disease registries or personal health trackers. This section focuses on patient registries. Patient-reported outcome (PRO) measures are discussed later in this chapter. Existing patient registries for Lyme IACI contain patient-generated and real-world data and are developed and maintained by patients. These include, but are not limited to, self-reported clinical data, such as diagnostic results, symptoms experienced and their severity over time, and experiences or results from a variety of interventions. Some registries are also tied to biological samples. Analysis of such datasets could help researchers identify and understand the characteristics of symptoms that matter most to people living with Lyme IACI, informing the planning and conduct of research. Common symptoms of those with Lyme IACI include fatigue, pain, and cognitive dysfunction (Rebman et al., 2017; Touradji et al., 2019). However, there appears to be a lack of quantitative or qualitative research on the symptoms people living with Lyme IACI deem most necessary to address to "return to functionality." Similarly, data from patient registries could be interrogated to derive the relevance of existing PROs or to help generate new ones. If the data do not already exist, registries can often be used to send out health surveys and questionnaires to derive the exact information desired from large sample sizes relatively quickly.

For patient registry data to be useful for research applications, the data must be representative of the heterogeneous Lyme IACI population. This standard may be difficult to meet for registries in which patients self-enroll due to the high potential for selection bias. Use of representative samples from within the registry or statistical methods such as weighting could help address this limitation. Further, to understand whether registry data are representative of the Lyme IACI population, the registry must collect and store data on the sociodemographic characteristics (e.g., age, sex, race and ethnicity) and health histories (e.g., diagnostic information, relevant exposures) of participants in sufficient detail.

There are inherent risks to using retrospective data contained in many patient registries without fully understanding and considering the data's quality. The quality of retrospective data relies upon accurate self-reporting based on an individual's memory, but in reality, they may be highly variable. Thus researchers must be mindful of learning about the registry's data-collection procedures and what filters are available for the data recording and extraction process in order to support the scientific rigor and reproducibility of the research using these data. Similarly, it is important for patient registries to implement standardized data collection procedures to minimize measurement bias. For example, the Patient-Centered Outcomes Research Institute outlines standards to improve the quality and transparency of patient registries (PCORI, 2024). Despite such risks, patient registries have the potential to provide important information about the symptoms and course of disease and to identify and elevate patient priorities, potentially accelerating research.

Another benefit to using patient registries is the opportunity they offer for people living with Lyme IACI and researchers to work collaboratively. For decades the Lyme IACI patient community has been raising awareness among researchers, clinicians, and policymakers about the toll of Lyme IACI. Yet, stigmatization of individuals with Lyme IACI has often persisted, in part due to a lack of understanding of both the disorder and patient experiences. Not only does stigmatization marginalize the Lyme IACI community, but it may also limit access to health care, potentially contributing to disability and death (e.g., suicide is a major cause of death in Lyme IACI) (Bransfield, 2017). Rebuilding the bonds of trust and communication, including offering acknowledgments of past harm, will be necessary for effective future collaborations. Working alongside patient communities requires and can help build respect for patients' perspectives and their decades of investments into the development of registries and the information these registries contain. Therefore, using patient registries in Lyme IACI research not only accelerates the search for symptom-based treatments that are most meaningful to the people living with Lyme IACI, but also can forge bonds between the medical, academic, and patient communities that strengthen trust and communication.

Patient registries can also be used as a recruitment platform for clinical trials, allowing researchers to meet enrollment targets more effectively. Developing and maintaining a patient registry can be expensive (Gliklich et al., 2020). Therefore, using the participants, infrastructure, and data that already exist within a patient registry to design and conduct clinical trials can make good use of the investment in the registry and save money compared to traditional trials (Anderson et al., 2020).

Biobanks

Biobanks are entities that collect and store human biological samples, such as tissue or blood, along with data associated with those samples for use in research. Biobanks are also often characterized by the presence of established governance structures that permit outside researchers access to the samples and data contained within them (Coppola et al., 2019). The biological specimens and data contained in biobanks are fundamental in biomedical research, enabling discoveries of the etiology, pathological mechanisms, risk factors, and molecular signatures of disease and treatment response (Annaratone et al., 2021; Harris et al., 2012). Researchers increasingly turn to biobanks to support a variety of applications, particularly for studies using human tissues, such as the creation of diagnostic tools, and the identification of biomarkers to guide treatment and diagnosis (Mackenzie, 2014). While their value to research is increasingly recognized, biobanks face financial strains from short-term funding and insufficient cost recovery that imperil their sustainability (Annaratone et al., 2021).

There are several active biobanks dedicated to Lyme disease. While this list is likely not comprehensive, these include:

- Columbia Lyme and Tick-Borne Diseases Research Center specimen bank
- Johns Hopkins SLICE biobank
- Lyme Disease Biobank
- Lyme serum repository
- Pediatric Lyme Biobank (Bay Area Lyme Research Foundation, n.d.; Boston Children's Hospital, n.d.; CUMC, 2025; Johns Hopkins Lyme Disease Research Center, 2025; Molins et al., 2014).

Still, the samples and data contained within these various biobanks could be used more consistently in Lyme IACI research. Out of 68 articles on Lyme IACI mechanism and diagnosis research included in the scoping review,

26 (38 percent) did not use any human biological samples. Of the other 42 articles that did report use of human biospecimens, three (7 percent) included samples from biobanks, while the other 39 articles reported using specimens that were collected during a previous study but not necessarily stored in a biobank. Most studies reviewed did not use biobanks despite their potential to optimize research for Lyme IACI by cutting down on enrollment times and improving data comparability.

To ensure the continued and expanded access to biobank samples in Lyme IACI research, it is imperative to address some of the challenges commonly encountered in biobanking. First, the quality of biobanks' biological samples and associated data, as well as the collection and storage methods are fundamental to their utility in clinical research (Dagher, 2022). Since many biobanks develop independently of one another, harmonizing collection and storage procedures can be difficult, affecting the validity and utility of collected samples and complicating research that aggregates or compares samples from multiple biobanks (Coppola et al., 2019). Similarly, standardizing metadata annotations, such as data provenance and experimental protocols, is important to promoting quality and interoperability of a biobank's data (Alkhatib and Gaede, 2024). Characterizing samples to an appropriate level of detail and specificity is another challenge that can threaten the utility of samples for research,[4] especially given the lack of established diagnostic criteria for Lyme IACI. Including well-characterized controls—such as healthy participants, samples collected before COVID, and participants with other IACI—within Lyme IACI biobanks will also be important for conducting comparative analyses. Several organizations have published best practices and standards in an effort to promote harmonization and quality in biobanking, including the International Society for Biological and Environmental Repositories and the International Organization for Standardization (International Standard, 2018; Snapes et al., 2023). Adherence to validated quality standards, such as those mentioned, is essential for Lyme IACI biobanks to be useful in research.

Biobank sustainability is yet another concern, given the open-endedness of their operation. Beyond ongoing funding, sustainability in terms of continuing to provide value to participants and researchers is a key consideration (Abdaljaleel et al., 2019; Coppola et al., 2019). To continue to provide value, it is critical for biobanks to adopt a reciprocal relationship with specimen donors, requiring collaboration with donors and relevant patient and advocacy groups. Moreover, it is important for biobanks and the researchers who use their samples to have a plan for returning aggregated research results to the individuals whose samples contributed to the research. There are also considerations unique to Lyme IACI for promoting

---

[4] As presented to the committee in open session by Liz Horn on July 11, 2024.

good stewardship of donor samples, including tiered informed consent approaches that enable donors to opt in to having samples used for research on other IACI and making accommodations during the informed consent process for prospective participants with neurocognitive symptoms as a result of Lyme IACI.[5] These considerations are important for building trust with the patient community.

Finally, access, governance, and transparency need to be considered in the development and operations of a biobank (Langhof et al., 2018). It is important that the governance structures of biobanks clearly outline the process for granting researchers access to samples and for participants to be informed of how their donated samples and data may be used. The development of a virtual catalog of biological samples and the data elements associated with those samples has been a successful strategy for improving awareness and accessibility of biological samples in research. Examples of where this strategy has been employed include the Stanford Biobank Laboratory Inventory Management System (Stanford Medicine, n.d.), OneDukebio Integrated Biospecimen Network (Duke University, n.d.), and National Heart, Lung, and Blood Institute Biologic Specimen and Data Repository Information Coordinating Center (NIH, n.d.). A similar approach could simplify and expand access to the patchwork network of Lyme IACI biobank samples.

Conclusion 4-2: Data from biobanks and registries can be highly informative and foundational for hypothesis generation and designing and carrying out treatment and mechanistic studies, but is currently underused due to a lack of awareness, coordination, governance, accessibility, sustainability, and standardization across biobanks and patient registries.

Conclusion 4-3: There is inconsistency in the provenance and standardization of registry data, biological samples, awareness of existing data domains, and quality of data generated through Lyme disease registries as well as heterogeneity in patients, which has limited the data's usefulness in research studies.

Diagnostic Tools

There is currently no diagnostic for Lyme IACI. However, currently available approaches to diagnose Lyme disease and co-infections, despite their limitations, could help designate relevant subpopulations for research. Additionally, emerging approaches to characterizing unique biomarker

---

[5] As presented to the committee in open session by Liz Horn on July 11, 2024.

profiles in Lyme IACI could, given additional research, assist in the diagnosis of Lyme IACI.

Diagnostics to Facilitate Stratification in Research

To investigate treatments for Lyme IACI, it is essential that patients be selected using accepted criteria of clinical diagnosis and it may be necessary to allocate patients to subgroups by scientifically valid criteria, which may include diagnostic testing. Ideally, the diagnostic tools would be widely available so that patients for prospective studies can be recruited widely from geographic areas beyond those located near major academic research centers.

To advance clinical trials of interventions treating Lyme IACI, it is important to use laboratory results from diagnostic assays for which the accuracy is known to stratify research participants in terms of those with and those without clear evidence of prior *Borrelia* spp. infection. Importantly, there are limitations to current Lyme disease diagnostics, given that standard two-tier serologic tests have a sensitivity of approximately 30 percent at the time of initial diagnosis of early Lyme disease (e.g., erythema migrans) and ranging from 34 percent to 61 percent in the 1–4 weeks after clinical diagnosis and initiation of antimicrobial therapy (Branda et al., 2011; Molins et al., 2014). The Tick-Borne Disease Working Group at the Department of Health and Human Services has submitted reports to Congress with recommendations regarding the improvement of both direct detection and indirect methods to provide laboratory evidence of Lyme disease, babesiosis, anaplasmosis, and deer tick virus. These reports—released in 2018, 2020, and 2022—are fundamental resources that identify the consensus for diagnosis of acute and early-stage tick-borne disease, topics that are out of scope for this committee (TBDWG, 2018, 2020, 2022).

In addition to classifying Lyme disease diagnosis history based on serologic evidence of *B. burgdorferi* infection and according to prior infection or coinfection with other tick-borne pathogens (e.g. babesiosis, anaplasmosis, Powassan virus), diagnostic tests and biomarkers for IACI, if they are identified, could be used to stratify patients into subgroups such as Lyme IACI only, Lyme IACI plus evidence of prior co-infections, Lyme IACI plus other IACI, and other relevant diagnoses

As described in Chapter 1, several diagnostic strategies are currently used to diagnose *B. burgdorferi* infection. Serological tools with multiplex capacity are currently available and can be designed to measure evidence of past exposure to the agents of multiple tick-borne infections, including Lyme disease, babesiosis, anaplasmosis, and deer tick virus, simultaneously. Microsphere immunoassay on the Luminex analyzer and line immunoblots with recombinant proteins of the target pathogens are currently available tools for both research and diagnostic testing (Porwancher et al., 2011; Shah et al., 2023). While these assays have not been reviewed by the FDA, there are proposed means to define accepted criteria for these assays. For example, the Clinical Laboratory Evaluation Program of the Wadsworth Center, New York State Department of Health, publishes their criteria for review and approval of laboratory-developed tests that can then be used for diagnosis and research purposes.[6] Laboratory-developed tests (i.e., not FDA-approved) that meet validation criteria for research purposes and as clinical diagnostics may in some cases be useful in allocating patients to Lyme IACI subgroups in the design of clinical research.

Diagnostics to Identify Co-Infections

Possible tick-borne coinfections that might be present from an *Ixodes* tick bite include babesiosis, anaplasmosis, and the deer tick lineage of Powassan viral encephalitis (Project Lyme, 2021). To date there is no strong evidence that bartonellosis results from tick bites (CDC, 2024). Simultaneous co-infections sometimes occur and may cause more severe disease than a single infection (Cutler et al., 2021). On the other hand, immune activation or immune priming may hasten the clearance of the pathogens. In terms of tick-transmitted illnesses, while simultaneous infection may occur, at other times a person is infected first by one pathogen and then weeks or months later by a second pathogen from another tick bite. If a person is at risk of one tick bite, it is possible that their environment or activities put them at risk of another tick bite.

While a review of diagnostics for various tick-borne infections is beyond the scope of this committee's task, the proper diagnosis of co-infections is important in Lyme IACI research. First, it is important to rule out an untreated co-infection as a cause of, or contributor to, persistent symptoms following Lyme disease. Second, characterizing whether people with Lyme IACI have also had certain tick-borne co-infections could be informative in better understanding Lyme IACI (NIAID, 2025), and may be important in considering design or interpretation of clinical studies. New technologies, such as multiplex diagnostics, may be able to advance accurate and timely diagnosis of co-infections (Nigrovic et al., 2023), but attention will need to be paid to the accuracy feasibility of these technologies before they can be more broadly adopted.

Importantly, if a person has Lyme IACI, it is likely that at least several months have passed since the original tick encounter, meaning that testing

---

[6] Relevant criteria published by the Wadsworth Center include the Diagnostic Immunology Checklist and the Microbiology Molecular Checklist, particularly the Validation of Next Generation Sequencing Methods for Identification and/or characterization of Infectious Agents. See: New York State, n.d.

for the presence of *Borrelia* infection by direct detection methods is highly likely to be negative. Serology is more likely to be positive, but antibody levels may have waned below a significant cutoff level for positivity. When several months have passed since the infected tick bite, infections may be at a point where no live organisms are present in the individual, and a positive result not only is unlikely (with the exception of joint fluid in active Lyme arthritis) but may not indicate the presence of active infection, but rather persistence of *B. burgdorferi* DNA (Marques, 2015).

If an individual with Lyme IACI symptoms is diagnosed with an ongoing tick-borne co-infection, it is important that the person receive treatment for the co-infection, if indicated. Fortunately, the generally recommended first-line therapy for Lyme disease, doxycycline, is also highly effective against *Anaplasma*. Doxycycline is not effective for babesiosis, for which the recommended therapy, if indicated, is atovaquone plus azithromycin or clindamycin plus quinine. There is only supportive therapy for infection with Powassan virus (Yale Medicine, n.d.).

Prospective observational studies are needed to ascertain the possible clinical impact of other concurrent or sequential tick-borne infections on the development, diagnosis, treatment, and prognosis of Lyme IACI. In parallel, trials for new treatments can determine and document participant status on prior infections (i.e., *Anaplasma*, babesiosis, and deer tick virus infection) at the time of enrollment and throughout the study so that this information can inform the categorization of subgroups and related data analyses for Lyme IACI research.

Diagnostic assays for the most common human disease-causing pathogens transmitted by *Ixodes scapularis* and *I. pacificus* are available and reviewed in depth elsewhere (Rowan et al., 2023; TBDWG, 2022). The development and use of diagnostic tests need to be fit for purpose, such as tracking disease epidemiology, guiding treatment, or research and discovery. Immunoassays are appropriate for prospective observational studies designed to gain understanding of the prevalence and influence of co-infections on Lyme IACI without seeking to provide treatment for acute infections and can be developed as multiplex tests for broad use.

Multiplex diagnostic tests can be used to identify multiple pathogens from the same sample within one reaction (e.g., molecular or immunoassay). One key technical challenge in multiplex diagnostic tests is the potential for cross-reactivity between the different antigens covered in the panel. The higher complexity of the reaction may also affect sensitivity and specificity for a multiplex panel (Otoo and Schlappi, 2022). There are no FDA-approved tick-borne diseases multiplex panels for use in humans, although research-use-only panels for common tick-borne pathogens have been published (Buchan et al., 2019; Nigrovic et al., 2023; Tokarz et al., 2018), and some laboratory-developed tests are in use (Mayo Clinic

Laboratories, n.d.). Future development of multiplex diagnostic panels for human use will need to clearly define the intended application of the test and balance benefits from the test with potential drawbacks such as costliness or inappropriate distress that could stem from false-positive results (Box 4-2). Metagenomic next-generation sequencing (NGS) is an emerging diagnostic approach that could enable the simultaneous analysis of genetic material from multiple pathogens (Chiu and Miller, 2019). While in early development, there is emerging evidence that metagenomic NGS could be a tool to conduct host transcriptomic analyses to detect altered gene expression within humans as an indicator of host response (Omura et al., 2025). Without a clear rationale, including use cases and market strategy, it may be difficult to justify the cost-effectiveness of development, manufacturing, and use of the diagnostic test with device developers and health care payors.

BOX 4-2
Considerations for Multiplex Tick-borne Disease Diagnostics to Understand the Impact of Co-Infections on Lyme IACI

Multiplex tests may be a helpful tool in gathering epidemiologic data on co-infections with Lyme disease to determine whether these affect the development and disease course of Lyme IACI. Ideally, these tests would use samples that are easy to obtain (e.g., serum instead of cerebrospinal fluid) and do not require highly specialized equipment or personnel to perform (e.g., standardized immunoassays without the need for a high-containment laboratory).

Multiplex panels are particularly useful when there are multiple likely causative agents for a syndrome. A review of FDA-approved multiplex diagnostic panels for common respiratory, gastrointestinal, and central nervous system infections reveals important caveats for use of these tests that may be relevant for future tick-borne disease multiplex tests. Multiplex tests may be more costly and have lower sensitivity or specificity than individual assays, so cost-effectiveness and appropriateness need to be carefully assessed to guide their use. For example, clear epidemiologic evidence that certain co-infections are risk factors for developing or worsening Lyme IACI could favor the use of a tick-borne diseases panel at initial diagnosis. However, as with existing diagnostics for Lyme disease, multiplex test results need to be interpreted carefully, since the detection of pathogen-specific antibodies or the presence of genomic material does not provide information on whether there is an active infection or the recency of past infection.

SOURCE: Hanson and Couturier (2016).

Emerging Approaches in Diagnostics for Lyme IACI

As noted in Chapter 2, no current diagnostic is capable of identifying individuals with Lyme IACI. However, novel technologies are being studied for the potential capability to detect changes in biomarkers that may be characteristic of Lyme IACI or other IACI. For example, one study using proteomics on cerebrospinal fluid (CSF) reported increases in several markers of complement activation that appeared to discriminate myalgic encephalitis/chronic fatigue syndrome (ME/CFS) from neurological post-treatment Lyme disease (PTLDS) (Schutzer et al, 2011). Similarly, another study suggested the ability of an ML algorithm to distinguish between individuals with Long COVID and Lyme IACI based on cytokine profiles (Patterson et al., 2024). In other studies, increases in cytokines such as IL-23 and interferon-alpha, and chemokines including CCL19, were reported that, if confirmed, may help discriminate individuals with Lyme IACI from persons who respond to therapy for Lyme disease (Aucott et al., 2016; Hernández et al., 2023; Strle et al., 2014). While in the early stages, the application of ML can be implemented to aid in developing new approaches to diagnosis. Significant advances have been made for cancer and rare disease genetic diagnostics and treatments using ML, but there has been little research conducted on its application in IACI. One study examining the proteomic profiles of individuals with Long COVID used ML to develop a random forest model, which was reported to accurately distinguish those with Long COVID from healthy controls (Gu et al., 2023). These and other promising approaches, particularly if confirmed, may also be tested in Lyme IACI.

Metabolomics analysis may also be useful in developing a diagnostic for Lyme IACI. One study observed notable differences between a group of Lyme disease patients who went on to develop PTLDS and those who returned to health after treatment, measured at the initial time point of diagnosis, at completion of antibiotics treatment (2 to 3 weeks after diagnosis), and one year after completion of treatment. Researchers identified and measured over 100 small molecule metabolites that formed the basis of biosignatures for the PTLDS and non-PTLDS groups. A smaller set of 72 small molecule metabolites demonstrated the strongest discriminatory effect between the two groups. The researchers validated their findings with a second cohort of people with and without PTLDS and observed similar longitudinal patterns (Fitzgerald et al., 2021).

Transcriptomics, which measures the expression of cellular mRNA to observe the effects of an infectious agent on host cell gene expression, is another method that may be promising for understanding and diagnosing Lyme or other IACI (Bouquet et al., 2016). Using RNA sequencing, a study compared the transcriptome profiles of 15 individuals with Lyme disease who returned to health with the profiles of 13 individuals with persistent symptoms after having Lyme disease. While no differentially expressed genes were observed between the two groups at individual time points (time of diagnosis, post-treatment, and 6-months post-treatment), combining the three time points revealed genes whose expression differed between those with resolved Lyme disease and those with persistent symptoms (Bouquet et al., 2016). Further examination in a larger study could help determine whether transcriptomic-based diagnostics may be capable of identifying individuals with Lyme IACI.

While promising, these tools are in the preliminary stages of validation for Lyme IACI diagnosis, are expensive, and are not widely accessible for primary care sites. Additional research into the candidate biomarkers identified through these emerging diagnostic approaches is needed to validate these tools. However, there are numerous opportunities to further evaluate these tools using prospective observational studies, specimens and data from biobanks, and other samples collected and stored in clinical trials.

DATA INTERPRETATION

Data can only be useful for solving scientific problems if they can be meaningfully interpreted. As more data are generated through improvements in research, it will be essential to develop novel approaches to interpret these larger quantities of data. One of the fundamental aspects of data interpretation is ensuring that the data are standardized with an emphasis on uniformity across different datasets.

Data Standardization

The use of common research tools and outcome measures across studies would facilitate direct study comparisons and data aggregation. Most data must be collected using identical and consistent methods and measures for comparisons across studies to be valid. Moreover, understanding the source of data is fundamental to accurately interpret and compare findings. Therefore, it is critical that certain data domains be routinely included in clinical research. These domains must be guided by patient-reported priorities to target the most important symptoms and quality-of-life issues and by the data quality needed for research. For example, standardized approaches to collecting and reporting disease and sociodemographic characteristics will be particularly important to defining the data's source population and promoting data quality in future analyses. CDEs, introduced in Chapter 3, encourage data standardization within a disease area across discrete research studies.

The development of CDEs for Lyme IACI may be guided by similar efforts in ME/CFS research. Defined CDEs for ME/CFS are encouraged to be used for studies on the condition and are classified into four categories: (1) Core, general information typically required for all studies funded by the National Institute of Neurological Disorders and Stroke, (2) Supplemental—Highly Recommended, specific to the disease, (3) Supplemental, common to clinical research but depends upon the protocol, and (4) Exploratory, which still requires validation. Due to the large degree of symptom overlap between Lyme IACI and ME/CFS, some elements may transfer directly (Bai and Richardson, 2023). In developing such CDEs, however, it will be important to develop Lyme-centric, patient-driven symptom measures for treatment endpoints.

CDEs will be particularly valuable if they are able to be tied into health care practice with the use of consistent coding conditions (e.g., to build accurate patient cohorts). As with the ME/CFS example, a committee that includes the research community and Lyme IACI patient representation may be helpful for determining CDEs for future Lyme IACI clinical research that will prioritize outcomes important to the Lyme IACI patient community.

The use of CDEs in Lyme IACI research would strengthen and accelerate research efforts in multiple ways, including data sharing, data mining, comparisons with other IACIs with overlapping CDEs, patient stratification (e.g., based on symptoms), identification of core data characteristics, and uniform classification of clinical markers. While the standardization offered by CDEs confers many benefits, it is important to allow for flexibility across study protocols, especially as exploratory treatments may not align precisely with CDE specifications. Separate CDEs for various study approaches would be helpful, enabling researchers to choose instruments best suited to their research question. For researchers new to the field, or those seeking guidance in a new area of Lyme IACI research, the publication of Lyme IACI CDEs could help identify which instruments to use and which variables to collect, expediting start-up time. Simple CDE sets that are not overly prescriptive would be easiest to implement, promoting early adoption.

The inclusion of standardized and validated PROs that are already known to be acceptable to regulators (e.g., the FDA) within CDEs could expedite approvals of new treatments. Of the 68 articles included in the treatment or mechanisms category of the scoping review, 34 did not report using any PRO tools in their study, 22 used structured PRO tools (e.g., SF-36, Fatigue Severity Scale), eight used unstructured methods (e.g., direct patient-reported symptoms), and four used data from MyLymeData, for which it was not possible to ascertain the types of tools used to collect data from individuals (Figure 4-2). Of the 22 articles that used structured PRO tools, six articles used tools specifically related to Lyme disease or Lyme IACI, such as the General Symptom Questionnaire-30 (GSQ-30) or

Post-Lyme Questionnaire of Symptoms (PLQS). From the evidence reviewed by the committee, it appears the use of standardized PRO tools, especially tools designed for Lyme disease or Lyme IACI, is limited within Lyme IACI research.

Currently, many Lyme IACI studies use the SF-36 as a measure of study outcomes. As a survey that assesses patient-reported quality-of-life measures related to physical health and mental health, the SF-36 is a generic tool used across many different disease areas and has not been specifically tailored to address multisystemic Lyme IACI symptoms. Several outcome measurement tools have been developed specifically to measure outcomes in people with Lyme IACI, including the GSQ-30 (Fallon et al., 2019) and the Multiple Systemic Infectious Disease Syndrome (MSIDS) model (Horowitz and Freeman, 2018). The GSQ-30 was specifically developed to assess patient-reported multisystem symptom burden in a brief format (Fallon et al., 2019), focusing on four core domains: pain/fatigue, neuropsychiatric, neurologic, and viral-like symptoms. However, these scoring domains have not been compared directly with other standard measuring tools. For instance, the GSQ-30 has not been compared with the SF-36 to address whether one may be more effective than the other for measuring treatment outcomes in a way that is meaningful to people living with Lyme IACI. Importantly, the GSQ-30 was modeled on existing scales and clinical experience rather than originating directly from patient input.

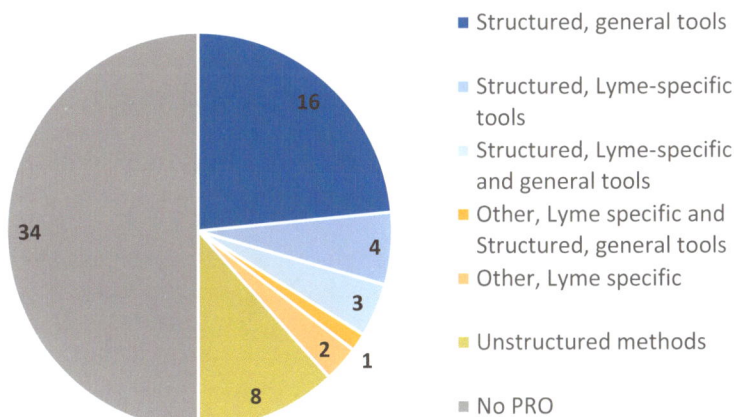

FIGURE 4-2 Types of patient-reported outcome tools used in Lyme IACI research articles identified in the committee's scoping review.
NOTES: IACI = infection-associated chronic illnesses; PRO = patient-reported outcome.

A validated outcome measurement tool that captures the symptoms most relevant to people with Lyme IACI is needed to improve comparisons across future studies and to steer those studies toward measuring the most pressing outcomes. The involvement of people with lived experience in the development of PROs is necessary to improve the relevance and comprehensibility of these tools, and to enhance the validity of studies that use the tools (Wiering et al., 2017). It is also essential for outcome measures and tools to be validated and acceptable to regulators so that their use can inform approval decisions. Moreover, outcome measurement tools have not generally been tailored to capture symptoms as experienced by pediatric patients. In developing such surveys, it will be vital to incorporate developmentally appropriate language or to create versions that could be completed by caregivers, or both.

Conclusion 4-4: There is a lack of standardized, validated measures for Lyme IACI study outcomes. It is unclear if existing measures adequately reflect patient well-being and clinical responses to treatment interventions. In particular, there are no validated tools developed for the pediatric population.

Outcome Evaluation

Determining the efficacy of a treatment is one of the core functions of clinical trials. This requires a comparison between the treatment's effects on a particular outcome or set of outcomes, compared with the effects of no active treatment or an alternative treatment. There are numerous statistical calculations that can determine the effect of an intervention on an outcome (e.g., relative risk, hazard ratio). Likewise, there are several statistical approaches to comparing the effects in different study arms to assess the likelihood that an intervention is associated with a specific outcome. However, the statistical significance of a result is not the same as clinical relevance—a large enough trial can produce a statistically significant result from just a small difference in outcomes that may not be clinically meaningful (Kieser et al., 2013). Conversely, due to issues in study design or size, some clinically meaningful effects may not reach commonly used levels of statistical significance. Therefore, measuring the effect size—or the magnitude of the treatment's effect—is important to understanding the clinical relevance of a treatment's effect (Aarts et al., 2014).

The minimal clinically important difference (MCID) is a concept that can help improve understanding of the clinical relevance of a treatment's effect, especially when PROs are used to assess outcomes. The MCID, which represents the smallest amount an outcome must change to be meaningful to patients, can contextualize an effect size within the values and priorities of patients (McGlothin and Lewis, 2014; Mouelhi et al., 2020). For example, a relatively small change in fatigue scores may represent meaningful relief for patients, or a large numerical change in an outcome measure may not affect how a patient feels. Ideally, evaluation studies would be conducted to determine the MCID for the particular outcome measure and patient population for which the MCID will be used, but they can be estimated using effect sizes or approximated by anchoring the outcome measure to an external measure—such as the global rating of change score—if a study is not feasible (Angst et al., 2017; Wright et al., 2012).

Artificial Intelligence[7]

Advances in AI models, which include ML approaches, can be applied to create tools that provide unique opportunities to advance Lyme IACI research. These models are particularly well suited to analyze disparate sources and types of data, including large and complex datasets, to identify new insights or generate hypotheses. Research tools that incorporate AI are relatively new technologies and will require significant human oversight, including from individuals with expertise in the development and use of these tools as well as in the underlying biological and clinical science.

Identifying Commonalities and Differences Between IACI

The need for expanding collection of data in research for complex IACI in order to distinguish commonalities and differences, discussed in Chapter 3, could involve deep phenotyping studies on defined disease (e.g., ME/CFS) or broadened inclusion for studies that allow enrollment from more than one disease (e.g., a clinical trial on fatigue that can include Lyme IACI and ME/CFS). Either approach will inevitably generate large amounts of data. AI tools could be used to make qualitative and quantitative comparisons and identify areas of similarity between Lyme IACI and other IACI. For example, AI tools could parse specific research findings, compare biomarkers and biometrics of interest, and generate testable hypotheses that predict relationships among IACI symptoms, pathogenesis, and etiology or risk factors. Immune profiling studies at single timepoints show common inflammatory markers across ages, including for individuals with autoimmune and neurological disorders (Chen et al., 2023; Nature Immunology, 2025; Wang et al., 2025; Zaslavsky et al., 2025). Time-based AI analyses that could be relevant to Lyme IACI also show early promise. Computational models predicting the dynamics of antibody memory formation from omics screens can help understand an individual's

---

[7] This section draws largely from a commissioned paper authored by Dr. Amina Qutub, a consultant to the committee.

immune cell exposures—potentially elucidating the environmental trigger of IACI symptoms (Cvijović et al., 2025). These tools may have applications in research on diagnostics that can distinguish between various IACI and identify potential treatment targets that several IACI have in common.

One specific application to facilitate usability for researchers is development of an integrative, searchable, AI-friendly database or federated data ecosystem that links IACI symptomatology, pathophysiology, and research categories and empowers researchers to identify connections. If a comprehensive Lyme IACI dataset is available, AI algorithms could quickly learn from it, drawing connections among the data that might otherwise be missed in manual evaluation. Among the benefits of using a well-established big data and an AI framework to host Lyme IACI data are the time saved in using robust database tools and the ability to quickly cross-reference new data for Lyme IACI with external public data resources. Connecting the Lyme IACI dataset with additional data from Long COVID, ME/CFS, and other conditions could allow identification of pathogenesis mechanisms that are shared across these diseases. There are existing examples of relevant, open public databases, including Google's COVID Symptoms dataset and the National Library of Medicine's COVID sequencing datasets.

Large language models (LLMs) are generative AI models that pre-train on massive amounts of textual or image data, or both (e.g., books, scientific literature, programming code) and then use statistical methods to predict relationships among letters, words, and sentences in the sequence of text or pixel relationships in an image. Since LLMs are adept at analyzing data and probabilistically inferring connections based on prior knowledge, they can generate hypotheses for Lyme IACI research if curated, high-quality data were available. Each of such AI-generated mechanistic hypothesis would still need to be tested, and any predictive models will need further validation from new patient datasets or clinical studies.

Challenges for the application of AI to Lyme IACI and other IACI include heterogeneity of the chronic symptoms; the combinatorial complexity of environmental, social, and psychological effects on the disease course; and lack of a single defining molecular feature (e.g., a single mutation present in some rare genetic diseases). One approach that has been taken to account for analogous challenges in other areas of biology research, such as experiments that measure a limited signal per molecule or drug development research with small effect sizes is the incorporation of weights for specific biomarkers and mathematical rules based on known immunological significance of a protein in predictive models. For example, a study on Long COVID developed the "long-hauler index," a formula that defines an algebraic relationship among the cytokines IFN-α, CCL4, and IL-2 (Patterson et al., 2024).

However, rule-based AI approaches will need to address the lack of a unified vetting process for data quality, inconsistency across research methods, and heterogeneity across patients and within patients over time. Similarly, without defined "gold standards" to delineate Lyme IACI and other IACI by molecular or phenotypic characteristics, the ability to apply supervised learning that predicts categories of IACI remains limited. Unsupervised approaches, including clustering, LLMs, and dimensional reduction methods that find patterns across datasets without needing labeled input data, offer alternatives that do not require known delineations of IACI, which may be particularly useful when the cause of IACI symptoms is unknown.

Subgroup Stratification

The heterogeneity of symptoms that people with Lyme IACI experience suggests that there may be distinct patient subgroups whose symptoms stem from different mechanisms or combinations of mechanisms. However, attempts to pinpoint specific biomarkers that classify such patient subgroups have so far been unsuccessful. Unsupervised ML approaches can be used within a well-curated IACI dataset to identify subgroups of patients based on one or many attributes of interest (e.g., symptoms, proteomics, genomics, brain-imaging abnormalities) (Hu et al., 2019; Petukhova et al., 2024; Zaslavsky et al., 2025). Such methods could limit the noise created by the heterogeneity within the Lyme IACI population, enabling more rapid discoveries of biomarkers and mechanisms for subgroups. This unbiased approach also allows the potential identification of individuals with Lyme IACI who group more closely with other IACI and may benefit from a different course of treatment.

In an example of this approach applied to Long COVID, semantic clustering was employed to identify six distinct clusters of people with Long COVID based on profiles of phenotypic abnormalities. Clusters identified people who closely shared phenotypic changes. One cluster had notably increased mortality, and others had distinct pulmonary, neuropsychiatric, and cardiovascular abnormalities (Reese et al., 2023). Another study applied a clustering-based method to a proteomic screen to conduct a molecular-based stratification and classify subsets of people with acute myeloid leukemia, which is also a highly heterogeneous disease. The ML method analyzed >300 protein expression levels plus clinical characteristics of 205 patients and identified expression patterns in protein functional groups and relationships among functional groups to discover global proteomic patterns (Hu et al., 2019). Neither of these examples was a completely unsupervised method, as both used publicly available reference databases to weight or structure the data. However, no labels were given to the patients a priori. These illustrative examples of ML applications demonstrate options that could be used to infer patient subgroups.

Increased availability of reference data could strengthen the capabilities of AI-driven analyses of multi-omics and mixed biological data in Lyme IACI. For example, interoperability of data gathered across various research studies in Lyme IACI, promoted through CDE adoption, would facilitate aggregation and comprehensive analysis of the Lyme IACI evidence base. Collection of relevant metadata in registries, biobanks, and other research repositories could also help inform AI analyses. Yet the potential for ML to amplify existing biases in the data necessitates the implementation of careful data-quality controls to minimize biases in the source data.

Enhancing Drug Development

AI could provide a deeper understanding of the relationships between therapeutic interventions and biomarkers or symptoms through computational methods and guide the design of new therapies or choice of FDA-approved drugs to test in a clinical trial. Examples include AI used to identify therapeutic targets in cancer from multi-omics biomarkers and drug screening efforts underway in many biotech companies—some with direct relevance to IACI. Unsupervised pattern-recognition methods may be a useful approach to finding relationships among symptoms, therapies, and molecular biomarkers. For example, clustering could be used to identify relationships between different symptoms or potential biomarkers against multiple therapeutic candidates. Temporal changes in symptoms and biomarkers in response to therapies could also be tracked by AI. AI methods including diffusion models and generative adversarial networks can predict changes in tissues as a function of a negative stress (e.g., inflammatory cytokines in the blood, spirochete bacteria) or therapeutic compound, and produce images and graphs that replicate what a medical test might produce. Overall, using these approaches could not only help identify therapeutic candidates, but also help inform disease mechanisms and identify quantitative endpoints for clinical trials.

Another route to identifying effective Lyme IACI treatments is through assessment of repurposing of existing therapies. Linking molecular targets and patient symptoms to known targets and clinical endpoints of FDA-approved drugs can help identify whether a drug can be repurposed for use in a subset of patients with Lyme IACI. A convergence of symptoms alone can help narrow the computational space needed to predict molecular targets and repurpose FDA-approved drugs for Lyme IACI. However, validation will require knowledge of target proteins or pathways that are not currently understood in Lyme IACI.

CONSIDERATIONS FOR IMPLEMENTATION

It is important that the evidence generated through clinical research informs future research and clinical practice. Even when clinical research demonstrates that an intervention is effective, a failure to consider how the intervention will be used in real-world settings can limit its adoption (Bauer and Kirchner, 2020). Careful consideration for the implementation of research findings while initial effectiveness data are being generated can increase the likelihood of a new intervention being adopted.

Dissemination

A robust dissemination strategy is fundamental to the successful and timely translation of research findings into clinical practice that is accessible to patients. This is underscored by the long lag times between medical discoveries and their implementation in the real world (Morris et al., 2011). Similarly, it is important to disseminate negative study results to prevent patients being given ineffective or unsafe treatments. Individuals with Lyme IACI and Lyme disease have organized a vibrant patient community and various advocacy groups (McPhail, 2017; Morrison et al., 2021). These existing networks of individuals living with Lyme IACI and their advocates are likely to champion the dissemination of promising research results on Lyme IACI treatments as well as to make others aware of negative findings. Yet dissemination cannot rest solely on the patient community.

There are several challenges that need to be addressed to improve the dissemination of results through the research ecosystem to the end users. First, many researchers lack the resources and capacity—or sometimes experience—to effectively convey their findings beyond traditional academic forums to lay audiences. Furthermore, clinicians may not be aware of the emerging evidence without targeted dissemination.

Many systematic challenges exist to the accurate dissemination of research to the public, but on an individual level researchers have a role to play in actively engaging the public, including through news and social media, and in scientific discourse, resisting pressure to hyperbolize results, and clearly describing the nuances and limitations of their findings (West and Bergstrom, 2021). Adopting better science communication practices can help researchers equip people with Lyme IACI and advocacy groups with accurate evidence to readily disseminate through their networks. Successful science communication strategies include transparently conveying uncertainty in scientific understanding and how scientific conclusions are drawn and tailoring messages to specific segments of the target audience based on values, beliefs, and information sources (NASEM, 2017). Researchers can access resources such as the American Association for the Advancement of

Sciences Communication Toolkit (AAAS, 2025) or the CDC Clear Communication Index (CDC, 2023) to help guide their communication strategies and messages.

Given that individuals with Lyme IACI can encounter dismissal and delegitimization of their symptoms and experiences from clinicians, it is also important to consider how best to disseminate Lyme IACI research results to treating clinicians. Lessons from HIV/AIDS advocacy may be particularly illuminating on how to bridge the gap between research and clinical practice. Similar to the case with Lyme IACI, people living with HIV were, and continue to be, vocal self-advocates who have enmeshed themselves in the scientific process, as exemplified through the creation of transnational advocacy networks that connected patients and researchers across the world (Colvin, 2014). Likewise, there are many other patient-centered groups that have advanced science and addressed unmet needs through dissemination, including groups dedicated to rare (e.g., cystic fibrosis) and common (e.g., breast cancer) diseases. In the case of HIV, for instance, scientific meetings and conferences offer an opportunity for advocates, researchers, and clinicians to share knowledge with one another and serve to keep clinicians and people living with HIV apprised of the latest research. HIV Source is another resource, maintained by NIH, which centrally collects resources on HIV research and treatment for clinicians, researchers, and the public (NIH OAR, n.d.). Within the realm of IACI, Project ECHO Global Health Initiatives has developed a course to share best practices in the care and treatment of Long COVID and ME/CFS (Project ECHO, n.d.). Clinician training is a key component of research dissemination, and programs that can help practitioners recognize IACI generally and distinguish between individual IACI will be valuable as more evidence is generated. Similar models of dissemination may be effective in aligning clinical practice with emerging research in Lyme IACI treatment. Additionally, implementation science could help further the understanding of dissemination processes that can facilitate the adoption of effective treatments for people with Lyme IACI.

Implementation Strategy

Engagement with the populations who will use an intervention is foundational to implementation. For this reason, patient engagement in clinical research must occur early and often and continue after research is completed. Even though this report highlights patient engagement as part of a research implementation strategy, patient engagement that starts after the research is completed is too late and often lacks authenticity. Intentional and sustained patient engagement enables lived experience to be embedded in research and can improve the responsiveness of research to patients' needs and values (Cavaller-Bellaubi et al., 2021). There are numerous opportunities to build in patient engagement across the research, development, and product life cycle, conferring benefits to patients, researchers, and developers throughout. Engagement in the early phases of research can involve identifying the research questions that matter most to patients and having patients provide input on the study design to improve accessibility and the capture of relevant data (Sacristán et al., 2016). Most relevant to the implementation phase is the potential for the patient engagement process to inform regulatory and coverage decisions about the product and to improve patient satisfaction with and use of the intervention (Puerini et al., 2024). Empowering expert patients through education on the clinical research process can further advance the goals of patient-centered and quality research throughout the product development life cycle (Sacristán et al., 2016). Examples of good practice in patient engagement published by Patient Focused Medicines Development can help guide patient engagement strategies in Lyme IACI research (PFMD, 2020).

A successful implementation strategy will also include engagement with industry and regulators. For interventions to be widely adopted, they need to achieve market viability (i.e., meet a demand in the market, be sold at an acceptable price, offer a return on investment, etc.). Collaborating with industry partners can thus strengthen the economic argument for implementation (Proctor et al., 2021). Early coordination with regulators, such as the FDA, is critical to the eventual adoption of Lyme IACI innovations. Discussions with FDA can help ensure that appropriate data of adequate quality are being collected in well-designed trials to inform and support regulatory decisions.

As evidence-based Lyme IACI treatments become available, it will become increasingly important to understand how they are used in clinical practice settings, especially given the heterogeneity of people living with Lyme IACI and the challenges that many individuals may have in receiving a timely and accurate diagnosis. The Agency for Healthcare Research and Quality could be well suited to conduct this research and to develop associated educational resources for clinicians.[8] Moreover, should various treatments be found to be effective, comparative effectiveness trials may be appropriate to determine the most effective Lyme IACI treatments and whether different patient subgroups respond better to certain treatments. These comparative effectiveness trials would align well with the research being funded by the Patient-Centered Outcomes Research Institute.

---

[8] As part of restructuring the Department of Health and Human Services announced on March 27, 2025, the Agency for Healthcare Research and Quality will be merged with the Assistant Secretary for Planning and Evaluation under a new Office of Strategy. See: HHS (2025).

REFERENCES

AAAS (American Association for the Advancement of Science). 2025. *AAAS communication toolkit.* https://www.aaas.org/resources/communication-toolkit (accessed January 28, 2025).

Aarts, S., M. van den Akker, and B. Winkens. 2014. The importance of effect sizes. *European Journal of General Practice* 20(1):61–64.

Abdaljaleel, M., E. J. Singer, and W. H. Yong. 2019. Sustainability in biobanking. *Methods in Molecular Biology* 1897:1–6.

Agarwal, A., P. M. Mehta, T. Jacobson, N. S. Shah, J. Ye, J. Zhu, Q. E. Wafford, E. Bahiru, A. N. de Cates, S. Ebrahim, D. Prabhakaran, A. Rodgers, and M. D. Huffman. 2024. Fixed-dose combination therapy for the prevention of atherosclerotic cardiovascular disease. *Nature Medicine* 30(4):1199–1209.

Anderson, B. R., E. G. Gotlieb, K. Hill, K. E. McHugh, M. A. Scheurer, C. M. Mery, G. J. Pelletier, J. R. Kaltman, O. J. White, F. L. Trachtenberg, D. Hollenbeck-Pringle, B. W. McCrindle, D. M. Sylvester, A. W. Eckhauser, S. K. Pasquali, J. B. Anderson, M. S. Schamberger, S. Shashidharan, J. P. Jacobs, M. L. Jacobs, M. Boskovski, J. W. Newburger, and M. Nathan. 2020. Registry-based trials: A potential model for cost savings? *Cardiology in the Young* 30(6):807–817.

Angst, F., A. Aeschlimann, and J. Angst. 2017. The minimal clinically important difference raised the significance of outcome effects above the statistical level, with methodological implications for future studies. *Journal of Clinical Epidemiology* 82:128–136.

Annaratone, L., G. De Palma, G. Bonizzi, A. Sapino, G. Botti, E. Berrino, C. Mannelli, P. Arcella, S. Di Martino, A. Steffan, M. G. Daidone, V. Canzonieri, B. Parodi, A. V. Paradiso, M. Barberis, and C. Marchiò. 2021. Basic principles of biobanking: From biological samples to precision medicine for patients. *Virchows Archiv* 479(2):233–246.

Ali, A., L. Vitulano, R. Lee, T. R. Weiss, and E. R. Colson. 2014. Experiences of patients identifying with chronic Lyme disease in the healthcare system: A qualitative study. *BMC Family Practice* 15(1):79.

Alkhatib, R., and K. I. Gaede. 2024. Data management in biobanking: Strategies, challenges, and future directions. *BioTech (Basel)* 13(3).

Aucott, J. N., M. J. Soloski, A. W. Rebman, L. A. Crowder, L. J. Lahey, C. A. Wagner, W. H. Robinson, and K. T. Bechtold. 2016. CCL19 as a chemokine risk factor for posttreatment Lyme disease syndrome: A prospective clinical cohort study. *Clinical and Vaccine Immunology* 23(9):757–766.

Aucott, J. N., T. Yang, I. Yoon, D. Powell, S. A. Geller, and A. W. Rebman. 2022. Risk of posttreatment Lyme disease in patients with ideally-treated early Lyme disease: A prospective cohort study. *International Journal of Infectious Diseases* 116:230–237.

Bai, N. A., and C. S. Richardson. 2023. Posttreatment Lyme disease syndrome and myalgic encephalomyelitis/chronic fatigue syndrome: A systematic review and comparison of pathogenesis. *Chronic Diseases and Translational Medicine* 9(3):183–190.

Bauer, M. S., and J. Kirchner. 2020. Implementation science: What is it and why should I care? *Psychiatry Research* 283:112376.

Bay Area Lyme Research Foundation. n.d. *Lyme disease biobank.* https://www.bayarealyme.org/biobank/ (accessed December 11, 2024).

Boston Children's Hospital. n.d. *Pedi Lyme Net.* https://www.childrenshospital.org/research/centers/pedi-lyme-net-research (accessed December 11, 2024).

Bouquet, J., M. J. Soloski, A. Swei, C. Cheadle, S. Federman, J.-N. Billaud, A. W. Rebman, B. Kabre, R. Halpert, M. Boorgula, J. N. Aucott, and C. Y. Chiu. 2016. Longitudinal transcriptome analysis reveals a sustained differential gene expression signature in patients treated for acute Lyme disease. *mBio* 7(1):10.1128/mbio.00100-00116.

Branda, J. A., K. Linskey, Y. A. Kim, A. C. Steere, and M. J. Ferraro. 2011. Two-tiered antibody testing for Lyme disease with use of 2 enzyme immunoassays, a whole-cell sonicate enzyme immunoassay followed by a VlsE C6 peptide enzyme immunoassay. *Clinical Infectious Diseases* 53(6):541–547.

Branda, J. A., and A. C. Steere. 2021. Laboratory diagnosis of lyme borreliosis. *Clinical Microbiology Reviews* 34(2).

Bransfield, R. C. 2017. Suicide and Lyme and associated diseases. *Neuropsychiatric Disease and Treatment* 13:1575–1587.

Brown, A. W., S. Aslibekyan, D. Bier, R. Ferreira da Silva, A. Hoover, D. M. Klurfeld, E. Loken, E. Mayo-Wilson, N. Menachemi, G. Pavela, P. D. Quinn, D. Schoeller, C. Tekwe, D. Valdez, C. J. Vorland, L. D. Whigham, and D. B. Allison. 2023. Toward more rigorous and informative nutritional epidemiology: The rational space between dismissal and defense of the status quo. *Crit Rev Food Sci Nutr* 63(18):3150–3167.

Buchan, B. W., D. A. Jobe, M. Mashock, D. Gerstbrein, M. L. Faron, N. A. Ledeboer, and S. M. Callister. 2019. Evaluation of a novel multiplex high-definition PCR assay for detection of tick-borne pathogens in whole-blood specimens. *Journal of Clinical Microbiology* 57(11):e00513–e00519.

Buchman, T. G., R. Draghia-Akli, S. J. Adam, N. R. Aggarwal, J. P. Fessel, E. S. Higgs, J. P. Menetski, S. W. Read, and E. A. Hughes. 2021. Accelerating coronavirus disease 2019 therapeutic interventions and vaccines-selecting compounds for clinical evaluation in coronavirus disease 2019 clinical trials. *Critical Care Medicine* 49(11):1963–1973.

Cavaller-Bellaubi, M., S. D. Faulkner, B. Teixeira, M. Boudes, E. Molero, N. Brooke, L. McKeaveney, J. Southerton, M. J. Vicente, N. Bertelsen, J. García-Burgos, V. Pirard, K. Reid, and E. Ferrer. 2021. Sustaining meaningful patient engagement across the lifecycle of medicines: A roadmap for action. *Therapeutic Innovation & Regulatory Science* 55(5):936–953.

CDC (Centers for Disease Control and Prevention). 2023. *The CDC Clear Communication Index*. https://www.cdc.gov/ccindex/index.html (accessed January 28, 2025).

CDC. 2024. *Bartonella infection*. https://www.cdc.gov/bartonella/about/index.html (accessed February 13, 2025).

Chen, Y., J. Dai, L. Tang, T. Mikhailova, Q. Liang, M. Li, J. Zhou, R. F. Kopp, C. Weickert, C. Chen, and C. Liu. 2023. Neuroimmune transcriptome changes in patient brains of psychiatric and neurological disorders. *Molecular Psychiatry* 28(2):710–721.

Chiu, C. Y., and S. A. Miller. 2019. Clinical metagenomics. *Nature Reviews Genetics* 20(6):341–355.

Colombel, J. F., W. J. Sandborn, W. Reinisch, G. J. Mantzaris, A. Kornbluth, D. Rachmilewitz, S. Lichtiger, G. D'Haens, R. H. Diamond, D. L. Broussard, K. L. Tang, C. J. van der Woude, and P. Rutgeerts. 2010. Infliximab, azathioprine, or combination therapy for Crohn's disease. *New England Journal of Medicine* 362(15):1383–1395.

Colvin, C. J. 2014. Evidence and AIDS activism: HIV scale-up and the contemporary politics of knowledge in global public health. *Global Public Health* 9(1–2):57–72.

Coppola, L., A. Cianflone, A. M. Grimaldi, M. Incoronato, P. Bevilacqua, F. Messina, S. Baselice, A. Soricelli, P. Mirabelli, and M. Salvatore. 2019. Biobanking in health care: Evolution and future directions. *Journal of Translational Medicine* 17(1):172.

CUMC (Columbia University Irving Medical Center). 2025. *Columbia specimen bank*. https://www.columbia-lyme.org/columbia-specimen-bank (accessed January 30, 2025).

Cutler, S. J., M. Vayssier-Taussat, A. Estrada-Peña, A. Potkonjak, A. D. Mihalca, and H. Zeller. 2021. Tick-borne diseases and co-infection: Current considerations. *Ticks and Tick-borne Diseases* 12(1):101607.

Cvijović, I., M. Swift, and S. R. Quake. 2025. Long-term B cell memory emerges at uniform relative rates in the human immune response. *Proceedings of the National Academy of Sciences* 122(9):e2406474122.

Dagher, G. 2022. Quality matters: International standards for biobanking. *Cell Proliferation* 55(8):e13282.
Duke University. n.d. *OneDukeBio Integrated Biospecimen Network (ODIN)*. https://medschool.duke.edu/research/research-support/core-facilities-service-centers/onedukebio-integrated-biospecimen-network (accessed December 11, 2024).
Duke-Margolis Center for Health Policy. 2019. *Determining real-world data's fitness for use and the role of reliability*. https://healthpolicy.duke.edu/sites/default/files/2019-11/rwd_reliability.pdf (accessed December 11, 2024).
Duke-Margolis Center for Health Policy. 2024. *Real-world evidence to support causal inference: Methodological considerations for non-interventional studies*. https://healthpolicy.duke.edu/publications/real-world-evidence-support-causal-inference (accessed January 28, 2025).
Dumes, A. A. 2020. Lyme disease and the epistemic tensions of "medically unexplained illnesses." *Medical Anthropology* 39(6):441–456.
Fallon, B. A., N. Zubcevik, C. Bennett, S. Doshi, A. W. Rebman, R. Kishon, J. R. Moeller, N. R. Octavien, and J. N. Aucott. 2019. The General Symptom Questionnaire-30 (GSQ-30): A brief measure of multi-system symptom burden in Lyme disease. *Frontiers in Medicine (Lausanne)* 6:283.
Fitzgerald, B. L., B. Graham, M. J. Delorey, A. Pegalajar-Jurado, M. N. Islam, G. P. Wormser, J. N. Aucott, A. W. Rebman, M. J. Soloski, J. T. Belisle, and C. R. Molins. 2021. Metabolic response in patients with post-treatment Lyme disease symptoms/syndrome. *Clinical Infectious Diseases* 73(7):e2342–e2349.
FDA (Food and Drug Administration). 2024. *Real-world evidence*. https://www.fda.gov/science-research/science-and-research-special-topics/real-world-evidence (accessed December 11, 2024).
Gu, X., S. Wang, W. Zhang, C. Li, L. Guo, Z. Wang, H. Li, H. Zhang, Y. Zhou, W. Liang, H. Li, Y. Liu, Y. Wang, L. Huang, T. Dong, D. Zhang, C. C. L. Wong, and B. Cao. 2023. Probing long COVID through a proteomic lens: A comprehensive two-year longitudinal cohort study of hospitalised survivors. *eBioMedicine* 98:104851.
Gliklich, R., M. Leavy, and N. Dreyer. 2020. *Registries for evaluating patient outcomes: A user's guide [internet]*: Agency for Healthcare Research and Quality. https://www.ncbi.nlm.nih.gov/books/NBK562567/ (accessed June 6, 2025).
Goodson, N., P. Wicks, J. Morgan, L. Hashem, S. Callinan, and J. Reites. 2022. Opportunities and counterintuitive challenges for decentralized clinical trials to broaden participant inclusion. *npj Digital Medicine* 5(1):58.
Hanson, K. E., and M. R. Couturier. 2016. Multiplexed molecular diagnostics for respiratory, gastrointestinal, and central nervous system infections. *Clinical Infectious Diseases* 63(10):1361–1367.
Harris, J. R., P. Burton, B. M. Knoppers, K. Lindpaintner, M. Bledsoe, A. J. Brookes, I. Budin-Ljøsne, R. Chisholm, D. Cox, M. Deschênes, I. Fortier, P. Hainaut, R. Hewitt, J. Kaye, J. E. Litton, A. Metspalu, B. Ollier, L. J. Palmer, A. Palotie, M. Pasterk, M. Perola, P. H. Riegman, G. J. van Ommen, M. Yuille, and K. Zatloukal. 2012. Toward a roadmap in global biobanking for health. *European Journal of Human Genetics* 20(11):1105–1111.
HHS (Department of Health and Human Services). 2025. *HHS announces transformation to make america healthy again*. https://www.hhs.gov/about/news/hhs-restructuring-doge.html (accessed March 27, 2025).
Hernández, S. A., K. Ogrinc, M. Korva, A. Kastrin, P. Bogovič, T. Rojko, K. W. Kelley, J. J. Weis, F. Strle, and K. Strle. 2023. Association of persistent symptoms after Lyme neuroborreliosis and increased levels of interferon-α in blood. *Emerging Infectious Diseases* 6(29):1091–1101.

Horowitz, R. I., and P. R. Freeman. 2018. Precision medicine: The role of the MSIDS model in defining, diagnosing, and treating chronic Lyme disease/post treatment Lyme disease syndrome and other chronic illness: Part 2. *Healthcare (Basel)* 6(4):129.

Houghton, C., M. Dowling, P. Meskell, A. Hunter, H. Gardner, A. Conway, S. Treweek, K. Sutcliffe, J. Noyes, D. Devane, and et al. 2020. Factors that impact on recruitment to randomised trials in health care: A qualitative evidence synthesis. *Cochrane Database of Systematic Reviews* 10(10):MR000045.

Hu, C. W., Y. Qiu, A. Ligeralde, A. Y. Raybon, S. Y. Yoo, K. R. Coombes, A. A. Qutub, and S. M. Kornblau. 2019. A quantitative analysis of heterogeneities and hallmarks in acute myelogenous leukaemia. *Nature Biomedical Engineering* 3(11):889–901.

International Standard. 2018. *Biotechnology-biobanking-general requirements for biobanking*. https://www.iso.org/standard/67888.html (accessed December 11, 2024).

IOM (Institute of Medicine). 2012. Facilitating collaborations to develop combination investigational cancer therapies: Workshop summary. Washington, DC: The National Academies Press. https://doi.org/10.17226/13262.

Jin, H., L. Wang, and R. Bernards. 2023. Rational combinations of targeted cancer therapies: Background, advances and challenges. *Nature Reviews Drug Discovery* 22(3):213–234.

Johns Hopkins Medicine Lyme Disease Research Center. 2025. *Research at the Lyme disease center*. https://www.hopkinslyme.org/research-at-the-lyme-disease-center/ (accessed February 26, 2025).

Kieser, M., T. Friede, and M. Gondan. 2013. Assessment of statistical significance and clinical relevance. *Statistics in Medicine* 32(10):1707–1719.

Langhof, H., H. Kahrass, T. Illig, R. Jahns, and D. Strech. 2018. Current practices for access, compensation, and prioritization in biobanks. Results from an interview study. *European Journal of Human Genetics* 26(11):1572–1581.

LaPoint. 2024. *Large-scale study will seek to unearth causes of persistent symptoms of Lyme disease*. https://medicine.tufts.edu/news-events/news/large-scale-study-will-seek-unearth-causes-persistent-symptoms-lyme-disease (accessed December 11, 2024)

Liu, F., and D. Panagiotakos. 2022. Real-world data: A brief review of the methods, applications, challenges and opportunities. *BMC Medical Research Methodology* 22(1):287.

Mackenzie, F. 2014. Biobanking trends, challenges, and opportunities. *Pathobiology* 81(5–6): 245–251.

Mahlich, J., A. Bartol, and S. Dheban. 2021. Can adaptive clinical trials help to solve the productivity crisis of the pharmaceutical industry? A scenario analysis. *Health Economics Review* 11(1):4.

Marques, A. R. 2015. Laboratory diagnosis of Lyme disease: Advances and challenges. *Infectious Disease Clinics of North America* 29(2):295–307.

Mayo Clinic Laboratories. n.d. *Tick-borne coinfection—Honing in on multiple infections*. https://news.mayocliniclabs.com/infectious-disease/vector-borne-diseases/tick-borne-coinfection/ (accessed January 30, 2025).

McGlothlin, A. E., and R. J. Lewis. 2014. Minimal clinically important difference: Defining what really matters to patients. *JAMA* 312(13):1342–1343.

McPhail, M. 2017. Making Lyme disease law: The role of patient advocacy in health law and policy. *Queen's Policy Review* 8(1):105–120.

Molins, C. R., C. Sexton, J. W. Young, L. V. Ashton, R. Pappert, C. B. Beard, and M. E. Schriefer. 2014. Collection and characterization of samples for establishment of a serum repository for Lyme disease diagnostic test development and evaluation. *Journal of Clinical Microbiology* 52(10):3755–3762.

Morris, Z. S., S. Wooding, and J. Grant. 2011. The answer is 17 years, what is the question: Understanding time lags in translational research. *Journal of the Royal Society of Medicine* 104(12):510–520.

Morrison, T., S. Madaras, C. Larson, and R. Harrison. 2021. Personal agency and community resilience: Narratives of women navigating health care with chronic Lyme disease. *Qualitative Health Research* 31(14):2706–2714.

Mouelhi, Y., E. Jouve, C. Castelli, and S. Gentile. 2020. How is the minimal clinically important difference established in health-related quality of life instruments? Review of anchors and methods. *Health and Quality of Life Outcomes* 18(1):136.

Naggie, S., D. R. Boulware, C. J. Lindsell, T. G. Stewart, N. Gentile, S. Collins, M. W. McCarthy, D. Jayaweera, M. Castro, M. Sulkowski, K. McTigue, F. Thicklin, G. M. Felker, A. A. Ginde, C. T. Bramante, A. J. Slandzicki, A. Gabriel, N. S. Shah, L. A. Lenert, S. E. Dunsmore, S. J. Adam, A. DeLong, G. Hanna, A. Remaly, R. Wilder, S. Wilson, E. Shenkman, A. F. Hernandez, and the Accelerating COVID-19 Therapeutic Interventions and Vaccines (ACTIV-6) Study Group and Investigators. 2022. Effect of ivermectin vs. placebo on time to sustained recovery in outpatients with mild to moderate COVID-19: A randomized clinical trial. *JAMA* 328(16):1595–1603.

NASEM (National Academies of Sciences, Engineering, and Medicine). 2017. *Communicating science effectively: A research agenda*. Washington, DC: The National Academies Press.

NASEM. 2022a. *Envisioning a transformed clinical trials enterprise for 2030: Proceedings of a workshop*. Edited by T. Wizemann, A. W. Gee and C. Shore. Washington, DC: The National Academies Press.

NASEM. 2022b. *Improving representation in clinical trials and research: Building research equity for women and underrepresented groups*. Washington, DC: The National Academies Press.

Natale, P., V. Saglimbene, M. Ruospo, A. M. Gonzalez, G. F. M. Strippoli, N. Scholes-Robertson, C. Guha, J. C. Craig, A. Teixeira-Pinto, T. Snelling, and A. Tong. 2021. Transparency, trust and minimizing burden to increase recruitment and retention in trials: A systematic review. *Journal of Clinical Epidemiology* 134:35–51.

Nature Immunology. 2025. Single-cell profiling of the immune landscape across the human lifespan. *Nature Immunology* 26(2):172–173.

New York State. n.d. Department of Health Wadsworth center test approval. https://www.wadsworth.org/regulatory/clep/clinical-labs/obtain-permit/test-approval (accessed March 13, 2025).

NIAID (National Institute of Allergy and Infectious Diseases). 2025. *Lyme disease co-infection*. https://www.niaid.nih.gov/diseases-conditions/lyme-disease-co-infection (accessed February 13, 2025).

Nigrovic, L. E., D. N. Neville, L. Chapman, F. Balamuth, M. N. Levas, A. D. Thompson, A. B. Kharbanda, D. Gerstbrein, J. A. Branda, and B. W. Buchan. 2023. Multiplex high-definition polymerase chain reaction assay for the diagnosis of tick-borne infections in children. *Open Forum Infectious Diseases* 10(4):ofad121.

NIH (National Institutes of Health). n.d. *Biologic Specimen and Data Repository Information Coordinating Center*. https://biolincc.nhlbi.nih.gov/about/ (accessed December 11, 2024).

NIH. 2016. *Final NIH policy on the use of a single institutional review board for multi-site research*. https://grants.nih.gov/grants/guide/notice-files/NOT-OD-16-094.html (accessed December 11, 2024).

NIH CC (National Institute of Health Clinical Center. n.d. *What is an IND?* https://www.cc.nih.gov/orcs/ind/what-is-an-ind (accessed January 20, 2025).

NIH OAR (National Institute of Health Office of AIDS Research). n.d. *HIV source*. https://hivinfo.nih.gov/hiv-source (accessed December 11, 2024).

Omura, C., M. de Lorenzi-Tognon, P. Benoit, V. Servellita, K. Foresythe, N. Brazer, M. Oseguera, D. Ingebrigtsen, J. Streithorst, D. Stryke, K. Zorn, M. Karalius, M. R. Wilson, and C. Chiu. 2025. Host response profiling from clinical metagenomic sequencing data for diagnosis of central nervous system infections. *Open Forum Infectious Disease* 12(Suppl 1).

Otoo, J. A., and T. S. Schlappi. 2022. REASSURED multiplex diagnostics: A critical review and forecast. *Biosensors (Basel)* 12(2):124.

Pallmann, P., A. W. Bedding, B. Choodari-Oskooei, M. Dimairo, L. Flight, L. V. Hampson, J. Holmes, A. P. Mander, L. Odondi, M. R. Sydes, S. S. Villar, J. M. S. Wason, C. J. Weir, G. M. Wheeler, C. Yap, and T. Jaki. 2018. Adaptive designs in clinical trials: Why use them, and how to run and report them. *BMC Medicine* 16(1):29.

Patterson, B. K., J. Guevara-Coto, J. Mora, E. B. Francisco, R. Yogendra, R. A. Mora-Rodríguez, C. Beaty, G. Lemaster, G. Kaplan Do, A. Katz, and J. A. Bellanti. 2024. Long COVID diagnostic with differentiation from chronic Lyme disease using machine learning and cytokine hubs. *Scientific Reports* 14(1):19743.

PCORI (Patient-Centered Outcomes Research Institute). 2024. *PCORI methodology standards*. https://www.pcori.org/research-related-projects/about-our-research/research-methodology/pcori-methodology-standards#Data%20Registries (accessed February 24, 2025).

Petukhova, A., J. P. Matos-Carcalho, and N. Fachada. 2024. Text clustering with large language model embeddings. *International Journal of Cognitive Computing in Engineering* 6:100–108.

PFMD (Patient Focused Medicines Development). 2020. *The PFMD book of good practices*. https://patientfocusedmedicine.org/bogp/2020/the-book-of-good-practices.pdf (accessed January 28, 2025).

Porwancher, R. B., C. G. Hagerty, J. Fan, L. Landsberg, B. J. Johnson, M. Kopnitsky, A. C. Steere, K. Kulas, and S. J. Wong. 2011. Multiplex immunoassay for Lyme disease using vlse1-igg and pepc10-igm antibodies: Improving test performance through bioinformatics. *Clinical Vaccine Immunology* 18(5):851–859.

Proctor, E. K., E. Toker, R. Tabak, V. R. McKay, C. Hooley, and B. Evanoff. 2021. Market viability: A neglected concept in implementation science. *Implementation Science* 16(1):98.

Project ECHO. n.d. *Long COVID and fatiguing illness recovery program echo*. https://iecho.org/public/program/PRGM1699044218879IERCAXHJ8Y (accessed February 25, 2025).

Project Lyme. 2021. *Introducing co-infections*. https://projectlyme.org/resource/introducing-co-infections/ (accessed February 13, 2025).

Puerini, R., A. Suthar, K. Forth, and K. Schneeman. 2024. *Defining and demonstrating the value of patient engagement in medtech research and product development*. https://milkeninstitute.org/sites/default/files/2024-10/PatientEngagementMedtech.pdf (accessed February 6, 2025).

Rebman, A. W., K. T. Bechtold, T. Yang, E. A. Mihm, M. J. Soloski, C. B. Novak, and J. N. Aucott. 2017. The clinical, symptom, and quality-of-life characterization of a well-defined group of patients with posttreatment Lyme disease syndrome. *Frontiers in Medicine (Lausanne)* 4:224.

RECOVERY Collaborative Group. 2021. Dexamethasone in hospitalized patients with COVID-19. *New England Journal of Medicine* 384(8):693–704.

Reese, J. T., H. Blau, E. Casiraghi, T. Bergquist, J. J. Loomba, T. J. Callahan, B. Laraway, C. Antonescu, B. Coleman, M. Gargano, K. J. Wilkins, L. Cappelletti, T. Fontana, N. Ammar, B. Antony, T. M. Murali, J. H. Caufield, G. Karlebach, J. A. McMurry, A. Williams, R. Moffitt, J. Banerjee, A. E. Solomonides, H. Davis, K. Kostka, G. Valentini, D. Sahner, C. G. Chute, C. Madlock-Brown, M. A. Haendel, P. N. Robinson, H. Spratt, S. Visweswaran, J. E. I. V. Flack, Y. J. Yoo, D. Gabriel, G. C. Alexander, H. B. Mehta, F. Liu, R. T. Miller, R. Wong, E. L. Hill, L. E. Thorpe, and J. Divers. 2023. Generalisable long COVID subtypes: Findings from the NIH N3C and RECOVER programmes. *eBioMedicine* 87:104413.

REMAP-CAP Investigators. 2021. Interleukin-6 receptor antagonists in critically ill patients with COVID-19. *New England Journal of Medicine* 384(16):1491–1502.

Rowan, S., N. Mohseni, M. Chang, H. Burger, M. Peters, and S. Mir. 2023. From tick to test: A comprehensive review of tick-borne disease diagnostics and surveillance methods in the United States. *Life (Basel)* 13(10).

Sacristán, J. A., A. Aguarón, C. Avendaño-Solá, P. Garrido, J. Carrión, A. Gutiérrez, R. Kroes, and A. Flores. 2016. Patient involvement in clinical research: Why, when, and how. *Patient Preference and Adherence* 10:631–640.

Schutzer, S. E., T. E. Angel, T. Liu, A. A. Schepmoes, T. R. Clauss, J. N. Adkins, D. G. Camp, B. K. Holland, J. Bergquist, P. K. Coyle, R. D. Smith, B. A. Fallon, and B. H. Natelson. 2011. Distinct cerebrospinal fluid proteomes differentiate post-treatment Lyme disease from chronic fatigue syndrome. *PLOS One* 6(2):e17287.

Schwartz, A. M., A. F. Hinckley, P. S. Mead, S. A. Hook, and K. J. Kugeler. 2017. Surveillance for Lyme disease—United States, 2008-2015. *MMWR Surveillance Summaries* 66(22):1–12.

Shah, J. S., J. J. Burrascano, and R. Ramasamy. 2023. Recombinant protein immunoblots for differential diagnosis of tick-borne relapsing fever and Lyme disease. *Journal of Vector Borne Diseases* 60(4):353-364.

Simon, G. E., R. Platt, J. H. Watanabe, A. B. Bindman, A. John London, M. Horberg, A. Hernandez, and R. M. Califf. 2022. When can we rely on real-world evidence to evaluate new medical treatments? *Clinical Pharmacology & Therapeutics* 111(1):30–34.

SLICE (Study of Lyme Disease Immunology and Clinical Events) Study. n.d. *The SLICE study.* http://www.slicestudies.org/ (accessed November 27, 2025).

Snapes, E., J. J. Astrin, N. Bertheussen Krüger, G. H. Grossman, E. Hendrickson, N. Miller, and C. Seiler. 2023. Updating International Society for Biological and Environmental Repositories Best Practices, fifth edition: A new process for relevance in an evolving landscape. *Biopreservation and Biobanking* 21(6):537–546.

Stanford Medicine. n.d. *Biobank services.* https://med.stanford.edu/biobank/services.html (accessed December 11, 2024).

Strle, K., D. Stupica, E. E. Drouin, A. C. Steere, and F. Strle. 2014. Elevated levels of IL-23 in a subset of patients with post-Lyme disease symptoms following erythema migrans. *Clinical Infectious Diseases* 58(3):372–380.

TBDWG (Tick-Borne Disease Working Group). 2018. *Tick-Borne Disease Working Group 2018 report to Congress.* https://www.hhs.gov/sites/default/files/tbdwg-report-to-congress-2018.pdf (accessed November 27, 2024).

TBDWG. 2020. *Tick-Borne Disease Working Group 2020 report to Congress.* https://www.hhs.gov/sites/default/files/tbdwg-2020-report_to-ongress-final.pdf (accessed November 27, 2024).

TBDWG. 2022. *Tick-Borne Disease Working Group 2022 report to Congress.* https://www.hhs.gov/sites/default/files/tbdwg-2022-report-to-congress.pdf (accessed November 27, 2024).

Tokarz, R., N. Mishra, T. Tagliafierro, S. Sameroff, A. Caciula, L. Chauhan, J. Patel, E. Sullivan, A. Gucwa, B. Fallon, M. Golightly, C. Molins, M. Schriefer, A. Marques, T. Briese, and W. I. Lipkin. 2018. A multiplex serologic platform for diagnosis of tick-borne diseases. *Scientific Reports* 8(1):3158.

Touradji, P., J. N. Aucott, T. Yang, A. W. Rebman, and K. T. Bechtold. 2019. Cognitive decline in post-treatment Lyme disease syndrome. *Archives of Clinical Neuropsychology* 34(4):455–465.

Tufts University. 2024. *Large-scale study will seek to unearth causes of persistent symptoms of lyme disease* https://medicine.tufts.edu/news-events/news/large-scale-study-will-seek-unearth-causes-persistent-symptoms-lyme-disease (accessed March 17, 2025).

Wang, Y., R. Li, R. Tong, T. Chen, M. Sun, L. Luo, Z. Li, Y. Chen, Y. Zhao, C. Zhang, L. Wei, W. Lin, H. Chen, K. Qian, A. F. Chen, J. Liu, L. Chen, B. Li, F. Wang, L. Wang, B. Su, and J. Pu. 2025. Integrating single-cell RNA and T cell/B cell receptor sequencing with mass cytometry reveals dynamic trajectories of human peripheral immune cells from birth to old age. *Nature Immunology* 26(2):308–322.
West, J. D., and C. T. Bergstrom. 2021. Misinformation in and about science. *Proceedings of the National Academy of Sciences* 118(15):e1912444117.
Wiering, B., D. de Boer, and D. Delnoij. 2017. Patient involvement in the development of patient-reported outcome measures: The developers' perspective. *BMC Health Services Research* 17(1):635.
Wolinetz, C. D., and F. S. Collins. 2017. Single-minded research review: The common rule and single IRB policy. *American Journal of Bioethics* 17(7):34–36.
Woodcock, J., and L. M. LaVange. 2017. Master protocols to study multiple therapies, multiple diseases, or both. *New England Journal of Medicine* 377(1):62–70.
Wormser, G. P., D. McKenna, C. L. Karmen, K. D. Shaffer, J. H. Silverman, J. Nowakowski, C. Scavarda, E. D. Shapiro, and P. Visintainer. 2020. Prospective evaluation of the frequency and severity of symptoms in Lyme disease patients with erythema migrans compared with matched controls at baseline, 6 months, and 12 months. *Clinical Infectious Diseases* 71(12):3118–3124.
Wright, W. F., D. J. Riedel, R. Talwani, and B. L. Gilliam. 2012. Diagnosis and management of Lyme disease. *American Family Physician* 85(11):1086–1093.
Yale Medicine. n.d. *Tick-borne illnesses.* https://www.yalemedicine.org/conditions/tick-borne-illnesses (accessed February 13, 2025).
Zaslavsky, M. E., E. Craig, J. K. Michuda, N. Sehgal, N. Ram-Mohan, J. Y. Lee, K. D. Nguyen, R. A. Hoh, T. D. Pham, K. Röltgen, B. Lam, E. S. Parsons, S. R. Macwana, W. DeJager, E. M. Drapeau, K. M. Roskin, C. Cunningham-Rundles, M. A. Moody, B. F. Haynes, J. D. Goldman, J. R. Heath, R. S. Chinthrajah, K. C. Nadeau, B. A. Pinsky, C. A. Blish, S. E. Hensley, K. Jensen, E. Meyer, I. Balboni, P. J. Utz, J. T. Merrill, J. M. Guthridge, J. A. James, S. Yang, R. Tibshirani, A. Kundaje, and S. D. Boyd. 2025. Disease diagnostics using machine learning of B cell and T cell receptor sequences. *Science* 387(6736):eadp2407.

5

Recommendations

The committee's charge for this report was to study the evidence base for treatments for Lyme infection-associated chronic illnesses (IACI). To this end, the committee reviewed the existing literature (see Appendix C) and obtained input from people living with Lyme IACI, clinicians, and researchers on current knowledge and gaps on the treatment, etiology, and diagnosis of Lyme IACI. Furthermore, the committee considered emerging lessons from Long COVID and other IACI, current knowledge on co-infections and implications for the development and diagnosis of Lyme IACI and explored advances in medicine and biotechnology that may provide solutions to the research gaps for Lyme IACI treatment. The findings and conclusions, based on the committee's evidence gathering and deliberations, are presented in the preceding chapters of this report. This includes a framework for evaluating and prioritizing clinical research intended to advance diagnostics and therapeutics for Lyme IACI.

In this chapter, the committee makes six recommendations to advance research on Lyme IACI, which will engage different collaborators throughout the research ecosystem, including policy makers, researchers, research institutions, and research funders (Box 5-1). These recommendations are designed to bridge the research gaps and challenges identified by the committee with strategies that have a high potential for accelerating discoveries. Common to all six recommendations is a call for increased coordination and more intentional collaboration, including with people living with Lyme IACI. Therefore, coordination and collaboration are foundational to the implementation of these recommendations. It is the committee's hope that

> **BOX 5-1**
> **Defining Research Funders**
>
> Research funders include any organization or entity that provides financial support for scientific research. This funding can be for preclinical or clinical research. A few examples of potential research funders in the Lyme IACI space include:
>
> **Public funders**
> - Department of Defense (Congressionally Directed Medical Research Programs)
> - Department of Health and Human Services (HHS), including the National Institutes of Health (NIH) and Centers for Disease Control and Prevention (CDC)
>
> **Private, for-profit funders**
> - Pharmaceutical industry
>
> **Private, nonprofit funders**
> - Bay Area Lyme Foundation
> - Global Lyme Alliance
> - LymeDisease.org
> - Steven & Alexandra Cohen Foundation
>
> **Public–private partnerships**
> - LymeX (HHS and the Steven & Alexandra Cohen Foundation)

this common foundation can help ensure that progress on any one recommendation will facilitate progress on others.

RESEARCH INTO NEW TREATMENTS THAT ALLEVIATE SYMPTOMS

In preparing this report, the committee investigated the existing evidence base on Lyme IACI treatments. The scoping review of that literature base is described in Chapter 2. The existing evidence is from randomized trials, single-arm trials, observational studies, and anecdotal reports. Among them, the committee found that only six trials for Lyme IACI treatment have been performed with the randomization needed to have high confidence in their results (Cameron, 2008; Fallon et al., 2008; Kaplan et al., 2003; Klempner et al., 2001; Krupp et al., 2003; Murray et al., 2022). Five of these six trials evaluated extended courses of antibiotic therapy, and one evaluated a yoga intervention (Murray et al., 2022). Unfortunately, these studies have not demonstrated a sustained improvement in patients' symptoms.

Through the scoping review, the committee found that the mechanisms of Lyme IACI remain poorly understood. However, most treatment trials tested interventions that target hypothesized, but currently unproven mechanisms of disease. Research on treatments that are reasonably likely to address the symptoms that contribute to the poor functionality and quality of life reported by people living with Lyme IACI will be critical as studies continue to evaluate the potential mechanisms of Lyme IACI.

To promote the patient-centeredness of future research, engagement with people living with Lyme IACI will be key throughout the process, from the identification of relevant research questions to the dissemination and implementation of results. Lyme IACI research could benefit from incorporating relevant practices and processes of organizations like the Patient-Centered Outcomes Research Institute, for example, as models for the meaningful engagement of patients in research decision-making. The Congressionally Directed Medical Research Programs (CDMRP) Tick-Borne Disease Research Program (TBDRP) has been a leader in patient engagement in Lyme disease research. In their work on tick-borne diseases, CDMRP includes patients and patient advocates in evaluating proposals and making recommendations for funding (CDMRP, 2024).

> **RECOMMENDATION 1:** Research funders should prioritize improving the function and quality of life for people living with Lyme infection-associated chronic illnesses, including the relief of common symptoms, with scientifically supported interventions. To ensure these interventions are supported by robust evidence, clinical studies should be well-designed, randomized trials with appropriate control groups and, whenever possible, include collection of data to help further understanding of disease mechanisms.

STANDARDIZED RESEARCH DEFINITIONS AND METRICS

In Chapter 2 the committee noted a general lack of standardization of research terminologies and approaches for Lyme IACI research. The lack of consensus definitions of the patient populations has resulted in the use of various terminologies and definitions to describe those with Lyme IACI. The PTLDS case definition, which is often used in research, requires that individuals meet specific criteria to establish a consistent and comparable patient group. However, the PTLDS definition excludes individuals in a broader population with similar symptoms, including some with possible Lyme-related IACI (Johnson et al., 2024). People who may have Lyme IACI

> **Considerations for Implementing Recommendation 1**
>
> **Engaging Individuals with Lived Experience**
>
> To improve the function and quality of life for people with Lyme IACI, it will be important to align research efforts with their experiences and priorities. One way to do so is by designing and supporting clinical studies to address the functional status and symptoms that matter most to people living with Lyme IACI. To accomplish this end, researchers and research funders would need to seek the engagement of people living with Lyme IACI early on to incorporate their input throughout the research and development process, including in the identification of research questions, study design and implementation, outcomes, and dissemination or research results. Research funders can also increase the responsiveness of research and focus the available resources by including, when feasible, input from people with lived experience during the funding decision making process.
>
> **Applying a Framework for Prioritization**
>
> For research funders, a framework to prioritizing research directions, such as one proposed in this report, can guide how new evidence is incorporated into the knowledge base and inform reevaluation of research priorities. Such a framework would clearly map out key criteria for incorporating a broad range of input (e.g., real-world data, observational trials, interventional trials, etc.), weighing the existing evidence, and decision-making to identify the most promising research directions to advance. Importantly, this strategic approach would lead to a comprehensive and transparent decision-making process that provides common ground for engagement among people with Lyme IACI, clinicians, researchers, and research funders.

but do not meet the PTLDS definition because of an unclear relationship to past Lyme disease or lack of functional impairment are typically excluded from studies, limiting the ability to recruit adequate numbers of representative study participants. Consequently, the relevance and impact of obtained research data may be unknown for the broader Lyme IACI population that does not meet PTLDS criteria. No objective biomarkers have been validated as prognostic or diagnostic tools for Lyme IACI (Fitzgerald et al., 2021). Yet, similar chronic illnesses with a potential infectious trigger, such as myalgic encephalomyelitis/chronic fatigue syndrome (ME/CFS), where the trigger is often unknown, and Long COVID have developed consensus syndromic definitions that can be useful for clinical research, including studies aimed at identifying effective therapies in the absence of objective diagnostic tools.

> RECOMMENDATION 2: The U.S. Department of Health and Human Services (HHS) should develop consensus research definitions for Lyme infection-associated chronic illnesses (IACI) that address the different strata of the broad range of people living with Lyme IACI.
>   a. HHS should develop a Lyme IACI definition and subgroup definitions that acknowledge the heterogeneity of these illnesses.
>   b. HHS should establish a mechanism to regularly review the Lyme IACI literature and update the consensus research definition and subgroup definitions as new evidence emerges.
>   c. The consensus research definition and subgroup definitions for Lyme IACI should be developed in such a way as to include a broad range of perspectives (e.g., lived experience, clinicians, researchers) and generally align with definitions for other similar conditions and facilitate coordination of research across the diseases.

In the absence of common standards, the committee found that individual Lyme IACI studies tend to evaluate treatments differently. For example, different studies may measure reductions in fatigue but use different

---

Considerations for Implementing Recommendation 2

Working with an Evolving Knowledge Base

With the consensus research definition and subgroup definitions being periodically assessed and updated to incorporate relevant new evidence, it is important for researchers to have a common approach on how to navigate this evolving knowledge base and maintain coordination across research studies. For example, without diagnostic and prognostic biomarkers specific for Lyme IACI, particularly those that distinguish the condition from other conditions with similar or overlapping symptoms (e.g., Long COVID), study enrollment and participant characterization can be based on clinical syndromes, patient histories, and the level of available clinical or laboratory evidence of prior *Borrelia* infection. When new diagnostic and prognostic biomarkers that better characterize people living with Lyme IACI emerge, those would be used in addition to help guide enrollment, participant characterization, and any stratification for clinical studies.

measurement instruments, measure different outcomes entirely, or examine different subsets of the Lyme IACI population. Additionally, existing standard general patient-reported health survey forms, such as the SF-36, have been used in research into Lyme IACI and other IACI with similar symptomatology, but may not always capture symptoms that are important to people living with Lyme IACI. Several symptom questionnaires have been specifically designed for Lyme IACI but have had limited patient involvement in their development. And there are currently no Lyme IACI-specific outcome measurement tools developed for use in children, while the pediatric population differs from adults in terms of physiological and mental development, including the ability to self-report health outcomes. The lack of standardization in outcome measures and tools hinders the ability to compare or combine results from multiple studies, often limiting their informativeness to individual studies. Common data elements (CDE) offer a solution to these challenges by aligning disparate researchers and institutions on outcomes, metrics, and data formats. The development of CDEs for Lyme IACI may be guided by similar efforts that are underway in the field of ME/CFS (NIH, n.d.).

RECOMMENDATION 3: The National Institutes of Health (NIH), in coordination with the Centers for Disease Control and Prevention (CDC), should define a set of standard research tools and metrics to advance research and development of new treatments for Lyme infection-associated chronic illnesses (IACI). These include common data elements (CDEs), sensitive outcome measures, and terminologies that reflect the lived experience of people with Lyme IACI.

    a. NIH and CDC should assess, with participation of all interested parties, whether existing patient-reported outcome measurement tools reliably and accurately capture the priority outcomes for people with Lyme IACI, or if new tools and measures are needed. This should include determining if there are groups (e.g., children) for which existing reporting tools do not capture necessary Lyme IACI constructs.

    b. NIH and CDC should evaluate existing CDEs from myalgic encephalomyelitis/chronic fatigue syndrome (ME/CFS) and Long COVID for components that can be incorporated into Lyme IACI CDEs to enable knowledge sharing among IACI, including through comparative studies of multiple disease areas. This could include adopting a core set of clinical characteristics for study participants, study methodologies, and symptom reporting questionnaires that mirror those already being used in ME/CFS or Long COVID research.

Considerations for Implementing Recommendation 3

Engaging New Insights

It is important for research tools and metrics that reflect the lived experience of people with Lyme IACI to accurately capture what they are meant to measure, and be easy to use by clinicians, researchers, patients, and, when appropriate, caregivers or other surrogates. To ensure incorporation of this broad range of perspectives, development of new research tools would include collaboration with the different entities that are interested in the use of these instruments. For example, Lyme IACI CDEs would be developed in consultation with a full range of interested parties, including researchers, clinicians, federal agencies, professional societies, and people with lived experience. Through establishing the CDEs, these perspectives are incorporated into the core research tools and metrics that set the standard for use across Lyme IACI research.

Taking a strategic, comprehensive approach to identify and engage a wide range of necessary perspectives in developing research tools and metrics would also facilitate the identification of underserved issues, such as the need for research instruments that are tailored to the pediatric population. Sometimes additional insights from outside the Lyme IACI research field will be necessary to inform specific aspects in developing these instruments. Some of these entities with relevant expertise include, but are not limited to, the Patient-Centered Outcomes Research Institute, U.S. Food and Drug Administration, and biotechnology and pharmaceutical industry (e.g., developers of drugs and medical devices).

Ensuring Reliability and Accuracy

Trust in the reliability and accuracy of patient-reported outcome measures across different populations will encourage uptake by researchers and support coordination across the field. Some of the variables to consider in conducting validation studies for the standardized set of patient-reported outcomes include measures of the sensitivity to capturing treatment responses, as well as their suitability for application across different languages, cultures, populations, and socioeconomic conditions.

SOURCE: Ramirez et al., 2024

IMPROVED ACCESS TO BIOBANKS AND REGISTRIES

The committee assessed the role and importance of biobanks and patient registries in facilitating Lyme IACI research. Samples and data from biobanks and registries can serve as valuable research elements for hypothesis generation and for performing treatment and mechanistic studies. Currently, several biobanks and registries exist that collect patient-derived biological samples and clinical and laboratory data from the Lyme IACI patient communities and investigators (Bay Area Lyme Research Foundation, n.d.; Boston Children's Hospital, n.d.; CUMC, 2025; Johns Hopkins Lyme Disease Research Center, 2025; Molins et al., 2014). However, these samples and data are currently not widely used in Lyme IACI research. Multiple factors likely contribute to the relatively rare use of biobanks and registries. The types of data collected by and contained in biobanks and registries are not consistently made transparent to potential participants and investigators. Furthermore, the heterogeneity of Lyme IACI along with the lack of diagnostic biomarkers increases the need for clear and consistent characterizations of participants and their samples. But the consistency that is needed is hindered by insufficient coordination between biobanks and registries. Promoting quality in the collection and storage of samples and data and paying attention to the responsibility that biobanks and registries owe to participants will play important roles in increasing the value these resources can add to clinical research.

An example from cancer research demonstrates how efforts to promote coordination and standardization among independent biobanks and research groups that collect samples have been an effective means of improving quality and visibility. A centralization initiative with the World Health Organization's International Agency for Cancer Research Biobank developed a common dataset, a platform of resources housed within the biobank, and a uniform governance structure. These centralization activities improved interoperability between samples and data collected at different sites and increased visibility and accessibility of resources that are stored at disparate sites (Mendy et al., 2019). Importantly, there are practical limitations to the adoption of a central governance structure for Lyme IACI biobanks that would enable a federated biobank network. Many Lyme IACI biobanks are managed by independent research groups, without a central authority to establish uniform governance. However, a federated Lyme IACI biobank is a worthy aspiration as coordination among biobanks takes hold.

RECOMMENDATION 4: To enhance impact in research, funders and managers of biobanks and patient registries for Lyme infection-associated chronic illnesses (IACI) should adopt the following practices that optimize the sustainability of these resources and the accessibility, quality, and utility of their samples.

a. Biobanks should promote awareness, coordination, governance, accessibility, sustainability, and standardization of data and samples from participants with Lyme IACI and those serving as appropriate control groups, including healthy controls and participants with similar conditions or symptoms.
b. Biobanks and patient registries should refine and make public the data domains they capture to increase accessibility and spur collaboration. In sample and data collection, the samples should be characterized in a manner that promotes data quality and confidence in their use. Biological collections associated with individual research studies should follow a standardized set of basic data and metadata domains to facilitate use across studies.
c. Biobanks and patient registries should develop and communicate protocols that describe the intended use of collected samples and data for participants who contribute their data and samples.

COORDINATED RESEARCH FUNDING AND COLLABORATION EFFORTS

Lyme IACI research relies on various funders and is conducted at diverse sites, often resulting in research silos with minimal coordination between different research efforts. The committee found that there is poor integration of research resources such as biobanks and registries with the traditional research infrastructure through which trials are conducted. The lack of coordination between disparate research endeavors hinders knowledge sharing and the ability to constructively build a synergistic evidence base (Coppola et al., 2019).

Other IACI, such as Long COVID and ME/CFS, have coordinating centers that promote research collaboration and knowledge sharing. Lyme IACI research could similarly benefit from promoting and supporting coordination between research sites and investigators to both build synergies and limit redundancy in research, helping make the most of the limited resources available to aid people living with Lyme IACI.

RECOMMENDATION 5: Research funders should support the development and sustainment of a Lyme infection-associated chronic illnesses (IACI) research data-coordinating center that facilitates resource and knowledge sharing across programs conducting Lyme IACI clinical research and incorporates input from people living with Lyme IACI.

a. To further the visibility of biobank resources, the research data coordinating center should collaborate with biobanks on the development of a central repository that catalogues the location and characteristics of available samples and data.

COLLABORATION ACROSS IACI RESEARCH

In Chapter 3, the committee explored research into mechanisms and treatments for other IACI, with a focus on symptom-based interventions. Several disease mechanisms driving IACI symptoms have been hypothesized, including infection-triggered immune dysfunction, pathogen or antigen

---

Considerations for Implementing Recommendation 4

Fostering Trust

While transparency and accessibility are important to enhance the research applications and impact of their samples and data, biobanks and patient registries are also stewards of their participants' privacy and their access to data. Fostering trust between participants, researchers, and the biobanks and registries that promote long-term engagement is fundamental to the sustainability of these resources. Principles to earning and maintaining the trust of people who contribute their data and samples include, but are not limited to, the following: informing donors of the results of research in which their samples were used, encouraging the collection and promoting the use of patient-generated data, and providing a clear framework for how the biobank or patient registry evaluates and prioritizes the use of their material in high-quality studies that can yield meaningful results.

Promoting Collaboration among Biobanks

Collaboration among Lyme IACI biobanks is fundamental to standardizing data and metadata, efforts that are needed to improve the quality of biobank samples and data, and their utility in research. A federated Lyme IACI biobank, under a unified governance structure, is an aspirational model to foster such collaboration. Other approaches to biobank collaboration that stop short of a federated system, such as common datasets and a shared inventory system, can also increase use of biobank samples and data in research.

Coordination between Lyme IACI biobanks and patient registries, and biobanks and registries for other IACI would help to standardize the characterization of samples and data in accordance with any relevant common data elements, and advance cross-IACI research.

> **Considerations for Implementing Recommendation 5**
>
> **Sharing Resources and Knowledge**
> There are many ways to facilitate coordination among clinical research programs for Lyme IACI, which can include clinical trial networks, individual research sites, and biobanks. Promoting the adoption of standardized case definitions, common data elements, and patient-centered research approaches (e.g., outcome measures, methodologies) can harmonize data collection across the different programs and activities. Taking one step further, the Lyme IACI research data coordinating center can facilitate learnings from other IACIs that share similar symptoms and disease mechanisms by reviewing and identifying areas of alignment in the approach to data collection, storage, and sharing with other research coordinating centers that have already been established for Long COVID and ME/CFS.

persistence, and microbiome dysbiosis. However, there is currently an insufficient understanding of the underlying mechanisms that cause Lyme IACI (Bai and Richardson 2023; Choutka et al., 2022). On the other hand, the overlap in common symptoms between Lyme IACI and other IACI and related conditions is well established, raising the question as to whether there might be commonalities in disease mechanisms underlying shared symptoms. To further explore this, some research is beginning to include multiple IACI populations within a single study (MIT, n.d.; PolyBio, n.d.). The committee considers this a potentially promising approach, as research on different IACI has generally been siloed.

Several initiatives have been implemented to align various partners in the research ecosystem on common goals. The federal government, in coordination with public and private partners—including patient communities—has developed action plans to address many conditions of public health concern and to align research efforts across government, academia, and industry, including the HHS National Action Plan on Long COVID. Further, NIH has recently funded a large prospective longitudinal trial to better understand progression from Lyme disease to Lyme IACI. However, these initiatives lack a cross-IACI collaborative approach that could yield findings that could advance research on multiple conditions simultaneously. As the HHS Office of Long COVID Research and Practice is set to close, a strategic plan will be critical to coordinate and monitor the many IACI research initiatives, and to ensure the efficiency of the complex IACI research ecosystem.

RECOMMENDATION 6: The Department of Health and Human Services (HHS) should develop an integrated strategic plan for infection-associated chronic illnesses (IACI) research that facilitates collaboration across the different disease research efforts. The strategic plan should improve the understanding of commonalities among IACI and identify and advance interventions to address specific conditions, including Lyme IACI. The strategic plan should balance the need for clinical research on treatments, basic and clinical research on disease mechanisms, and incorporation of real-world evidence (RWE).

   a. The strategic plan should prioritize the development and support of substantive efforts to improve the treatment and management of IACI symptoms.
   b. The strategic plan should include continued investment in large-scale, prospective, multicenter observational studies designed to generate evidence on the mechanistic similarities and differences between Lyme IACI and other IACI, including clinical and laboratory characteristics.
   c. To complement prospective studies, the strategic plan should address the opportunity to use RWE, including information based on patient registry data and findings from observational studies.

Considerations for Implementing Recommendation 6

Integrating Learnings from Across IACI

Prior experience from efforts to address ME/CFS and Long COVID can inform the range of partners to be involved in the development, communication, and execution of an integrated strategic plan for collaboration across multiple IACI, such as the NIH, CDC, industry and other research funders, organizations of people living with Lyme IACI, and other nonprofit organizations. There are several opportunities to improve understanding of commonalities among IACI and advance development of new treatments through this integrated strategic plan. It will be important for this strategic plan to outline an approach for conducting studies that enroll participants from multiple IACI populations and enable comparisons between the syndromes. Furthermore, learning from the approach to address Long COVID, the strategic plan can incorporate support for randomized trials and prospective observational studies that are specifically designed and statistically powered to enable subgroup analyses to elucidate subgroup differences within the Lyme IACI population, such as sex-based and age-related differences, the level of clinical and diagnostic evidence of prior Lyme disease, and defined common clinical syndromes. Observational studies can also be designed to collect samples and data to look for distinguishing biomarkers, and serve as recruitment platforms for clinical trials.

CLOSING THOUGHTS

In this report, the committee has described its findings, conclusions, and recommendations, which were developed based on its review of the literature, internal discussions, and valuable input from patient representatives, clinicians, and researchers. While Lyme IACI is poorly understood and heterogeneous, patients currently considered under the umbrella of Lyme IACI have a significant burden of symptoms and disability that requires urgent attention.

To get to effective treatments, there is a need for coordinated definitions, research efforts, and resources. While continuing research into the triggers and mechanisms responsible for the development of Lyme IACI is essential, the urgent need for effective interventions requires an enhanced focus on developing therapies to treat those symptoms most debilitating and important to people living with Lyme IACI. Innovative approaches to the design, conduct, and interpretation of studies could be more broadly adopted in Lyme IACI research to expand the breadth and depth of the evidence base. Furthermore, similarities between Lyme IACI and other IACI offer untapped opportunities for Lyme IACI research to build on the successes of research on Long COVID and ME/CFS. These commonalities also warrant coordination and collaboration between researchers studying these various conditions to constructively develop and evaluate their evidence bases together. The committee hopes that their recommendations and proposed research framework can accelerate new developments in the field of Lyme IACI and contribute to the discovery of effective treatments for the many living with this syndrome.

REFERENCES

Bai, N. A., and C. S. Richardson. 2023. Posttreatment Lyme disease syndrome and myalgic encephalomyelitis/chronic fatigue syndrome: A systematic review and comparison of pathogenesis. *Chronic Diseases and Translational Medicine* 9(3):183–190.

Bay Area Lyme Research Foundation. n.d. *Lyme disease biobank*. https://www.bayarealyme.org/biobank/ (accessed January 27, 2025).

Boston Children's Hospital. n.d. *Pedi Lyme Net*. https://www.childrenshospital.org/research/centers/pedi-lyme-net-research (accessed December 11, 2024).

Cameron, D. 2008. Severity of Lyme disease with persistent symptoms. Insights from a double-blind placebo-controlled clinical trial. *Minerva Medica* 99(5):489–496.

CDMRP (Congressionally Directed Medical Research Programs). 2024. *Tick-borne disease*. https://cdmrp.health.mil/tbdrp/default (accessed December 11, 2024).

Choutka, J., V. Jansari, M. Hornig, and A. Iwasaki. 2022. Unexplained post-acute infection syndromes. *Nature Medicine* 28(5):911–923.

Coppola, L., A. Cianflone, A. M. Grimaldi, M. Incoronato, P. Bevilacqua, F. Messina, S. Baselice, A. Soricelli, P. Mirabelli, and M. Salvatore. 2019. Biobanking in health care: Evolution and future directions. *Journal of Translational Medicine* 17(1):172.

CUMC (Columbia University Irving Medical Center). 2025. *Columbia specimen bank.* https://www.columbia-lyme.org/columbia-specimen-bank (accessed January 30, 2025).

Fallon, B. A., J. G. Keilp, K. M. Corbera, E. Petkova, C. B. Britton, E. Dwyer, I. Slavov, J. Cheng, J. Dobkin, D. R. Nelson, and H. A. Sackeim. 2008. A randomized, placebo-controlled trial of repeated IV antibiotic therapy for Lyme encephalopathy. *Neurology* 70(13):992–1003.

Fitzgerald, B. L., B. Graham, M. J. Delorey, A. Pegalajar-Jurado, M. N. Islam, G. P. Wormser, J. N. Aucott, A. W. Rebman, M. J. Soloski, J. T. Belisle, and C. R. Molins. 2021. Metabolic response in patients with post-treatment Lyme disease symptoms/syndrome. *Clinical Infectious Diseases* 73(7):e2342–e2349.

Johns Hopkins Medicine Lyme Disease Research Center. 2025. Research at the Lyme disease center. https://www.hopkinslyme.org/research-at-the-lyme-disease-center/ (accessed February 27, 2025).

Johnson, L., M. Shapiro, D. Needell, and R. B. Stricker. 2024. Optimizing exclusion criteria for clinical trials of persistent Lyme disease using real-world data. *Healthcare (Basel)* 13(1):20.

Kaplan, R. F., R. P. Trevino, G. M. Johnson, L. Levy, R. Dornbush, L. T. Hu, J. Evans, A. Weinstein, C. H. Schmid, and M. S. Klempner. 2003. Cognitive function in post-treatment Lyme disease: Do additional antibiotics help? *Neurology* 60(12):1916–1922.

Klempner, M. S., L. T. Hu, J. Evans, C. H. Schmid, G. M. Johnson, R. P. Trevino, D. Norton, L. Levy, D. Wall, J. McCall, M. Kosinski, and A. Weinstein. 2001. Two controlled trials of antibiotic treatment in patients with persistent symptoms and a history of Lyme disease. *New England Journal of Medicine* 345(2):85–92.

Krupp, L. B., L. G. Hyman, R. Grimson, P. K. Coyle, P. Melville, S. Ahnn, R. Dattwyler, and B. Chandler. 2003. Study and treatment of post Lyme disease (STOP-LD): A randomized double masked clinical trial. *Neurology* 60(12):1923–1930.

Mendy, M., E. Caboux, C. P. Wild, R. Herrero, R. Accardi-Gheit, G. Clifford, E. Françon, A. Kesminiene, J. McKay, S. Rinaldi, A. Scalbert, G. Scélo, E. Seleiro, and J. Zavadil. 2019. Centralization of the iarc biobank: Combining multiple sample collections into a common platform. *Biopreservation and Biobanking* 17(5):433–443.

MIT (Massachusetts Institute of Technology). n.d. *MIT MAESTRO Study.* https://talresearchgroup.mit.edu/mitmaestro (accessed January 30, 2025).

Molins, C. R., C. Sexton, J. W. Young, L. V. Ashton, R. Pappert, C. B. Beard, and M. E. Schriefer. 2014. Collection and characterization of samples for establishment of a serum repository for Lyme disease diagnostic test development and evaluation. *Journal of Clinical Microbiology* 52(10):3755–3762.

Murray, L., C. Alexander, C. Bennett, M. Kuvaldina, G. Khalsa, and B. Fallon. 2022. Kundalini yoga for post-treatment Lyme disease: A preliminary randomized study. *Healthcare (Basel)* 10(7):1314.

NIH (National Institute of Health). n.d. *Myalgic encephalomyelitis/chronic fatigue syndrome.* https://www.commondataelements.ninds.nih.gov/Myalgic%20Encephalomyelitis/Chronic%20Fatigue%20Syndrome (accessed January 27, 2025).

PolyBio. n.d. *Lumbrokinase LongCOVID & ME/CFS clinical trial.* https://polybio.org/projects/lumbrokinase-longcovid-me-cfs-clinical-trial/ (accessed January 30, 2025).

Ramirez, L. G., M. Louisias, P. U. Ogbogu, A. Stinson, R. Gupta, S. Sansweet, T. Singh, A. Apter, B. L. Jones, and S. M. Nyenhuis. 2024. Understanding health equity in patient-reported outcomes. *The Journal of Allergy and Clinical Immunology: In Practice* 12(10):2617–2624.

Appendix A

Committee Meeting Agendas

Meeting 1—Virtual
April 22, 2024

CLOSED SESSION—COMMITTEE MEMBERS ONLY

12:30–2:35 PM CLOSED SESSION

OPEN SESSION

2:45 PM Sponsors remarks and committee questions
BEN NEMSER
Steven & Alexandra Cohen Foundation

3:15 PM Federal agencies remarks and committee questions
LYLE PETERSEN
National Center for Emerging and Zoonotic Infectious Diseases
Centers for Disease Control and Prevention

NADINE BOWDEN
National Institute of Allergy and Infectious Diseases
National Institutes of Health

KRISTEN HONEY
Office of Assistant Secretary of Health
Department of Health and Human Services

CLOSED SESSION—COMMITTEE MEMBERS ONLY

4:00–5:00 PM	CLOSED SESSION
5:00 PM	END OF MEETING

Meeting 1.5—Virtual
May 14, 2024

CLOSED SESSION—COMMITTEE MEMBERS ONLY

12:00 PM	CLOSED SESSION
3:30 PM	ADJOURN

Meeting 2—Hybrid Workshop
July 11–12, 2024

DAY 1—THURSDAY, JULY 11, 2024

CLOSED SESSION

9:00 AM	CLOSED SESSION

OPEN SESSION

9:30 AM	Welcome KENT KESTER, *Committee Chair* IAVI

APPENDIX A   *191*

Opening Session: An Overview of Challenges in Lyme IACI Research

Objectives
- Understand Lyme IACI disease impact; and
- Present overview of current status of ongoing research for Lyme IACI.

Framing Questions
- What is the impact of Lyme IACI in the U.S. and globally?
- What is the current evidence base toward understanding and developing treatments for Lyme IACI?
- What are key scientific or technical barriers in addressing challenges to develop new treatments?
- How are patient perspectives and input incorporated into prospective research studies?

9:35 AM	Patient perspective: Impact of Lyme IACI Rhisa Parera Your Labs Are Normal
9:45 AM	Overview: Current status and challenges in research for Lyme IACI treatment John Aucott Johns Hopkins University
10:05 AM	Building on current progress: Reflections from the HHS Tick-Borne Diseases Working Group C. Benjamin Beard Division of Vector-Borne Diseases Centers for Disease Control and Prevention
10:15 AM	Q&A
10:45 AM	BREAK

SESSION 1: Potential Commonalities Across Other Fields and Implications for Lyme IACI

Objectives
- Examine the commonalities between Lyme IACI and other diseases and potential shared mechanisms of pathology; and
- Evaluate the relative strength of evidence for the potential mechanisms of Lyme IACI pathology
- Discuss implications and unique considerations for Lyme IACI.

Framing Questions
- What similarities or differences exist between Lyme IACI and other IACI with neurologic, cognitive, or psychiatric symptoms?
- What does the current evidence suggest about the biological plausibility of the neurologic, cognitive, and psychiatric symptoms of Lyme IACI being caused by different mechanisms of pathology?
- What factors should be considered in prospective studies that seek to identify whether there are inflammatory and/or autoimmune biomarkers associated with Lyme IACI?
- Is research on pathogen persistence from other IACI translatable to developing potential treatment for Lyme IACI?

11:00 PM	**Autoimmune mechanisms of IACI** WILLIAM ROBINSON Stanford University
11:10 PM	**Inflammatory responses in IACI** DANIEL CLAUW University of Michigan
11:20 PM	**Current evidence for mechanisms of colonization and pathogenesis** JOHN LEONG Tufts University
11:30 PM	**Elucidating pathophysiology: lessons from ME/CFS** AVINDRA NATH National Institute of Neurological Disorders and Stroke, NIH
11:40 PM	Discussion and Q&A
12:15 PM	LUNCH

SESSION 2: Advances in Diagnostics Research

Objectives
- o Explain the relationships between diagnostics research and research on Lyme IACI etiology and treatment;
- o Provide an overview of current approaches to diagnostics that may hold promise for Lyme IACI diagnosis;
- o Identify current challenges in advancing diagnostics to support development of Lyme IACI treatment and emerging technologies that may mitigate these challenges; and
- o Discuss opportunities for implementation of these emerging technologies and other mitigating factors.

Framing Questions
- o What are challenges in developing diagnostics for Lyme IACI?
- o How do these challenges impact development of treatments?
- o What scientific advances exist that may address these challenges?
- o What are barriers (technical and/or market forces) to implementing these technologies for Lyme IACI?

1:00 PM	Current diagnostic approaches and emerging technologies CHARLES CHIU University of California, San Francisco
1:10 PM	Challenges in diagnostics research NANCY KLIMAS Nova Southeastern University
1:20 PM	Challenges in advancing new diagnostics development RAYMOND DATTWYLER New York Medical College
1:30 PM	Challenges in regulatory considerations of new diagnostics ELLIOT COWAN Partners in Diagnostics
1:40 PM	Discussion and Q&A

SESSION 3: Strategies to Improve the Applicability of Research

Objectives
- o Explore elements of study designs that enable collection of data from more inclusive patient samples;
- o Discuss strategies to standardize research questions and outcome measures; and
- o Assess the feasibility of implementing data sharing practices across Lyme IACI research studies.

Framing Questions
- o What are key factors to model or consider in large or in-depth prospective studies designed to interrogate potential pathways to developing treatments for Lyme IACI?
- o What challenges may have been encountered or can be anticipated in collecting and sharing data across different studies?

2:10 PM	Patient-generated data BETH JAWORSKI *All of Us* Research Program, National Institutes of Health
2:20 PM	Patient registries and biobanks for Lyme IACI LIZ HORN Lyme Disease Biobank
2:30 PM	Platform trial designs toward standardization and quality across studies ROGER LEWIS University of California, Los Angeles
2:40 PM	Research trials network and data sharing RACHELE HENDRICKS-STURRUP Duke-Margolis Institute for Health Policy
2:50 PM	Discussion and Q&A
3:20 PM	BREAK

APPENDIX A   *195*

SESSION 4:   Bridging Opportunities and Action

Session Objectives
- o Identify additional barriers that restrict progress on Lyme IACI research;
- o Consider how patient-defined research priorities and patient-reported outcomes can inform future research; and
- o Discuss opportunities to advance translation of Lyme IACI research into development.

Framing Questions
- o What mechanisms or processes are need to incorporate patient priorities into the research agenda in a more systematic way?
- o How can barriers to the conduct of Lyme IACI research be overcome? Who needs to be involved in developing solutions to address those barriers?
- o What opportunities already exist to advance Lyme IACI research toward the development of treatments and diagnostics, and how can those opportunities be better utilized?
- o What would success look like if different stakeholders were able to align on research priorities for Lyme IACI treatment? Are there any examples of successful collaboration for Lyme IACI research?

3:30 PM	**Panel Discussion: Patient-defined priorities for research**
	Patient-centered outcomes
	LORRAINE JOHNSON
	LymeDisease.org
	Patient participation in research and data collection
	WENDY ADAMS
	Bay Area Lyme Foundation
	Bridging between funder and patient priorities
	TIMOTHY SELLATI
	Global Lyme Alliance
4:00 PM	**Funder perspective**
	LEITH STATES
	Office of the Assistant Secretary for Health, HHS

4:10 PM	Industry perspective MATT TINDALL FlightPath Biosciences
4:20 PM	Regulatory perspective STACIE HUDGENS Clinical Outcomes Solutions
4:30 PM	Discussion and Q&A

Day 1 Wrap-Up

4:55 PM	Final Remarks KENT KESTER, *Committee Chair* IAVI
5:00 PM	ADJOURN DAY 1

DAY 2—FRIDAY, JULY 12, 2024

CLOSED SESSION

9:00 AM	Committee meets in closed session
3:30 PM	ADJOURN MEETING

Meeting 3—Virtual
August 12-13, 2024

DAY 1—MONDAY, AUGUST 12, 2024

CLOSED SESSION

9:00 AM	Committee meets in closed session

APPENDIX A   *197*

OPEN SESSION

WELCOME

9:45 AM   Welcome and opening remarks
           KENT KESTER, *Committee Chair*
           CEPI

SESSION 1 Moving toward Treatments: Remaining Questions in Lyme
           IACI Research

Session Objective:
   o Identify unresolved research questions on the etiology of Lyme IACI
     that can inform treatment development and discuss key actions
     necessary to fill this knowledge gap.

9:50 AM   Evidence for central nervous system involvement in
           Lyme IACI
           BRIAN FALLON
           Lyme and Tick-Borne Diseases Research Center
           Columbia University Vagelos College of Physicians and
           Surgeons

10:00 AM   Pathogen persistence and host immune response
           MONICA EMBERS
           Tulane School of Medicine

           LINDA BOCKENSTEDT
           Yale School of Medicine

10:20 AM   Microbiome dysbiosis
           ILHEM MESSAOUDI POWERS
           University of Kentucky, College of Medicine

10:30 AM   Discussion: Clinician perspective on challenges in clinical
           diagnosis and treatment outcomes
           RAVINDRA GANESH
           Post COVID Care Clinic at Mayo Clinic

           RYAN HURT
           Mayo Clinic

           LISA SANDERS
           Yale New Haven Health Systems Long COVID Consultation
           Clinic

10:45 AM	Open discussion with committee
11:30 AM	BREAK

CLOSED SESSION

12:00 PM	Committee meets in closed session
2:00 PM	ADJOURN DAY 1

DAY 2—TUESDAY, AUGUST 13, 2024

OPEN SESSION

WELCOME

9:00 AM Welcome and opening remarks
KENT KESTER, *Committee Chair*
CEPI

SESSION 2 Health Equity Considerations for Future Research Agenda

Objectives:
- Examine unique challenges in working with underserved populations for research studies on Lyme IACI treatment and discuss mitigation strategies.
- Examine what is known about co-infections with other tick-borne pathogens and the relevance for developing new treatments and diagnostics for Lyme IACI.
- Elucidate current understanding of additional risk factors in developing Lyme IACI from acute Lyme disease and identify promising research directions.

9:05 AM Underserved populations
ROBERTA DEBIASI
Children's National Research Institute

BETHANY ALCAUTER
National Center for Farmworker Health

APPENDIX A   199

9:25 AM   Additional risk factors in developing Lyme IACI

           Host risk factors including sex differences
           MICHAL TAL
           Massachusetts Institute of Technology

           Role of environmental exposures
           ESTHER MELAMED
           University of Texas at Austin, Dell Medical School

           Co-infections and potential interplay of immune responses
           EROL FIKRIG
           Yale School of Medicine
9:55 AM   Open discussion with committee

10:15 AM   BREAK

                          CLOSED SESSION

10:30 AM   Committee meets in closed session

2:30 PM   ADJOURN

                       Meeting 3.5—Virtual
                       September 10, 2024

              CLOSED SESSION—COMMITTEE MEMBERS ONLY

2:00 PM   CLOSED SESSION

5:00 PM   ADJOURN

Meeting 4—Hybrid
October 1–2, 2024

DAY 1 | TUESDAY, OCTOBER 1, 2024 (all times EDT)

CLOSED SESSION—COMMITTEE MEMBERS ONLY

10:00 AM	CLOSED SESSION
5:00 PM	ADJOURN

DAY 2 | WEDNESDAY, OCTOBER 2, 2024 (all times EDT)

CLOSED SESSION—COMMITTEE MEMBERS ONLY

9:00 AM	CLOSED SESSION
3:00 PM	ADJOURN

Meeting 5—Virtual
November 6, 2024

CLOSED SESSION—COMMITTEE MEMBERS ONLY

1:30 PM	CLOSED SESSION
5:30 PM	ADJOURN

Meeting 6—Virtual
January 7, 2025

CLOSED SESSION—COMMITTEE MEMBERS ONLY

2:00 PM	CLOSED SESSION
5:00 PM	ADJOURN

Appendix B

Committee Member and Staff Biographies

Kent Kester, M.D. (Chair), is currently the executive director of vaccine research and development at the Coalition for Epidemic Preparedness Innovations (CEPI). During a 24-year career in the U.S. Army, he worked extensively in clinical vaccine development and led multiple research platforms at the Walter Reed Army Institute of Research, the Department of Defense's largest and most diverse biomedical research laboratory, with a major emphasis on emerging infectious diseases; he later led that institution as its commander. His final military assignment was as the associate dean for clinical research in the School of Medicine at the Uniformed Services University of the Health Sciences (USUHS). During his military service, Dr. Kester was appointed as the lead policy advisor to the U.S. Army Surgeon General in both infectious diseases and in medical research and development. More recently, he served as the head of translational medicine and biomarkers at Sanofi Pasteur. Dr. Kester holds an undergraduate degree from Bucknell University and an M.D. from Jefferson Medical College. Currently a member of the Department of Veterans Affairs Health Services Research and Development Service Merit Review Board, the National Academy Standing Committee on Emerging Infectious Diseases and 21st Century Health Threats, and the CEPI scientific advisory committee, he previously chaired the steering committee of the National Institute of Allergy and Infectious Diseases (NIAID)/USUHS Infectious Disease Clinical Research Program, and he has served as a member of the Presidential Advisory Council on Combating Antibiotic-Resistant Bacteria, the Food and Drug Administration's Vaccines and Related Biologics Products Advisory Committee, the NIAID advisory council, and board of scientific counselors for the Office of Infectious Diseases at the Centers for Disease Control and Prevention. He is the vice chair of the National Academy of Medicine Forum on Microbial Threats. Board-certified in both internal medicine and infectious diseases, Dr. Kester holds faculty appointments at USUHS and the University of Maryland. He is a fellow of the American College of Physicians, the Royal College of Physicians of Edinburgh, the Infectious Disease Society of America, and the American Society of Tropical Medicine and Hygiene. He is a member of the clinical faculty at the University of Maryland Shock Trauma Center in Baltimore and the Wilkes-Barre Veterans' Administration Medical Center in Wilkes-Barre, Pennsylvania.

John A. Branda, M.D., is an associate professor of pathology at Harvard Medical School and an associate pathologist at Massachusetts General Hospital. He specializes in medical microbiology and has broad expertise in infectious disease diagnostic testing methods. His primary academic focus has been the development of improved diagnostic tests for Lyme disease and other tick-borne infections. He was co-recipient of the 2015 Bay Area Lyme Foundation Emerging Leader Award and a 2022 Phase 1 LymeX Diagnostics Prize through the Lyme Innovation Accelerator (administered independently in a public-private partnership between the Department of Health and Human Services and the Steven & Alexandra Cohen Foundation). Prior to 2020, he received research funding support from Lyme Disease Biobank Foundation, the Fairbairn Family Lyme Research Initiative at Harvard Medical School, and diagnostic companies for the detection of acute Lyme disease. Dr. Branda is currently a principal investigator for the Pfizer-Valneva vaccine trial for Lyme disease. He received his medical degree in 2000 from Harvard Medical School, after which he completed a clinical pathology residency and a medical microbiology fellowship at Massachusetts General Hospital. Dr. Branda is co-inventor on a patent pending for a serologic diagnostic assay to detect *Borrelia burgdorferi* sensu lato complex. He previously served on the scientific advisory boards of DiaSorin (2019), Roche Diagnostics (2019), FlightPath Biosciences (2023), and Tarsus Pharmaceuticals (2023) and received compensation for these services. He is also a coauthor on the 2020 IDSA/AAN/ACR Lyme disease treatment and diagnosis guidelines and was a member of the Federal Tick-borne Disease Working Group.

Betty A. Diamond, M.D., is the director of the Institute of Molecular Medicine in the Feinberg Institute for Medical Research at Northwell Health. Her research has focused on the induction and pathogenicity of autoantibodies in systemic lupus erythematosus (SLE), especially in the brain. Most recently, she has become interested in the anti-inflammatory effects of the immune protein C1q. In recent years, she has also become involved in clinical trials in SLE and has led several clinical trials of novel therapeutics. Dr. Diamond currently receives compensation as a consultant for biotech companies that are developing CAR-T cell therapies, including iCell Gene Therapeutics, Atara Biotherapeutics, Adicet Bio, and Sail Biomedicines. She also serves as an editor for *eLife* and *Frontiers* journals. Dr. Diamond is a member of both the National Academy of Medicine and the National Academy of Sciences and previously served on National Academies committees Examining the Working Definition for Long COVID and Diagnostic Criteria for Myalgic Encephalomyelitis/Chronic Fatigue Syndrome. She is a past president of the American Association of Immunologists and has received the Distinguished Investigator award and the Presidential Gold Medal from the American College of Rheumatology. She received her M.D. from Harvard Medical School, performed a residency in internal medicine at Columbia Presbyterian Medical Center, and then trained in immunology at the Albert Einstein College of Medicine

Jesse L. Goodman, M.D., M.P.H., is a professor of medicine at Georgetown University and the director of the Center on Medical Product Access, Safety and Stewardship, which focuses on science and policy to address public health needs. He is an attending physician in infectious diseases at Georgetown University, Washington D.C., Veterans Administration, and Walter Reed medical centers. He was previously the chief scientist of the Food and Drug Administration (FDA), serving in the government's senior leadership for the 2009 influenza pandemic and other public health responses. Prior to that, he served as a senior advisor to the FDA Commissioner where he co-chaired the U.S. Task Force to Combat Antimicrobial Resistance before going on to direct FDA's Center for Biologics Evaluation and Research. Previously he was a professor of medicine and the chief of infectious diseases at the University of Minnesota, where his laboratory isolated *Anaplasma phagocytophilum*, the cause of human granulocytic anaplasmosis, and studied Lyme disease, including dissemination of the organism in early disease and persistent infection as the primary cause of arthritis. Dr. Goodman currently serves as a member of the board of directors and recently completed his term as chair of the science committee at GlaxoSmithKline, for which he receives compensation. He also currently serves as a scientific advisory board member at Intellia and Adaptive Phage Therapeutics, both with compensation. He received his M.D. from the Albert Einstein College of Medicine and his M.P.H. from the University of Minnesota. He has served on advisory committees at the Centers for Disease Control and Prevention, the National Institutes of Health, the Department of Defense, the Coalition for Epidemic Preparedness Innovations, and the World Health Organization and as past president and board member of the United States

Pharmacopeia. He is a member of the National Academy of Medicine and was previously a member of the Forum on Microbial Threats.

Miguel A. Hernán, M.D., Dr.P.H., M.P.H., is the Kolokotrones Professor of Biostatistics and Epidemiology and the director of CAUSALab at the Harvard T.H. Chan School of Public Health. He uses health data and causal inference methods to learn what works. Dr. Hernán and his collaborators repurpose real-world data into evidence for the prevention and treatment of infectious diseases, cancer, cardiovascular disease, and mental illness. This work has contributed to the shaping of health policy and research methodology worldwide. Dr. Hernán has received several awards, including the Rousseeuw Prize for Statistics, the Rothman Epidemiology Prize, and a MERIT award from the U.S. National Institutes of Health. He has also received research funding from the National Institutes of Health, the Veteran Administration, Patient-Centered Outcome Research Institute, and the Department of Defense. He is fellow of the American Association for the Advancement of Science and the American Statistical Association and the associate editor of *Annals of Internal Medicine*. He has served on multiple committees of the National Academies. Dr. Hernán received an M.D. from the Universidad Autónoma de Madrid and an M.P.H., Dr.P.H., and M.S. from Harvard University.

Adrian F. Hernandez, M.D., M.H.S., is the vice dean of the Duke School of Medicine and the executive director of the Duke Clinical Research Institute (DCRI). He is a cardiologist who aims to improve health by accelerating clinical evidence through outcomes research, clinical trials, comparative effectiveness, and health policy. He has led multiple large-scale patient-centered research programs, registries, and clinical trials across multiple health conditions, including the Health System Collaboratory of the National Institutes of Health (NIH) and PCORnet, funded by the Patient-Centered Outcomes Research Institute, and he is involved in the NIH Researching COVID to Enhance Recovery initiative. He has served as the steering committee chair or principal investigator on multiple studies and has authored over 800 publications. Dr. Hernandez received his medical degree from the University of Texas–Southwestern at Dallas and completed his residency in internal medicine at the University of California San Francisco School of Medicine before completing a fellowship in cardiology at Duke University. He is an elected member of the American Society for Clinical Investigation and the Association of American Physicians and serves on the board of directors of the Reagan-Udall Foundation. Dr. Hernandez frequently consults with and receives research support from pharmaceutical companies, none of which have active portfolios in the treatment or diagnosis of Lyme disease.

Brandon L. Jutras, Ph.D., is an associate professor in the Microbiology–Immunology Department at the Feinberg School of Medicine at Northwestern University. His laboratory is focused on understanding the basic biology of *Borrelia burgdorferi* with emphasis on using the bacterial cell wall to understand everything from the cell cycle to developing novel Lyme disease treatments and diagnostics. Dr. Jutras's laboratory currently receives grants from the National Institutes of Health, the Department of Defense, Global Lyme Alliance, the Bay Area Lyme Foundation, and the LymeX Diagnostics Innovation Prize. His laboratory previously received funding from the Steven & Alexandra Cohen Foundation, which concluded in 2023. Dr. Jutras earned his Ph.D. at the University of Kentucky, where he studied molecular mechanisms of gene regulation in *B. burgdorferi* prior to being a Howard Hughes postdoctoral fellow in the field of Lyme disease bacterial cell biology. He has more than 18 years of Lyme disease research experience and has published dozens of peer-reviewed publications in the field.

Nicole Malachowski, COL, USAF (ret.), is the Founder and Chief Executive Officer of Nicole Malachowski & Associates, LLC. A 2019 National Women's Hall of Fame inductee and recent Presidential appointee, Col. Malachowski has more than 21 years of experience as an officer, leader, and fighter pilot in the United States Air Force. Upon her commission into the military, she was competitively selected to fly combat aircraft and embarked on an adventure among the first group of women to fly modern fighter jets. Col. Malachowski served as a mission-ready fighter pilot in three operational F-15E squadrons and accumulated over 2,300 flight hours, including 188 hours in combat. She has had the honor of commanding a fighter squadron, flying as a USAF Thunderbird pilot, and serving as a White House Fellow and as an advisor to the First Lady of the United States. Col. Malachowski has forged a successful path through immense cultural changes in the military as well as significant adversity in her personal life. Following her medical retirement from the Air Force due to the severe impacts of late-stage tick-borne illness, she reinvented herself as a highly successful entrepreneur, professional speaker, and leadership consultant. Col. Malachowski is a sought-after keynote speaker and shares her experience with Lyme disease to inspire resilience and reinvention with many companies, such as Endo Pharmaceuticals. She served on the Tick-Borne Diseases Panel for the Department of Defense Congressionally Directed Medical Research Program and as a subcommittee member of the Federal Tick-Borne Diseases Working Group. She continues to hold volunteer positions as an ambassador with the Bay Area Lyme Foundation, patient advocate speaker with the Center for Lyme Action, and as a mentor and ambassador in the Wounded Warriors program. Col. Malachowski currently serves on the advisory board of Invisible International and as a board member of the LivLyme Foundation. She has previously volunteered as an advisory board member at the Dean Center for Tick Borne Illness,. Col. Malachowski has been honored with the IMPACT Award by the White House Fellow Foundation. She finds immense meaning in traveling and advocating for those affected by tick-borne illnesses.

Cherie Marvel, Ph.D., is a cognitive neuroscientist and an associate professor of neurology at the Johns Hopkins University School of Medicine. She uses brain imaging methods such as magnetic resonance imaging (MRI) to examine brain function in healthy and clinical populations. Her research in Lyme disease applies MRI methods to characterize brain changes in people with acute Lyme and post-treatment Lyme disease and relate these changes to cognition, mood, and clinical outcomes. Dr. Marvel served as the president of the International Society of Behavioural Neuroscience from 2021 to 2025 and served as the chair of the National Institutes of Health (NIH) study section NIH Fellowships: Learning and Memory, Language, Communication, and Related Neurosciences (F01B) from 2022 to 2023. She is funded by the NIH, the Department of Defense, and private foundations for her research in Lyme disease. Dr. Marvel obtained her Ph.D. in neuroscience from Georgetown University. She completed a fellowship in clinical neuroscience at the University of Iowa and then completed a second fellowship in Cognitive Neuroscience at Johns Hopkins University.

Debjani Mukherjee, Ph.D., M.A., is an associate professor of medical ethics in clinical medicine and clinical rehabilitation medicine at Weill Cornell Medical College and senior clinical ethicist at New York Presbyterian/Weill Cornell Medical Center. Dr. Mukherjee is a clinical/community psychologist and clinical ethicist with expertise in disability and rehabilitation ethics. She was invited to help start the first Center for Clinical Ethics in Paris, France, and was awarded a Fulbright Scholarship to India to study long-term adjustment to brain injury. In 2023 she was elected a Hastings Center Fellow. Her scholarly interests are in the ethical dilemmas posed by neurological impairments, the emotional impact of medical decisions, the practice of clinical ethics consultation, and ethical concerns in rehabilitation medicine. Dr. Mukherjee received her bachelor's degree in psychology from Cornell University and her M.A. and Ph.D. in clinical/community psychology from the University of Illinois at Urbana–Champaign. She then completed two years of postdoctoral fellowship at the Maclean Center for Clinical Medical Ethics at the University of Chicago. Before joining the faculty of Weill Cornell Medical College in 2020, she was the director of the Donnelley Ethics Program at the Shirley Ryan AbilityLab and faculty at Northwestern University Feinberg School of Medicine.

Lise E. Nigrovic, M.D., M.P.H., is a professor of pediatrics at Harvard Medical School and practices as a pediatric emergency physician at Boston Children's Hospital. She serves as the Boston Children's Hospital principal investigator for the National Center for Advancing Translational Sciences–supported Harvard Catalyst program. Dr. Nigrovic is the founding chair of the Pedi Lyme Net research network, the only multicenter pediatric Lyme disease clinical research network, with more than 5,000 adults and children undergoing evaluation for Lyme disease enrolled to collect clinical phenotype and matched biosamples. With support from the National Institute of Allergy and Infectious Diseases, she is leading a 21-center study to compare short- and long-term outcomes for children with Lyme meningitis by antibiotic treatment regimen. Dr. Nigrovic previously served as a consultant with Adaptive Biotechnologies and as an advisory board member with Tarsus Pharmaceutical and received compensation for these services in assisting with the development of diagnostic tests, preventatives, and prophylaxis. She currently serves on the clinical research advisory committee at Global Lyme Alliance. Her current research support includes funding from the National Institutes of Health, the Department of Defense, and Global Lyme Alliance. Dr. Nigrovic has also received funding in the past from the Global Lyme Alliance, the Bay Area Lyme Foundation, the Milton Foundation, and the Fairbairn Family Lyme Research Initiative at Harvard Medical School. Of her more than 200 peer-reviewed publications, 50 are related to Lyme disease and other tick-borne infections in children. Dr. Nigrovic received her M.D. from Harvard Medical School and her M.P.H from the Harvard School of Public Health. In recognition of her expertise, Dr. Nigrovic was selected as an inaugural member of the Federal Tick-Borne Illness Working Group as well as a working group member of IDSA/AAN/ACR Lyme disease clinical guideline panel.

Simone A. Seward, Dr.P.H., M.P.H., is currently an assistant professor in public health and preventive medicine at SUNY Upstate Medical University in Syracuse, New York. As an educator, community health advocate, and mixed methods researcher, Dr. Seward has developed strategic approaches that center on social justice and racial equity. Using community engagement as a vehicle for systemic change, Dr. Seward builds interdisciplinary, collaborative partnerships that are sensitive to diverse perspectives and population needs. With over 15 years of extensive training and diverse practice-based experiences at the federal, state, and local levels and in academia, Dr. Seward ensures that community health interventions and programs include the voices and lived experiences of the target community. As a dedicated researcher and advocate specializing in maternal and child health disparities, Dr. Seward has devoted her career to understanding and addressing the unique challenges facing Black mothers and infants. Her research and scholarly area of interest focuses on examining the root causes of racial disparities in maternal and infant health outcomes, including the impact of systemic racism as a contributing factor to healthcare disparities. Dr. Seward obtained a master of public health degree from Boston University School of Public Health, followed by a doctor of public health degree from the University at Albany School of Public Health. Dr. Seward has received numerous awards for her work and leadership, including the Faculty Gold Standard Award, Upstate President Award for Community Service Team, and Faculty and Staff Association for Diversity Award. In addition, Dr. Seward is a scholar of the Public Health Leadership Institute of Florida, the SUNY SAIL Leadership Institute, and a former Presidential Health Disparities Fellow of the Center for the Elimination of Minority Health Disparities at the University at Albany. Dr. Seward also has several professional affiliations where she donates her time. She currently serves as vice chair of the board of directors for the Central New York Lyme and Tickborne Disease Alliance and is a member of the Blueprint 15 board of directors, the Onondaga County Health Advisory Council whose responsibilities include Lyme disease reporting as well as a member of the community action network for the Syracuse Healthy Start initiative. She was also previously a public health fellow for Onondaga County focusing on maternal and child health.

Robert P. Smith, M.D., M.P.H., is an infectious disease physician who currently directs research studies into the ecology, epidemiology, and clinical recognition of tick-borne diseases at the MaineHealth Institute for Research. His team at the Vector-Borne Disease Laboratory there includes scientists with training in medical entomology, biostatistics/mathematical modeling, vector ecology, and clinical research. Current projects include tick-borne disease surveillance/epidemiology, strategies for vector control, phylogenetics and ecology of Powassan virus, and novel diagnostic approaches for early Lyme disease. He is a member of the Division of Infectious Diseases at Maine Medical Center and served as the director of the Division of Infectious Diseases there from 2014 to 2022. Dr. Smith has been a regional leader in professional and public outreach regarding the recognition and treatment of tick-borne diseases and often gives talks and publishes on Lyme disease. He also served from its inception in 1992 until 2022 as the director of an interdisciplinary specialty clinic at Maine Medical Center focused on the care of persons with HIV and other viral infections. Dr. Smith has received research support from the National Institutes of Health, including two Small Business Innovation Research awards, from the Centers for Disease Control and Prevent and from the State of Maine Department of Health and Human Services related to Lyme disease research. Dr. Smith also served as co-investigator as part of the Pfizer–Valneva vaccine trial research site at

MaineHealth. Dr. Smith received his medical degree from Johns Hopkins University School of Medicine and is a professor of medicine at Tufts University School of Medicine. He has widely published on served on numerous federal panels and work groups related to tick-borne diseases, the Federal Tick-Borne Disease Working Group (2018), and was an invited reviewer of the (then) Institute of Medicine 2011 report Critical Needs and Gaps in Understanding, Amelioration and Prevention of Lyme disease and Other Tick-borne Infections. He is a fellow of the American College of Physicians and of the Infectious Disease Society of America.

Qing-Mei Wang, M.D., Ph.D., is a physician–scientist and physiatrist at Spaulding Rehabilitation Hospital, the teaching affiliate of Harvard Medical School. She is an assistant professor in the Department of Physical Medicine and Rehabilitation at Harvard Medical School. She is also the director of the Stroke Biological Recovery Laboratory and conducts translational research in neuro-rehabilitation. She has been providing rehabilitation care to patients with post-treatment Lyme disease syndrome (PTLDS) since 2020. This devastating disease and the lack of effective treatment led her to conduct clinical studies using non-invasive vagal nerve stimulation technology. The results from her study suggest that transcutaneous auricular vagal nerve stimulation may improve neurocognitive impairment in PTLDS. This study may provide a novel approach to treat PTLDS. She is the recipient of the Rehabilitation Medicine Scientist Training Program (K12) and NIH K08 awards. Dr. Wang obtained her Ph.D. and M.D. at the University of Medicine and Dentistry of New Jersey and completed residency training in physical medicine and rehabilitation at Mount Sinai Medical Center in New York. She is a member of the American Association of Physiatrists.

Susan J. Wong, Ph.D., M.Sc., was the director of diagnostic immunology at the Wadsworth Center (New York State Department of Health, NYSDOH) for 26 years before retiring in 2020. While at the Wadsworth Center, Dr. Wong set up the first tests for *Anaplama phagocytophilum* and *Babesia microti* serology for New York State. She has evaluated microsphere immunoassays using recombinant proteins of *Borrelia*, *Babesia*, and *Anaplasma* for multiplex serology of tickborne infections; established microsphere immunoassays to detect Powassan virus, deer tick virus, and tick-borne encephalitis virus; and applied microsphere immunoassays to differentiate flavivirus infections (West Nile, St. Louis encephalitis, Zika, and dengue). Dr. Wong earned a bachelor of science in molecular biology from the University of Wisconsin and then went on to receive a master of science in biochemistry from the University of New Hampshire and a Ph.D. in biochemistry from the University of Saskatchewan. Dr. Wong has been honored with the Wadsworth Center Recognition Award in 1999, the NYSDOH

Commissioner's Recognition Award for response to the West Nile Virus and SARS, and the Thomas Nakano Commendation from the Centers for Disease Control and Prevention (CDC) and U.S. Public Health Service (USPHS), and a nominee for the Charles Shepard Science Award from the CDC and USPHS. Dr. Wong also has experience working globally, serving as a consultant to the Ethiopian Health and Nutrition Research Institute in Addis Ababa through the Association of Public Health Laboratories, and she worked as a consultant to the Iraq Science Engagement Program in Baghdad, Iraq, with the Civilian Research and Development Foundation.

STAFF

Julie Liao, Ph.D. (*Study Co-Director*), is a senior program officer with the Board on Global Health of the National Academies of Sciences, Engineering, and Medicine, where she directs the Forum on Microbial Threats. In 2023 the Forum on Microbial Threats co-convened a public workshop, *Toward a Common Research Agenda for Infection-Associated Chronic Illnesses*, which highlighted current research progress and opportunities for coordination between these chronic conditions including myalgic encephalomyelitis (chronic fatigue syndrome), Long COVID, and Lyme disease. Before joining the National Academies in 2020, she was involved in pre-clinical vaccine development research in the biotechnology industry. She received a Ph.D. in molecular science and microbiology from Binghamton University and completed postdoctoral training at Boston Children's Hospital.

Andrew March, M.P.H. (*Study Co-Director*), is a program officer with the Board on Health Sciences Policy of the National Academies of Sciences, Engineering, and Medicine. Most recently, he served as the co-director for the consensus study, *Developing a Framework to Address Legal, Ethical, Regulatory, and Policy Issues for Research Specific to Pregnant and Lactating Persons*. He has contributed to consensus studies on diverse topics in health policy, including medical product supply chains, dementia care interventions, and the safety and effectiveness of compounded drug preparations. Before joining the National Academies in 2018, he conducted research on the intersection of maternal and occupational health at the Center for Research in Occupational Health in Barcelona, and he worked in the Department of Clinical Epidemiology and Public Health at the Hospital de la Santa Creu i Sant Pau. Mr. March obtained his M.P.H. at the Universitat Pompeu Fabra and his B.S. degree in biology and Spanish from Roanoke College.

Emily McDowell, M.P.H., is a research associate with the Board on Health Sciences Policy of the National Academies of Sciences, Engineering, and

Medicine. Most recently, she assisted with a consensus study, *Advancing Clinical Research in Pregnant and Lactating Populations Overcoming Real and Perceived Liability Risks*, and she has contributed to other projects at the National Academies relating to health equity and policy. She is a M.P.H. graduate from George Washington University concentrating her studies on epidemiology and environmental health. Before joining the National Academies, Ms. McDowell worked for a nonprofit emergency management organization, Healthcare Ready, and assisted with the reauthorization of the Pandemic and All-Hazards Advancing Innovation Act (PAHPAIA). Her studies at George Washington University concluded with the presentation of her thesis entitled "Microplastics and Human Health: An Inescapable Exposure." Ms. McDowell received her B.S. in community health, concentrating in global health at George Mason University.

Julie Pavlin, M.D., Ph.D., M.P.H., is the director of the Board on Global Health at the National Academies of Sciences, Engineering, and Medicine, where she coordinates analyses of health developments beyond U.S. borders and areas of international health investment that promote global well-being, security, and economic development. Prior to this position, she was a research area director at the Infectious Disease Clinical Research Program and the deputy director of the Armed Forces Health Surveillance Center. She is a retired Colonel in the U.S. Army with previous assignments including the Armed Forces Research Institute of Medical Sciences in Bangkok, Thailand, the Walter Reed Army Institute of Research, and the U.S. Army Medical Research Institute for Infectious Diseases. She concentrated most of her time with the Department of Defense in the design of real-time disease surveillance systems and was a co-founder of the International Society for Disease Surveillance. Dr. Pavlin received her A.B. from Cornell University, M.D. from Loyola University, M.P.H. from Harvard University and Ph.D. in emerging infectious diseases at the Uniformed Services University.

Rayane Silva-Curran is a senior program assistant on the Board on Health Sciences Policy, with the Forum on Medical and Public Health Preparedness for Disasters and Emergencies. Before joining the National Academies, Ms. Silva-Curran worked as a COVID-19 contact tracer for the Fairfax County Health Department. She received her B.S., in community health with a concentration in global health from George Mason University. She also holds a B.S. in biology from the Universidade Estadual de Goias (Brazil).

Carolyn Shore, Ph.D., directs the Forum on Drug Discovery, Development, and Translation and serves as Global Health Lead for the National Academies of Sciences, Engineering, and Medicine (National Academies). Before joining the National Academies, Carolyn was an officer on Pew's antibiotic resistance project, leading work on research and policies to spur the discovery and development of urgently needed antibacterial therapies. She previously served as a foreign affairs officer at the U.S. Department of State, where she led an initiative on open data and innovation-based solutions to global challenges. She also served as the State Department's representative to intergovernmental organizations focusing on food safety, plant and animal health, biosecurity, and agricultural trade policy. Carolyn was an American Society for Microbiology congressional fellow, working on science-based policy related to antibiotic stewardship and other public health issues. She holds a doctoral degree in Microbiology and Molecular Genetics from Harvard University. As a graduate student, she studied antimalarial drug resistance in Senegal and worked jointly between the Medicines for Malaria Venture, Genzyme Corporation, and the Broad Institute of Harvard and MIT to discover new anti-malarial compounds. Carolyn was awarded a Fulbright Fellowship for work at the University of Queensland in Brisbane, Australia, and a National Institutes of Health Training Grant for postdoctoral work at the University of Iowa.

Clare Stroud, Ph.D., is the senior board director for the Board on Health Sciences Policy at the National Academies of Sciences, Engineering, and Medicine. In this capacity she oversees a program of activities aimed at fostering the basic biomedical and clinical research enterprises; addressing the ethical, legal, and social contexts of scientific and technologic advances related to health; and strengthening the preparedness, resilience, and sustainability of communities. Previously, she served as director of the National Academies' Forum on Neuroscience and Nervous System Disorders, which brings together leaders from government, academia, industry, and nonprofit organizations to discuss key challenges and emerging issues in neuroscience research, the development of therapies for nervous system disorders, and related ethical and societal issues. She also led consensus studies and contributed to projects on such topics as pain management, medications for opioid use disorder, traumatic brain injury, preventing cognitive decline and dementia, supporting persons living with dementia and their caregivers, the health and well-being of young adults, and disaster preparedness and response. Dr. Stroud first joined the National Academies as a Mirzayan Science and Technology Policy Graduate Fellow. She has also been an associate at AmericaSpeaks, a nonprofit organization that engaged citizens in decision making on important public policy issues. Dr. Stroud received her Ph.D. from the University of Maryland, College Park, with research focused on the cognitive neuroscience of language, and her bachelor's degree from Queen's University in Canada.

Appendix C

Methodology of Literature Review

There are currently no safe and effective treatments or diagnostics for Lyme infection-associated chronic illnesses (IACI). Research remains necessary to elucidate the underlying mechanisms and develop new treatments and diagnostic tests for Lyme IACI patients. These efforts may be buoyed by exploring research approaches and findings from commonalities with other similar conditions such as Long COVID and myalgic encephalomyelitis/chronic fatigue syndrome (ME/CFS).

At the request of the Steven & Alexandra Cohen Foundation, an ad hoc committee convened by the National Academies was tasked to examine the existing evidence and knowledge gaps on the etiology and treatment of Lyme IACI and to identify opportunities for learning from similar conditions that can accelerate development of new treatments for Lyme IACI. To explore opportunities where new knowledge can be applied toward accelerating treatment development for Lyme IACI, the committee determined that it was necessary to have an overview of the current evidence and gaps in the Lyme IACI research landscape. The committee structured their approach to addressing this charge into three components:

- Landscape mapping of research related to understanding the etiology and diagnosis of Lyme IACI in humans.
- Landscape mapping of clinical trials from Lyme IACI that tested treatments for persistent symptoms with the greatest impact for those living with Lyme IACI.

- Landscape mapping of clinical trials from other similar conditions, with a focus on Long COVID and ME/CFS, that address the priority symptoms that Lyme IACI shares with these conditions.

To address the first two components, the committee conducted a scoping review of the literature. To address the third component, and in line with the research prioritization principles discussed in Chapter 4, where potential treatments for Lyme IACI that draw from another disease area should be supported by established evidence of efficacy, the committee surveyed recent systematic reviews (since 2020) to identify treatments for ME/CFS and Long COVID that have shown efficacy in randomized controlled clinical trials.

A scoping review is an efficient and appropriate approach to assess the existing evidence base and analyze knowledge gaps. A preliminary search of PubMed did not reveal current scoping reviews on the etiology, treatment, or diagnosis of Lyme IACI in North America; the only available and relevant record is a scoping review that examined the prevalence of reporting on neuropsychiatric manifestations and cognitive decline and the association of delayed diagnosis with symptom severity, in patients with longstanding Lyme disease (Brackett et al., 2024).

The scoping review was carried out by research librarians at the National Academies with consultant research methodologists from PICO Portal and the National Academies study staff, in accordance with the Preferred Reporting Items for Systematic Reviews and Meta-Analyses Extension for Scoping Reviews (PRISMA-ScR). The survey of systematic reviews for ME/CFS and Long COVID was performed by the National Academies study staff and research librarians with assistance from the PICO Portal software service for records de-duplication and management. The method for the scoping review and strategy for survey of systematic reviews are detailed below.

SCOPING REVIEW

Literature Search Strategy

The purpose of this scoping review is to identify and characterize peer-reviewed primary research published between 1970 and May 2024 that attempted to elucidate potential pathophysiology mechanisms that underlie symptoms of Lyme IACI or to assess the efficacy of treatments and diagnostics for adults and children with Lyme IACI in North America. A supplemental search was conducted in August 2024 to expand the search terms to include those used in older publications and to identify articles published since the initial search using the updated set of search terms.

Due to the differences in the causative agents and potential implications for disease presentation and long-term manifestations, the committee limited the literature review to North America and excluded studies of Lyme IACI in Europe and elsewhere in the world. Articles were limited to the English language. Databases searched include PubMed, Medline (Ovid), Embase (Ovid), and Scopus.

A standard definition for Lyme IACI does not exist, but it is essential to describe the population that would be included in this literature review. For the purpose of this study, the committee describes the population included in the literature review under this operational scope: that "Lyme infection-associated chronic illnesses" are considered as otherwise unexplained symptoms that persist for at least 6 months following antibiotic treatment for either proven or presumed infection with *Borrelia* spp. that cause Lyme disease. Keywords applied to the literature search were deliberately broadly inclusive, followed by abstracts and full-text screening to remove irrelevant articles (Table C-1). While it is possible that some studies still may not be captured by these search terms, the committee believes this approach balanced efficiency with the retrieval of a sufficiently representative collection of the evidence base.

Abstract and Full-Text Screening

The results from the search were imported into the PICO Portal online software service and de-duplicated. Abstracts were screened for inclusion eligibility (Table C-2) through dual review (National Academies staff), with a third member of the study staff to adjudicate differences. During abstract screening, articles were sorted into one of three categories for full-text review (disease mechanism, treatment, diagnosis). The inclusion criteria for each of the three categories were applied for full text screening (Table C-3).

TABLE C-1 Keywords Used to Describe Lyme IACI for Title and Abstract Literature Search

Initial literature search
• Post-Lyme disease syndrome
• Post-treatment Lyme disease
• Post-treatment Lyme disease syndrome
• Chronic Lyme disease
• Persistent Lyme disease
Supplemental literature search
• Lyme neuroborreliosis
• Lyme AND "chronic disease" or "persist*"

NOTE: IACI = infection-associated chronic illnesses.

TABLE C-2 Inclusion and Exclusion Criteria for Abstracts Screening

Category	Inclusion	Exclusion
Date	• 1970 to present (August 2024)	• Before 1970
Location	• North America	• Outside of North America
Language	• Publication in English	• Original text not in English
Study design	• Any primary research design with human participants (adults, children)	• Studies that only report on microbiology, in vitro assays, animal, or in silico models
Publication type	• Primary literature, full text available	• Reviews and meta-analyses, books, grey literature, opinions, abstract-only articles, conference abstracts, dissertations
Outcomes	• Any study outcomes	• None excluded

TABLE C-3 Inclusion and Exclusion Criteria for Full-Text Screening

Category	Inclusion	Exclusion
Disease mechanisms	• Observational studies • Research population includes individuals with Lyme IACI	• Case reports, case series • Research only on Lyme disease, not Lyme IACI
Treatment	• Observational clinical trials • Interventional clinical trials • Research population includes individuals with Lyme IACI	• Not clinical trial (case reports, case series, retrospective chart review) • Research only on Lyme disease, not Lyme IACI
Diagnosis	• Observational studies • Case reports and case series • Research population includes individuals with Lyme IACI	• None • Research only on Lyme disease, not Lyme IACI

NOTE: IACI = infection-associated chronic illnesses.

Data Extraction and Summary of Evidence

Select data variables from the included full text articles were obtained by dual extraction with two methodologists at PICO Portal and verified to resolve misalignments and ensure completeness by a senior methodologist from PICO Portal (Table C-4). A total of 1,579 records were obtained from the literature search and imported into the PICO Portal system. After the removal of 755 duplicates, 824 abstracts were screened for eligibility by two reviewers and one adjudicator. Of the 232 titles included for review, one article could not be retrieved and an additional 146 were excluded

APPENDIX C

upon screening to yield 85 full text articles. The committee reviewed the articles and extracted data for each of the three categories. Summary findings and conclusions drawn based on this scoping review are presented throughout the report.

TABLE C-4 Data Extraction for Each Full-Text Category

Variable	Disease Mechanism	Treatment	Diagnosis
Study design	✓	✓	✓
Controls	✓	✓	✓
Blinding	Not required	✓	✓
Intervention tested	Not required	✓	✓
Sample size	✓	✓	✓
Outcomes	✓	✓	✓

SCOPING REVIEW: FULL TEXT ARTICLES INCLUDED

TABLE C-5 Articles Included in Scoping Review

Reference	Category
Aucott et al. (2013)	Mechanisms
Aucott et al. (2016)	Mechanisms
Aucott et al. (2022)	Mechanisms, Diagnosis
Bayer et al. (1996)	Diagnosis
Bouquet et al. (2017)	Mechanism
Bouquet et al. (2016)	Mechanism
Bransfield et al. (2020)	Diagnosis
Cameron (2008)	Treatment
Chandra et al. (2010)	Mechanism
Chandra et al. (2011)	Mechanism
Chung et al. (2023)	Mechanism
Citera et al. (2017)	Diagnosis
Clarke et al. (2021)	Mechanism
Clarke et al. (2022)	Mechanism
Coughlin et al. (2018)	Mechanism, Diagnosis
Coyle et al. (1994)	Diagnosis
D'Adamo et al. (2015)	Treatment
Dattwyler et al. (1988)	Mechanism, Diagnosis
Derderian and Otenbaker (2024)	Treatment

continued

TABLE C-5 Continued

Reference	Category
Donta (1997)	Treatment
Donta (2003)	Treatment
Donta, Noto, and Vento (2012)	Diagnosis
Elkins et al. (1999)	Mechanism
Fallon, B.A. et al. (1999)	Treatment
Fallon, B.A. et al. (2003)	Mechanism
Fallon, B.A. et al. (2008)	Treatment
Fallon, B.A. et al. (2009)	Mechanism
Fallon, B.A. et al. (2019)	Diagnosis
Fallon, B.A. et al. (2020)	Mechanism
Fallon, J. et al. (1999)	Diagnosis
Fitzgerald et al. (2021)	Mechanism, Diagnosis
Fleming et al. (2004)	Diagnosis
Fried et al. (2002)	Mechanism
Gaudino, Coyle, and Krupp (1997)	Mechanism
Gorlyn, Keilp, and Fallon (2023)	Mechanism
Greco, Conti-Kelly, and Greco (2011)	Diagnosis
Hassett et al. (2008)	Mechanism
Horowitz and Freeman (2016)	Treatment
Horowitz and Freeman (2018)	Diagnosis
Horowitz and Freeman (2019)	Treatment
Horowitz, Fallon, and Freeman (2023)	Treatment
Jacek et al. (2013)	Mechanism, Diagnosis
Jernigan et al. (2021)	Treatment
Johnson et al. (2020)	Treatment
Johnson et al. (2023)	Mechanism
Johnson, Shapiro, and Mankoff (2018)	Mechanism
Kaplan et al. (2003)	Treatment
Keilp et al. (2006)	Mechanism
Keshtkarjahromi et al. (2024)	Mechanism
Kim et al. (2022)	Mechanism
Klempner et al. (2001)	Treatment
Klempner et al. (2005)	Mechanism

TABLE C-5 Continued

Reference	Category
Krupp et al. (2003)	Treatment
Logigian et al. (1990)	Treatment
Logigian and Steere (1992)	Mechanism
Lyon and Seung (2019)	Mechanism
Marques et al. (2014)	Diagnosis
Marques, Brown, and Fleisher (2009)	Mechanism
Marvel et al. (2022)	Mechanism, Diagnosis
Middelveen et al. (2018)	Mechanism
Miller et al. (2024)	Mechanism, Diagnosis
Morgen et al. (2001)	Mechanism
Morrissette et al. (2020)	Mechanism, Diagnosis
Murray et al. (2022)	Treatment
Mustafiz et al. (2022)	Mechanism
Nicolson, Settineri, and Ellithorpe (2012)	Treatment
Novak et al. (2019)	Mechanism
Patrick et al. (2015)	Mechanism
Phillips et al. (1998)	Diagnosis
Plutchok et al. (1999)	Diagnosis
Rebman et al. (2017)	Mechanism
Sapi et al. (2019)	Diagnosis
Schutzer et al. (2011)	Mechanism
Shere-Wolfe et al. (2024)	Treatment
Solomon et al. (1998)	Mechanism
Stricker, Burrascano, and Winger (2002)	Diagnosis
Stricker et al. (2009)	Diagnosis
Tang et al. (2015)	Mechanism
Touradji et al. (2019)	Mechanism
Turk et al. (2019)	Diagnosis
Uhde et al. (2016)	Mechanism, Diagnosis
Weitzner et al. (2015)	Mechanism
Wormser et al. (2015)	Mechanism
Wormser et al. (2021)	Mechanism, Diagnosis

REFERENCES

Aucott, J. N., A. W. Rebman, L. A. Crowder, and K. B. Kortte. 2013. Post-treatment Lyme disease syndrome symptomatology and the impact on life functioning: Is there something here? *Qual Life Res* 22(1):75-84.

Aucott, J. N., M. J. Soloski, A. W. Rebman, L. A. Crowder, L. J. Lahey, C. A. Wagner, W. H. Robinson, and K. T. Bechtold. 2016. Ccl19 as a chemokine risk factor for posttreatment Lyme disease syndrome: A prospective clinical cohort study. *Clin Vaccine Immunol* 23(9):757-766.

Aucott, J. N., T. Yang, I. Yoon, D. Powell, S. A. Geller, and A. W. Rebman. 2022. Risk of post-treatment Lyme disease in patients with ideally-treated early Lyme disease: A prospective cohort study. *Int J Infect Dis* 116:230-237.

Bayer, M. E., L. Zhang, and M. H. Bayer. 1996. Borrelia burgdorferi DNA in the urine of treated patients with chronic Lyme disease symptoms. A PCR study of 97 cases. *Infection* 24(5):347-353.

Bouquet, J., J. L. Gardy, S. Brown, J. Pfeil, R. R. Miller, M. Morshed, A. Avina-Zubieta, K. Shojania, M. McCabe, S. Parker, M. Uyaguari, S. Federman, P. Tang, T. Steiner, M. Otterstater, R. Holt, R. Moore, C. Y. Chiu, D. M. Patrick, and the Complex Chronic Disease Study Group. 2017. RNA-seq analysis of gene expression, viral pathogen, and b-cell/t-cell receptor signatures in complex chronic disease. *Clinical Infectious Diseases* 64(4):476-481.

Bouquet, J., J. Soloski Mark, A. Swei, C. Cheadle, S. Federman, J.-N. Billaud, W. Rebman Alison, B. Kabre, R. Halpert, M. Boorgula, N. Aucott John, and Y. Chiu Charles. 2016. Longitudinal transcriptome analysis reveals a sustained differential gene expression signature in patients treated for acute Lyme disease. *mBio* 7(1):10.1128/mbio.00100-00116.

Bransfield, R. C., D. M. Aidlen, M. J. Cook, and S. Javia. 2020. A clinical diagnostic system for late-stage neuropsychiatric Lyme borreliosis based upon an analysis of 100 patients. *Healthcare (Basel)* 8(1).

Brackett, M., J. Potts, A. Meihofer, Y. Indorewala, A. Ali, S. Lutes, E. Putnam, S. Schuelke, A. Abdool, E. Woldenberg, and R. J. Jacobs. 2024. Neuropsychiatric manifestations and cognitive decline in patients with long-standing Lyme disease: A scoping review. *Cureus* 16(4):e58308.

Cameron, D. 2008. Severity of Lyme disease with persistent symptoms. Insights from a double-blind placebo-controlled clinical trial. *Minerva Med* 99(5):489-496.

Chandra, A., G. P. Wormser, M. S. Klempner, R. P. Trevino, M. K. Crow, N. Latov, and A. Alaedini. 2010. Anti-neural antibody reactivity in patients with a history of Lyme borreliosis and persistent symptoms. *Brain, Behavior, and Immunity* 24(6):1018-1024.

Chandra, A., G. P. Wormser, A. R. Marques, N. Latov, and A. Alaedini. 2011. Anti-borrelia burgdorferi antibody profile in post-Lyme disease syndrome. *Clinical and Vaccine Immunology* 18(5):767-771.

Chung, M. K., M. Caboni, P. Strandwitz, A. D'Onofrio, K. Lewis, and C. J. Patel. 2023. Systematic comparisons between Lyme disease and post-treatment Lyme disease syndrome in the U.S. with administrative claims data. *eBioMedicine* 90:104524.

Citera, M., P. R. Freeman, and R. I. Horowitz. 2017. Empirical validation of the horowitz multiple systemic infectious disease syndrome questionnaire for suspected Lyme disease. *Int J Gen Med* 10:249-273.

Clarke, D. J. B., A. W. Rebman, A. Bailey, M. L. Wojciechowicz, S. L. Jenkins, J. E. Evangelista, M. Danieletto, J. Fan, M. W. Eshoo, M. R. Mosel, W. Robinson, N. Ramadoss, J. Bobe, M. J. Soloski, J. N. Aucott, and A. Ma'ayan. 2021. Predicting Lyme disease from patients' peripheral blood mononuclear cells profiled with RNA-sequencing. *Front Immunol* 12:636289.

Clarke, D. J. B., A. W. Rebman, J. Fan, M. J. Soloski, J. N. Aucott, and A. Ma'ayan. 2022. Gene set predictor for post-treatment Lyme disease. *Cell Reports Medicine* 3(11).

Coughlin, J. M., T. Yang, A. W. Rebman, K. T. Bechtold, Y. Du, W. B. Mathews, W. G. Lesniak, E. A. Mihm, S. M. Frey, E. S. Marshall, H. B. Rosenthal, T. A. Reekie, M. Kassiou, R. F. Dannals, M. J. Soloski, J. N. Aucott, and M. G. Pomper. 2018. Imaging glial activation in patients with post-treatment Lyme disease symptoms: A pilot study using [(11)c]DPA-713 PET. *J Neuroinflammation* 15(1):346.

Coyle, P. K., L. B. Krupp, C. Doscher, and K. Amin. 1994. Borrelia burgdorferi reactivity in patients with severe persistent fatigue who are from a region in which Lyme disease is endemic. *Clin Infect Dis* 18 Suppl 1:S24-27.

D'Adamo, C. R., C. R. McMillin, K. W. Chen, E. K. Lucas, and B. M. Berman. 2015. Supervised resistance exercise for patients with persistent symptoms of Lyme disease. *Medicine & Science in Sports & Exercise* 47(11):2291-2298.

Dattwyler, R. J., D. J. Volkman, B. J. Luft, J. J. Halperin, J. Thomas, and M. G. Golightly. 1988. Seronegative Lyme disease. *New England Journal of Medicine* 319(22):1441-1446.

Derderian, G. P., and N. Otenbaker. 2024. A prospective study of patients with post treatment Lyme disease syndrome treated with modified VFEM energy. *Journal of Cosmetic Dermatology* 23(6):2044-2048.

Donta, S. T. 1997. Tetracycline therapy for chronic Lyme disease. *Clinical Infectious Diseases* 25(Supplement_1):S52-S56.

Donta, S. T. 2003. Macrolide therapy of chronic Lyme disease. *Med Sci Monit* 9(11):Pi136-142.

Donta, S. T., R. B. Noto, and J. A. Vento. 2012. Spect brain imaging in chronic Lyme disease. *Clin Nucl Med* 37(9):e219-222.

Elkins, L. E., P. D. A., S. S. R., and L. B. and Krupp. 1999. Psychological states and neuropsychological performances in chronic Lyme disease. *Applied Neuropsychology* 6(1):19-26.

Fallon, B. A., J. Keilp, I. Prohovnik, R. V. Heertum, and J. J. Mann. 2003. Regional cerebral blood flow and cognitive deficits in chronic Lyme disease. *J Neuropsychiatry Clin Neurosci* 15(3):326-332.

Fallon, B. A., J. G. Keilp, K. M. Corbera, E. Petkova, C. B. Britton, E. Dwyer, I. Slavov, J. Cheng, J. Dobkin, D. R. Nelson, and H. A. Sackeim. 2008. A randomized, placebo-controlled trial of repeated iv antibiotic therapy for Lyme encephalopathy. *Neurology* 70(13):992-1003.

Fallon, B. A., R. B. Lipkin, K. M. Corbera, S. Yu, M. S. Nobler, J. G. Keilp, E. Petkova, S. H. Lisanby, J. R. Moeller, I. Slavov, R. Van Heertum, B. D. Mensh, and H. A. Sackeim. 2009. Regional cerebral blood flow and metabolic rate in persistent Lyme encephalopathy. *Archives of General Psychiatry* 66(5):554-563.

Fallon, B. A., B. Strobino, S. Reim, J. Stoner, and M. W. Cunningham. 2020. Anti-lysoganglioside and other anti-neuronal autoantibodies in post-treatment Lyme disease and erythema migrans after repeat infection. *Brain, Behavior, & Immunity - Health* 2:100015.

Fallon, B. A., F. A. Tager, J. G. Keilp, N. Weiss, L. Fein, and K. B. Liegner. 1999. Repeated antibiotic treatment in chronic Lyme disease. *Journal of Spirochetal and Tick-Borne Diseases* 6:94-102.

Fallon, B. A., N. Zubcevik, C. Bennett, S. Doshi, A. W. Rebman, R. Kishon, J. R. Moeller, N. R. Octavien, and J. N. Aucott. 2019. The general symptom questionnaire-30 (gsq-30): A brief measure of multi-system symptom burden in Lyme disease. *Front Med (Lausanne)* 6:283.

Fallon, J., D. I. Bujak, S. Guardino, and A. Weinstein. 1999. The fibromyalgia impact questionnaire: A useful tool in evaluating patients with post–Lyme disease syndrome. *Arthritis Care & Research* 12(1):42-47.

Fitzgerald, B. L., B. Graham, M. J. Delorey, A. Pegalajar-Jurado, M. N. Islam, G. P. Wormser, J. N. Aucott, A. W. Rebman, M. J. Soloski, J. T. Belisle, and C. R. Molins. 2021. Metabolic response in patients with post-treatment Lyme disease symptoms/syndrome. *Clinical Infectious Diseases* 73(7):e2342-e2349.

Fleming, R. V., A. R. Marques, M. S. Klempner, C. H. Schmid, L. G. Dally, D. S. Martin, and M. T. Philipp. 2004. Pre-treatment and post-treatment assessment of the c(6) test in patients with persistent symptoms and a history of Lyme borreliosis. *European Journal of Clinical Microbiology & Infectious Diseases* 23(8):615-618.

Fried, M. D., D. Pietrucha, G. Madigan, and A. Bal. 2002. Borrelia burgdorferi persists in the gastrointestinal tract of children and adolescents with Lyme disease. *Journal of Spirochetal and Tick-Borne Diseases* 9:11-15.

Gaudino, E. A., P. K. Coyle, and L. B. Krupp. 1997. Post-Lyme syndrome and chronic fatigue syndrome: Neuropsychiatric similarities and differences. *Archives of Neurology* 54(11):1372-1376.

Gorlyn, M., J. G. Keilp, and B. A. Fallon. 2022. Language fluency deficits in post-treatment Lyme disease syndrome. *Archives of Clinical Neuropsychology* 38(4):650-654.

Greco, T. P., Jr., A. M. Conti-Kelly, and T. P. Greco. 2011. Antiphospholipid antibodies in patients with purported "chronic Lyme disease." *Lupus* 20(13):1372-1377.

Hassett, A. L., D. C. Radvanski, S. Buyske, S. V. Savage, M. Gara, J. I. Escobar, and L. H. Sigal. 2008. Role of psychiatric comorbidity in chronic Lyme disease. *Arthritis Rheum* 59(12):1742-1749.

Horowitz, R., and P. R. Freeman. 2016. Are mycobacterium drugs effective for treatment resistant Lyme disease, tick-borne co-infections, and autoimmune disease? *JSM Arthritis* 1(2):1008.

Horowitz, R. I., J. Fallon, and P. R. Freeman. 2023. Comparison of the efficacy of longer versus shorter pulsed high dose dapsone combination therapy in the treatment of chronic Lyme disease/post treatment Lyme disease syndrome with bartonellosis and associated coinfections. *Microorganisms* 11(9):2301.

Horowitz, R. I., and P. R. Freeman. 2018. Precision medicine: The role of the MSIDS model in defining, diagnosing, and treating chronic Lyme disease/post treatment Lyme disease syndrome and other chronic illness: Part 2. *Healthcare (Basel)* 6(4).

Horowitz, R. I., and P. R. Freeman. 2019. Precision medicine: Retrospective chart review and data analysis of 200 patients on dapsone combination therapy for chronic Lyme disease/post-treatment Lyme disease syndrome: Part 1. *International Journal of General Medicine* 12:101-119.

Jacek, E., B. A. Fallon, A. Chandra, M. K. Crow, G. P. Wormser, and A. Alaedini. 2013. Increased IFNα activity and differential antibody response in patients with a history of Lyme disease and persistent cognitive deficits. *J Neuroimmunol* 255(1-2):85-91.

Jernigan, D. A., M. C. Hart, K. K. Dodd, S. Jameson, and T. Farney. 2021. Induced native phage therapy for the treatment of Lyme disease and relapsing fever: A retrospective review of first 14 months in one clinic. *Cureus* 13(11):e20014.

Johnson, L., M. Shapiro, S. Janicki, J. Mankoff, and R. B. Stricker. 2023. Does biological sex matter in Lyme disease? The need for sex-disaggregated data in persistent illness. *Int J Gen Med* 16:2557-2571.

Johnson, L., M. Shapiro, and J. Mankoff. 2018. Removing the mask of average treatment effects in chronic Lyme disease research using big data and subgroup analysis. *Healthcare (Basel)* 6(4).

Johnson, L., M. Shapiro, R. B. Stricker, J. Vendrow, J. Haddock, and D. Needell. 2020. Antibiotic treatment response in chronic Lyme disease: Why do some patients improve while others do not? *Healthcare* 8(4):383.

Kaplan, R. F., R. P. Trevino, G. M. Johnson, L. Levy, R. Dornbush, L. T. Hu, J. Evans, A. Weinstein, C. H. Schmid, and M. S. Klempner. 2003. Cognitive function in post-treatment Lyme disease: Do additional antibiotics help? *Neurology* 60(12):1916-1922.

Keilp, J. G., K. Corbera, I. Slavov, M. J. Taylor, H. A. Sackeim, and B. A. Fallon. 2006. Wais-iii and wms-iii performance in chronic Lyme disease. *Journal of the International Neuropsychological Society* 12(1):119-129.

Keshtkarjahromi, M., A. W. Rebman, A. A. R. Antar, Y. C. Manabe, L. Gutierrez-Alamillo, L. A. Casciola-Rosen, J. N. Aucott, and J. B. Miller. 2024. Autoantibodies in post-treatment Lyme disease and association with clinical symptoms. *Clinical and Experimental Rheumatology* 42(7):1487-1490.

Kim, Y., A. W. Rebman, T. P. Johnson, H. Wang, T. Yang, C. Colantuoni, P. Bhargava, M. Levy, P. A. Calabresi, J. N. Aucott, M. J. Soloski, and E. Darrah. 2022. Peptidylarginine deiminase 2 autoantibodies are linked to less severe disease in multiple sclerosis and post-treatment Lyme disease. *Frontiers in Neurology* 13.

Klempner, M. S., L. T. Hu, J. Evans, C. H. Schmid, G. M. Johnson, R. P. Trevino, D. Norton, L. Levy, D. Wall, J. McCall, M. Kosinski, and A. Weinstein. 2001. Two controlled trials of antibiotic treatment in patients with persistent symptoms and a history of Lyme disease. *New England Journal of Medicine* 345(2):85-92.

Klempner, M. S., G. H. Wormser, K. Wade, R. P. Trevino, J. Tang, R. A. Kaslow, and C. Schmid. 2005. A case-control study to examine HLA haplotype associations in patients with posttreatment chronic Lyme disease. *Journal of Infectious Diseases* 192(6):1010-1013.

Krupp, L. B., L. G. Hyman, R. Grimson, P. K. Coyle, P. Melville, S. Ahnn, R. Dattwyler, and B. Chandler. 2003. Study and treatment of post Lyme disease (stop-LD): A randomized double masked clinical trial. *Neurology* 60(12):1923-1930.

Logigian, E. L., R. F. Kaplan, and A. C. Steere. 1990. Chronic neurologic manifestations of Lyme disease. *New England Journal of Medicine* 323(21):1438-1444.

Logigian, E. L., and A. C. Steere. 1992. Clinical and electrophysiologic findings in chronic neuropathy of Lyme disease. *Neurology* 42(2):303-303.

Lyon, J., and H. Seung. 2019. Genetic variation in the ABCB1 gene associated with post treatment Lyme disease syndrome status. *Meta Gene* 21:100589.

Marques, A., M. R. Brown, and T. A. Fleisher. 2009. Natural killer cell counts are not different between patients with post-Lyme disease syndrome and controls. *Clinical and Vaccine Immunology* 16(8):1249-1250.

Marques, A., S. R. Telford, III, S.-P. Turk, E. Chung, C. Williams, K. Dardick, P. J. Krause, C. Brandeburg, C. D. Crowder, H. E. Carolan, M. W. Eshoo, P. A. Shaw, and L. T. Hu. 2014. Xenodiagnosis to detect borrelia burgdorferi infection: A first-in-human study. *Clinical Infectious Diseases* 58(7):937-945.

Marvel, C. L., K. H. Alm, D. Bhattacharya, W. Rebman Alison, A. Bakker, O. P. Morgan, J. A. Creighton, E. A. Kozero, A. Venkatesan, P. A. Nadkarni, and J. N. Aucott. 2022. A multimodal neuroimaging study of brain abnormalities and clinical correlates in post treatment Lyme disease. *PLOS One* 10(17).

Middelveen, M. J., E. Sapi, J. Burke, K. R. Filush, A. Franco, M. C. Fesler, and R. B. Stricker. 2018. Persistent borrelia infection in patients with ongoing symptoms of Lyme disease. *Healthcare* 6(2):33.

Miller, J. B., A. W. Rebman, M. D. V. de Flores, H. Wang, E. Darrah, and J. N. Aucott. 2024. Annexin a2 antibodies in post-treatment Lyme disease. *Therapeutic Advances in Infectious Disease* 11:20499361241242971.

Morgen, K., R. Martin, R. D. Stone, J. Grafman, N. Kadom, H. F. McFarland, and A. Marques. 2001. Flair and magnetization transfer imaging of patients with post-treatment Lyme disease syndrome. *Neurology* 57(11):1980-1985.

Morrissette, M., N. Pitt, A. González, P. Strandwitz, M. Caboni, A. W. Rebman, R. Knight, A. D'Onofrio, J. N. Aucott, M. J. Soloski, and K. Lewis. 2020. A distinct microbiome signature in posttreatment Lyme disease patients. *mBio* 11(5).

Murray, L., C. Alexander, C. Bennett, M. Kuvaldina, G. Khalsa, and B. Fallon. 2022. Kundalini yoga for post-treatment Lyme disease: A preliminary randomized study. *Healthcare (Basel)* 10(7).

Mustafiz, F., J. Moeller, M. Kuvaldina, C. Bennett, and B. A. Fallon. 2022. Persistent symptoms, Lyme disease, and prior trauma. *Journal of Nervous and Mental Disorders* 210(5):359-364.

Nicolson, G., R. Settineri, and R. Ellithorpe. 2012. Glycophospholipid formulation with NADH and COQ10 significantly reduces intractable fatigue in western blot-positive 'chronic Lyme disease' patients: Preliminary report. *Functional Foods in Health and Disease* 2:35-47.

Novak, P., D. Felsenstein, C. Mao, N. R. Octavien, and N. Zubcevik. 2019. Association of small fiber neuropathy and post treatment Lyme disease syndrome. *PLOS One* 14(2): e0212222.

Patrick, D. M., R. R. Miller, J. L. Gardy, S. M. Parker, M. G. Morshed, T. S. Steiner, J. Singer, K. Shojania, P. Tang, for the Complex Chronic Diseases Study Group. 2015. Lyme disease diagnosed by alternative methods: A phenotype similar to that of chronic fatigue syndrome. *Clinical Infectious Diseases* 61(7):1084-1091.

Phillips, S. E., L. H. Mattman, D. Hulínská, and H. Moayad. 1998. A proposal for the reliable culture of borrelia burgdorferi from patients with chronic Lyme disease, even from those previously aggressively treated. *Infection* 26(6):364-367.

Plutchok, J. J., R. S. Tikofsky, K. B. Liegner, J. M. Kochevan, B. A. Fallon, and R. L. Van Heertum. 1999. TC-99M HMPAO brain spect imaging in chronic Lyme disease. *Journal of Spirochetal and Tick-Borne Diseases* 6:117-122.

Rebman, A. W., K. T. Bechtold, T. Yang, E. A. Mihm, M. J. Soloski, C. B. Novak, and J. N. Aucott. 2017. The clinical, symptom, and quality-of-life characterization of a well-defined group of patients with posttreatment Lyme disease syndrome. *Frontiers in Medicine (Lausanne)* 4:224.

Sapi, E., R. S. Kasliwala, H. Ismail, J. P. Torres, M. Oldakowski, S. Markland, G. Gaur, A. Melillo, K. Eisendle, K. B. Liegner, J. Libien, and J. E. Goldman. 2019. The long-term persistence of borrelia burgdorferi antigens and DNA in the tissues of a patient with Lyme disease. *Antibiotics (Basel)* 8(4).

Schutzer, S. E., T. E. Angel, T. Liu, A. A. Schepmoes, T. R. Clauss, J. N. Adkins, D. G. Camp, B. K. Holland, J. Bergquist, P. K. Coyle, R. D. Smith, B. A. Fallon, and B. H. Natelson. 2011. Distinct cerebrospinal fluid proteomes differentiate post-treatment Lyme disease from chronic fatigue syndrome. *PLOS One* 6(2):e17287.

Shere-Wolfe, K. D., N. George, G. M. Al Kibria, R. Silk, and C. S. Alexander. 2023. A multimodal ayurveda and mind–body therapeutic intervention for chronic symptoms attributed to a postinfectious syndrome: A pilot study. *Journal of Integrative and Complementary Medicine* 30(5):450-458.

Solomon, S. P., E. Hilton, B. S. Weinschel, S. Pollack, and E. Grolnick. 1998. Psychological factors in the prediction of Lyme disease course. *Arthritis & Rheumatism* 11(5):419-426.

Stricker, R. B., J. Burrascano, and E. Winger. 2002. Longterm decrease in the CD57 lymphocyte subset in a patient with chronic Lyme disease. *Ann Agric Environ Med* 9(1):111-113.

Stricker, R. B., V. R. Savely, N. C. Motanya, and P. C. Giclas. 2009. Complement split products C3A and C4A in chronic Lyme disease. *Scandinavian Journal of Immunology* 69(1):64-69.

Tang, K. S., M. S. Klempner, G. P. Wormser, A. R. Marques, and A. Alaedini. 2015. Association of immune response to endothelial cell growth factor with early disseminated and late manifestations of Lyme disease but not posttreatment Lyme disease syndrome. *Clinical Infectious Diseases* 61(11):1703-1706.

Touradji, P., J. N. Aucott, T. Yang, A. W. Rebman, and K. T. Bechtold. 2019. Cognitive decline in post-treatment Lyme disease syndrome. *Arch Clin Neuropsychol* 34(4):455-465.

Turk, S. P., K. Lumbard, K. Liepshutz, C. Williams, L. Hu, K. Dardick, G. P. Wormser, J. Norville, C. Scavarda, D. McKenna, D. Follmann, and A. Marques. 2019. Post-treatment Lyme disease symptoms score: Developing a new tool for research. *PLOS One* 14(11):e0225012.

Uhde, M., M. Ajamian, X. Li, G. P. Wormser, A. Marques, and A. Alaedini. 2016. Expression of C-reactive protein and serum amyloid A in early to late manifestations of Lyme disease. *Clin Infect Dis* 63(11):1399-1404.

Weitzner, E., D. McKenna, J. Nowakowski, C. Scavarda, R. Dornbush, S. Bittker, D. Cooper, R. B. Nadelman, P. Visintainer, I. Schwartz, and G. P. Wormser. 2015. Long-term assessment of post-treatment symptoms in patients with culture-confirmed early Lyme disease. *Clin Infect Dis* 61(12):1800-1806.

Wormser, G. P., D. McKenna, K. D. Shaffer, J. H. Silverman, C. Scavarda, and P. Visintainer. 2021. Evaluation of selected variables to determine if any had predictive value for, or correlated with, residual symptoms at approximately 12 months after diagnosis and treatment of early Lyme disease. *Diagn Microbiol Infect Dis* 100(3):115348.

Wormser, G. P., E. Weitzner, D. McKenna, R. B. Nadelman, C. Scavarda, and J. Nowakowski. 2015. Long-term assessment of fatigue in patients with culture-confirmed Lyme disease. *The American Journal of Medicine* 128(2):181-184.